AF745102

University of Edinburgh

30150 024905413

PSYCHOLOGY
LIBRARY
CANCELLED

A Special Issue of
Visual Cognition

Binding

Guest Editors

James R. Brockmole
University of Edinburgh

and

Steven L. Franconeri
Northwestern University

WITHDRAWN

Psychology Press
Taylor & Francis Group
HOVE AND NEW YORK

First published 2009 by Psychology Press
27 Church Road, Hove, East Sussex, BN3 2FA

http://www.psypress.co.uk

Simultaneously published in the USA and Canada
by Psychology Press
270 Madison Avenue, New York, NY 10016

Psychology Press is part of the Taylor & Francis Group, an Informa business

© 2009 by Psychology Press

All rights reserved. No part of this book may be reprinted or
reproduced or utilised in any form or by any electronic,
mechanical, or other means, now known or hereafter invented,
including photocopying and recording, or in any information
storage or retrieval system, without permission in writing from the publishers.

British Library Cataloguing in Publication Data
A catalogue record for this book is available from the British Library

ISBN 13: 978-1-84169-865-6
ISSN 1350-6285

Cover design by Design Deluxe
Typeset by Datapage (India) Private Limited, Chennai, India
Printed in the UK by Henry Ling Limited at the Dorset Press, Dorchester
Bound in the UK by TJ International Ltd, Padstow
The publication has been produced with paper manufactured to strict
environmental standards and with pulp derived from sustainable forests.

Contents*

---

* This book is also a special issue of the journal Visual Cognition, and forms issues 1 & 2 of Volume 17 (2009).

VISUAL COGNITION, 2009, 17 (1/2), 1–9

Psychology Press
Taylor & Francis Group

Introduction

James R. Brockmole
University of Edinburgh, Edinburgh, UK

Steven L. Franconeri
Northwestern University, Evanston, IL, USA

In many ways visual processing acts as a prism, splitting visual information from the retinal image into separately processed visual features such as colours, shapes, sizes, or orientations. *Binding* refers to the set of cognitive and neural mechanisms that reintegrate these features to create a holistic representation of the objects in the visual field. The *binding problem* in vision refers to how this integration is achieved. Because binding processes must be applied to virtually every level of visual processing, the binding problem is a ubiquitous one that applies to perception, attention, working memory, and long-term memory systems. It is more appropriate, therefore, to conceptualize the binding problem not as a singular problem, but as a constellation of interrelated problem*s*. For example, how does one perceive and represent the fact that features *a*, *b*, and *c* belong to object *X*, whereas features *q*, *r*, and *s* belong to object *Y*? How does one perceive and represent the relationships among objects such as the fact that object *Y* is to the left of object *X* and to the right of object *Z*? How does one perceive and represent that events *x* and *y* are temporally related to each other, but are distinct from events *p* and *q*? What happens to bound representations when the relations among features, objects, or events change? How functional are these representations in the service of visually guided tasks?

This special issue of *Visual Cognition* provides a sampling of current work being done in visual perception and visual memory to understand how human observers accomplish the appropriate binding of features within objects, the relational binding among objects, and the binding between temporally related events. Within these broad areas, the papers cover a wide

Please address all correspondence to James R. Brockmole, Psychology Department, University of Edinburgh, 7 George Square, Edinburgh EH8 9JZ, UK. E-mail: James.Brockmole@ed.ac.uk

© 2008 Psychology Press, an imprint of the Taylor & Francis Group, an Informa business
http://www.psypress.com/viscog DOI: 10.1080/13506280802333211

range of topics including the role of attention in feature binding, the representation of static and moving multifeature objects in memory, the binding of objects to scenes, binding processes involved in learning and long-term memory, binding of information about objects perceived in visual and nonvisual modalities, the development of binding abilities, and the neural substrates involved in binding processes. The goal of this special issue is not to disseminate conclusive solutions to the various instantiations of the binding problem. Although this collection of papers converges on several theoretical points, there are also examples of clear divergence. It is our hope, rather, that this collection of work will describe the current state-of-the-science regarding binding processes in visual perception and memory, outline the critical issues that have yet to be resolved, and highlight the interconnections between the binding problems and the approaches taken to solve them. In this single volume readers will encounter work with children, young adults, and patients, and work that uses traditional behavioural measures, eye movement recording, functional imaging, and transcranial magnetic stimulation.

The special issue begins by examining the role attention plays in binding. Although attention will be important in many of the papers in this volume, the first set of papers make it their primary focus and take up the classic and hotly debated question regarding the degree to which, and conditions under which, binding relies on focused attention.

Hyun, Woodman, and Luck examine the attentional requirements of explicitly binding surface features to their spatial locations in visual perception. The authors asked observers to either indicate whether a target colour was present in a display, or to report the location of the target colour. The first task simply required observers to detect a feature, and the second task additionally required observers to bind a feature to a location. The principle measure of participants' relative allocation of attention resources was the lateralized N2pc ERP component, which shows a larger amplitude when a relatively greater share of spatial attention is allocated to objects in the visual field contralateral to certain posterior electrodes. A larger N2pc component was observed in the localization condition, suggesting that greater attentional resources are required to discriminate colour–location bindings than to detect individual colours. Thus, attention plays a special role in the binding of features to locations and the attentional mechanism responsible for this binding operates at a level indexed by the N2pc, which includes intermediate and high levels of extrastriate visual cortex.

Braet and Humphreys also emphasize the role of attention in a two-stage account of binding. In the first stage, they argue that features are weakly bound to objects and that these bindings are noisy and potentially fleeting. The second stage is the application of top-down attentional feedback, which consolidates and stabilizes visual representations. After an initial feedforward sweep of activation in visual pathways, reentrant processes stemming from higher visual areas such as the Posterior Parietal Cortex (PPC) tune the incoming signals. If this tuning includes the stabilization of representations of bound objects, then selectively disrupting these late processes might selectively disrupt binding and produce, for example, illusory conjunctions. To test the importance of the proposed reentrant processes in binding, the authors asked a patient with bilateral PPC damage to perform a rapid binding task in which she was to identify the colour and identity of a target letter that was presented alongside a different (in both colour and identity) distractor letter. In this patient, presenting the objects for long durations (300 ms)—when reentrant feedback processes should normally help to consolidate binding—led to more binding errors (illusory conjunctions) than short presentations (100 ms). This pattern contrasted with performance for reporting individual features, which improved with longer presentation times. In addition, the authors disrupted reentrant binding processes in normal observers using transcranial magnetic stimulation of the PPC. The pulse only disrupted binding performance at an above-chance level when it was delivered 150–200 ms after the presentation of the binding task, suggesting that it disrupted reentrant processes directed by the PPC. The data lend support to a multistage model of binding where attentional feedback, specifically from PPC, plays an important role in relatively late perceptual processes related to feature binding.

As in perception, Fougnie and Marois argue that spatial attention also plays an important role in maintaining bound *memory* representations of objects. The authors critique several recent papers demonstrating that observers can retain feature bindings in memory even in the face of attentional distraction. The authors suggest that the visual attention tasks used in past studies were not difficult enough, and instead use a taxing multiple object tracking (MOT) task during the retention interval of a working memory task. The MOT task impaired performance far more when the memory task required binding compared to when binding was not required, suggesting that spatial attention is indeed necessary for maintaining bindings in memory. Interestingly, however, spatial attention was only critical for binding when the objects in the memory task were presented simultaneously in different spatial locations. When the objects were presented sequentially at the centre of the screen, the object tracking task had a much smaller impact on performance in the binding condition. The authors conclude that spatial attention plays an important, although perhaps not an exclusive, role for binding in visual memory.

Oakes, Messenger, Ross-Sheehy, and Luck take a developmental approach to investigating the attentional control mechanisms underlying binding in visual working memory. When shown alternating displays of coloured squares, 6-month-old infants are able to detect changes to a square's colour when only one is present, as demonstrated by a looking preference for the changing stream, relative to a nonchanging stream. However, once multiple squares of heterogeneous colour are present, and colours cycle among the squares on each new display, 6-month-old infants do not demonstrate a preference for the changing stream, suggesting that the 6-month-olds fail to bind or appropriately compare object feature information from one display to the next. Surprisingly, even when shown displays of heterogeneously coloured squares that are replaced with a set of entirely new colours, 6-month-olds continued to show no preference for the changing stream. This finding is counterintuitive because the same population of infants can detect colour changes to single object arrays, and successful binding of a single colour to location would allow detection of the changes in these displays containing three times the opportunity to notice an identical change. Thus, although the infants have the ability to remember a single colour and compare it to a later colour, increasing display complexity leads to a failure of binding, even though many more changes may occur within the display. After only one more month of development, 7-month-old infants are able to complete all of these tasks. The authors argue that this in this extra month the infants might benefit from maturation of the parietal areas important for the control of attention, and these same areas are argued by Braet and Humphreys (this issue) to support binding.

In contrast to the apparent convergence on the role of attention in feature binding in the preceding papers, the final three papers in this set challenge the conclusion that attention is necessarily required for binding. In the first of these, Allen, Hitch, and Baddeley, examined the role of attention in the generation and maintenance of working memory representations that must bind object features that are directly perceived and those that are described verbally. Observers were asked to retain object representations in memory for either unified visual stimuli (for example, seeing a red circle), or cross-modal stimuli in which one feature was presented visually and the other auditorily (for example, seeing the outline of a circle and hearing the word "red"). Performance in a visual discrimination task, in which observers judged whether a coloured shape was part of the to-be-remembered set, was broadly equivalent across the presentation conditions, indicating that purely visual and cross-modal representations are equally effective in supporting the recognition of visual objects. Concurrent tasks that led to performance decrements equally affected the visual and cross-modal binding conditions, suggesting that the act of binding cross-modal information is no more attention demanding than binding within visual memory. The authors argue that bindings are held in a general passive store (the episodic buffer) that may be fed from a range of features and modalities with the role of focused attention limited to controlling the relative contribution made by different features to memory.

In the next paper of this set, van Rullen challenges the idea that all complex object recognition requires attention to bind the object's features. Instead, he proposes that two modes of binding may exist. The first is a "hardwired binding", which operates when an observer is confronted with frequently encountered natural objects. With frequent exposure, networks might develop that include detectors for common feature conjunctions, eliminating the need for selective attention to perform the binding. But a second type of "on-demand" binding, mediated by attention, is needed for arbitrary or less frequently encountered feature conjunctions. This framework can explain many results that seem inconsistent with the need for attention in binding, such as the rapid categorization of real-world objects and natural scenes.

A distinction between "hardwired" and "on-demand" binding is also discussed by Hommel and Colzato. Observers were presented with two objects in sequence. Each object was either a strawberry or a banana. Upon presentation of the first object observers were only required to press a predefined key. Upon presentation of the second object, observers made a speeded judgement of the object's identity (i.e., shape), regardless of the object's colour (which varied). Although the first object was irrelevant to this classification task, response times to the second shape were fastest when shape and colour of both objects matched, demonstrating priming from the first shape. Interestingly, response times were also faster when neither shape nor colour matched, relative to when only one dimension matched. That is, preceding the shape judgment with an object that matches in only one dimension actually caused a relative slowing of response time to the target object. The authors interpret this effect as demonstrating that the colour and shape of the first strawberry or banana are automatically bound, because long-term memory for these objects emphasizes the importance of shape and colour information for recognition of these frequently encountered objects (as opposed to location information, which is not as important for identifying fruit). Critically, when the fruit were replaced with circles and triangles, which should not produce a strong LTM influence over the relevant dimensions for recognition, this one-dimension priming cost was minimized. Together, these results suggest that experience with frequently encountered objects builds schemas of the types of features that are important to bind in the recognition of those objects.

The next two papers consider the fragility of bindings in visual working memory. When perceptual input changes, how easily can existing bindings be maintained? Alvarez and Thompson showed observers a set of coloured dots which rotated around a central fixation point, occasionally disappearing behind and reappearing from occluders. Observers were to keep track of where each colour was located throughout the trial. At the end of a trial the dots stopped behind the occluders and observers were asked to report either the colour behind a specific occluder or the location of a specific colour. Performance on these tasks was relatively high, compared to when observers were instead asked to indicate whether, during the trial, two colours had switched locations. These results suggest that past work measuring binding memory, which largely relies on asking observers to detect swapped features, may have underestimated one's ability to maintain object–feature bindings for moving objects. To account for this difference, the authors further show that when feature-switches are missed, observers base their recall on the updated object–feature bindings rather than the original bindings, suggesting that failures to detect feature-switches arise because updated perceptual input leads to the automatic rewriting and rebinding of otherwise fragile information.

Logie, Brockmole, and Vandenbroucke continue with this line of enquiry by using working memory tasks to explore whether memory traces of individual features and feature conjunctions are completely lost from trial to trial, or whether they can be retained in long-term memory. Across trials, either the same to-be-remembered colour–shape (integrated object) combinations were consistently repeated or one feature was repeated while the other randomly varied. Performance on change-detection and cued recall tasks improved when the same integrated objects were repeatedly presented on every trial, indicating long-term retention of bindings in memory. For repeated single features, learning effects were markedly weaker than those observed for integrated objects. All learning effects were eliminated if just two novel object arrays were inserted between each repeated array. Consistent with the results presented by Alvarez and Thompson (this issue), these results suggest that bindings in memory are fragile and are readily displaced in memory when new bindings are created. Despite this fragility, however, longer term residual traces can be generated to support learning, although any learning that does occur is largely based on bound objects, not individual features.

The next four papers consider binding mechanisms across time as well as space. In the first of these papers, Makovski and Jiang considered whether tracking multiple moving objects is easier when the target objects can be distinguished by simple features or combinations of features. Although better tracking performance was observed when at least one single feature differentiated all objects (e.g., all objects had different colours or different identities), no benefit was observed when a combination of features differentiated the objects. These results suggest that object features are not properly conjoined during attentive tracking. The authors argue binding may be particularly difficult for moving objects because motion causes the basis for binding—shared location—to be an unstable object property.

Mitroff, Arita, and Fleck explore the rules that determine whether visual entities are bound into a singular representation that is maintained and updated across object motion. In their first experiment observers saw two squares, defined by a physical contour or an illusory contour. A letter was briefly presented in each square, and then both squares moved to new locations. Following this motion, a single probe letter was displayed in one of the squares and observers judged whether or not it matched either of the preview letters. When squares were defined by physical contours, these judgements were faster if the probe letter reappeared in the same square in which it was previewed, suggesting that the letters were bound to specific squares and that this binding persisted across the object's motion. Illusory contoured objects also generated this object-specific preview benefit but only if all object contours were illusory. If physical and illusory contoured entities were intermixed, the preview benefit was eliminated for the illusory stimuli. In a second experiment, the authors presented preview letters either within or adjacent to each square. Containment always led to an object-specific preview benefit, whereas adjacently presented letters could remain bound to objects only if all letters were presented outside the objects. From these results the authors propose that "boundedness" and "containment" are important principles used by the visual system to determine which entities should be bound into a single representation, and whether these bindings should be maintained when one of these entities is set into motion. Importantly, however, the observed contextual influences demonstrate for the first time that the binding of object features and properties are sensitive to more than just the physical properties contained within any given visual display.

In the third paper of this set, Saiki investigated the degree to which memory for an object's features can efficiently substitute for missing perceptual information. In this study, a set of elongated coloured bars moved horizontally until they became occluded behind squares. The remerging portion of each bar was either the same or a different colour as it had been prior to occlusion. In one condition the head of the bar remerged before the tail was occluded so that the colour change was perceptible. In another condition the occlusion was complete so that detection of the colour change required memory. With only one bar in the display, observers performed both tasks equal well, however, when presented with two or more bars, performance in the memory condition dropped quickly, even though the number of presented objects was well within the capacity of working memory. Thus, when only one colour was relevant so that binding was not necessary, memory information could be used to support task performance. Once multiple objects had to be monitored so that the binding of colours to objects was required, the use of working memory to find the nonmatching object became less efficient. The results suggest that although multiple bound object representations may be maintained in working memory, very few (perhaps only one) of these traces can efficiently function as a replacement for missing perceptual information.

Finally, Holcombe considers the problem of temporal binding in which features that cooccur in time must be linked. Specifically, he addresses the mechanisms used to bind the features of a single object as it changes over time. Holcombe used displays where objects rapidly alternated across two feature dimensions, colour and motion direction. For example, an object might turn green at the same time as its internal texture moves to the left, and then turn red when its texture begins to move to the right. Correctly binding the colour and its associated motion direction requires that the two features be marked as occurring at the same time, despite potential differences in processing latency. However, this marking does not coincide with precise temporal pairing of the features, as binding is best when changes in motion direction actually precede changes in colour. The paper presents a series of studies suggesting that the visual system samples the features at a temporal marker caused by transient changes in the features, and argues that the colour–motion asymmetry is caused by differences in the way that this transient change of colour and motion direction unfold over time.

The special issue closes with two papers that extend consideration of binding from features within single objects to the relations among multiple objects. First, Ryan and Villate examined the construction of, and subsequent access to, representations regarding the relative spatial and temporal relations among serially presented objects. Participants were sequentially shown three objects in separate spatial locations. Subsequently, a test display revealed all three objects simultaneously and participants judged whether the relative relations among the objects were maintained. The authors used observers' eye movements as their primary dependent variable. During the presentation phase, observers' eye movements transitioned between the location of the presented object and the locations that previously housed the prior study images, revealing the implicit generation and rehearsal of relational bindings in memory. During the test phase, eye movements distinguished intact displays from those in which the relations had been altered. For example, eye movements were directed towards the locations that would have contained an object had the relative spatial relations been maintained. Furthermore, objects in unaltered test displays tended to be fixated in the same temporal order in which they had been studied, an effect not observed with manipulated test images. These results demonstrate that visual representations include information regarding the relative spatial and temporal relations among objects and that eye movements may be one means by which information is bound into a lasting representation, and by which current information is compared to stored representations.

Hollingworth extends consideration of relational binding to real-world scenes and asks whether episodic scene memory includes information regarding the binding of objects to the scene's layout. Observers saw an image of a scene followed by a target probe object which was displayed in isolation at the centre of the display. The scene was presented again and observers were to search for a probe object and indicate whether its orientation in the scene was the same as depicted in the probe display, or whether it was mirror reversed. Compared to a baseline condition in which no preview was given, both preview conditions (target-absent and target-present) resulted in more efficient search, indicating that memory for general context and layout facilitates search. Critically, Hollingworth also varied whether or not the target object was in the original scene. Search was more efficient if the preview scene contained the target than if it did not, demonstrating that scene memory representations that are functional in guiding search further preserve the specific binding of objects in a scene to their locations. Memory for context and memory for object–location bindings are at least partially independent.

In closing, we would like to express our thanks to all of the contributors for choosing to publish their fine work in this special issue of *Visual Cognition*. We would also like to extend our thanks to all those who so graciously provided expert reviews and commentaries on these papers. Because of their efforts, this special issue is a collection of interesting cutting-edge research papers, which blend a variety of experimental approaches and theoretical points of view that we hope will stimulate the field for years to come.

VISUAL COGNITION, 2009, 17 (1/2), 10–24

Psychology Press
Taylor & Francis Group

The role of attention in the binding of surface features to locations

Joo-seok Hyun
Volen Center for Complex Systems, Brandeis University, Boston, MA, USA

Geoffrey F. Woodman
Department of Psychology, Vanderbilt University, Nashville, TN, USA

Steven J. Luck
Department of Psychology and Center for Mind and Brain, University of California, Davis, CA, USA

Previous studies have proposed that attention is not necessary for detecting simple features but is necessary for binding them to spatial locations. The present study tested this hypothesis, using the N2pc component of the event-related potential waveform as a measure of the allocation of attention. A simple feature detection condition, in which observers reported whether a target colour was present or not, was compared with feature-location binding conditions, in which observers reported the location of the target colour. A larger N2pc component was observed in the binding conditions than in the detection condition, indicating that additional attentional resources are needed to bind a feature to a location than to detect the feature independently of its location. This finding supports theories of attention in which attention plays a special role in binding features.

This study examines the role of attention in binding surface feature information to spatial locations in visual perception. Treisman's feature integration theory proposes that spatially focused attention is necessary to localize and bind the features of an object to the locus of focused attention, but that simple, salient features can be detected without focusing attention onto their locations (Treisman, 1988; Treisman & Gelade, 1980; Treisman & Sato, 1990). Many studies have tested this proposal by comparing the

Please address all correspondence to Steven J. Luck, UC-Davis Center for Mind & Brain, 267 Cousteau Place, Davis, CA 95618, USA. E-mail: sjluck@ucdavis.edu

This research was made possible by grants MH63001 and MH65034 from the National Institute of Mental Health.

© 2008 Psychology Press, an imprint of the Taylor & Francis Group, an Informa business
http://www.psypress.com/viscog DOI: 10.1080/13506280802113894

attentional requirements of conjunction discrimination with the attentional requirements of feature detection (Cohen & Ivry, 1989, 1991; Luck, Girelli, McDermott, & Ford, 1997b; Luck & Hillyard, 1994a, 1994b, 1995; Prinzmetal, Presti, & Posner, 1986; Treisman & Sato, 1990; Treisman & Schmidt, 1982). However, there have been no truly direct tests of the hypothesis that perceiving the spatial location of a feature—which requires binding feature and location information—is more attention demanding than the perception of feature presence.

The most relevant studies tested the hypothesis that single-feature targets can be detected even when they cannot be localized, whereas conjunction targets cannot be detected unless they are localized. Treisman and Gelade (1980) found exactly this pattern of results. However, Johnston and Pashler (1990) argued that these results could have been a result of a guessing strategy and minor errors in location reporting. They designed an experiment to eliminate these possibilities, and they found that observers were unable to correctly report the presence of a feature target unless they were able to at least coarsely localize it. Thus, they concluded that feature detection is accompanied by at least coarse feature localization.

Other studies have indirectly assessed the role of attention in localizing features by comparing performance for feature-defined and conjunction-defined targets in a variety of tasks. In some sense, features must be localized to be correctly bound together, and several studies have found evidence for a greater role of attention for conjunction targets than for feature targets (e.g., Luck & Ford, 1998; Luck, Girelli, et al., 1997b; Prinzmetal et al., 1986; Treisman & Gelade, 1980; Treisman & Sato, 1990). However, it is possible that the binding of multiple surface features such as colour and location is achieved on the basis of implicit location information rather than an explicit perception of the feature locations. Indeed, patients with parietal lesions and disrupted attention and spatial abilities have been shown to exhibit implicit localization of features (Robertson, Treisman, Friedman-Hill, & Grabowecky, 1997). The present study was designed to provide a direct test of the attentional requirements of the explicit binding of surface features to their locations in space.

To assess the attentional requirements of feature detection and feature localization, we recorded event-related potentials (ERPs) and focused on the N2pc (N2-posterior-contralateral) component. This ERP component reflects the focusing of attention onto the location of a target item in a visual search array (Eimer, 1996; Luck, Chelazzi, Hillyard, & Desimone, 1997a; Luck & Hillyard, 1994a, 1994b; Woodman & Luck, 1999, 2003). It is generated primarily in ventral stream visual areas, including area V4 and the lateral occipital complex (Hopf, Boehler, et al., 2006a; Hopf, Luck, et al., 2006b; Hopf et al., 2000). The N2pc appears to be an ERP analog of single-unit attention effects that have been observed in monkeys (Chelazzi,

Duncan, Miller, & Desimone, 1998; Chelazzi, Miller, Duncan, & Desimone, 1993; Chelazzi, Miller, Duncan, & Desimone, 2001; Luck, Girelli, et al., 1997b), and N2pc-like activity has been observed in ERP recordings from monkeys (Woodman, Kang, Rossi, & Schall, 2007).

Previous research indicates that the amplitude of the N2pc component elicited by a given visual search target reflects the attentional requirements of performing the task for that target. For example, a large N2pc component is elicited both by targets and by nontargets that closely resemble the targets, but little or no N2pc activity is elicited by objects that can be rejected on the basis of salient feature information (Luck & Hillyard, 1994a, 1994b, 1995). In addition, conjunction targets elicit larger N2pc components than simple feature targets (Luck, Girelli, et al., 1997b). Thus, N2pc amplitude is a sensitive measure of the extent to which attention is allocated to a target item in a visual search task.

The goal of the present study was to use N2pc amplitude to determine whether discriminating feature-location bindings (i.e., localizing features) is more attention demanding than detecting features independent of their locations. Previous N2pc and single-unit studies have provided suggestive evidence supporting this hypothesis. Specifically, when observers were required to make an eye movement toward a target, a larger N2pc was elicited than when they were required to simply press a button upon detecting the presence of the target (Luck, Girelli, et al., 1997b). The same pattern of results was obtained in single-unit recordings from monkeys: Neural activity in inferotemporal cortex exhibited larger attentional modulations when the monkeys made eye movement responses to a target than when they made lever-release responses (Chelazzi & Desimone, 1994; Chelazzi et al., 1993). Making an eye movement to a target requires localization of the target, so this pattern of results suggests that the requirement to localize a target increases the attentional demands of the task. However, this result is merely suggestive, because target localization is not the only factor that differs between eye movement tasks and manual response tasks.

To address this issue more directly, we measured the N2pc component while observers performed visual search tasks that required detection, coarse localization, or fine localization of a target defined by a simple feature. Our primary interest was to determine whether N2pc amplitude would be greater in the localization conditions than in the detection condition, consistent with the proposed role of attention in feature localization. We compared the coarse and fine localization conditions to rule out the possibility that N2pc amplitude reflects the general level of task difficulty rather than a specific role of attention in binding features to locations. That is, N2pc amplitude might be larger for the coarse localization condition than for the detection condition simply because the coarse localization task is more difficult. If

N2pc amplitude is simply related to the overall difficulty of the task, then it should be greater for the fine localization task than for the coarse localization task as well as being greater for the coarse localization task than for the detection task. If, however, N2pc amplitude is equivalent for the coarse and fine localization conditions but is greater for these conditions than for the detection condition, this will indicate that the N2pc effect is due to the specific need to bind feature and location information in the localization conditions rather than a general difference in task difficulty.

METHOD

Task overview

Because ERPs are highly sensitive to the physical properties of the eliciting stimulus, all three conditions of the experiment used the same stimulus arrays, and only the instructions varied. The stimuli are illustrated in Figure 1. In the *detection* condition, observers were instructed to report the presence or absence of a square drawn in a particular colour, irrespective of its location. In the *coarse localization* condition, observers were instructed to indicate whether this coloured square was above or below the horizontal meridian; it was always well above or well below, so this task required very little spatial resolution. In the *fine localization* condition, observers were instructed to indicate whether this coloured square was above or below a nearby reference line; it was only slightly above or slightly below, so this condition required relatively high spatial resolution.

Subjects

The subjects in this experiment were 20 neurologically normal students at the University of Iowa, between 18 and 26 years old. They were paid for

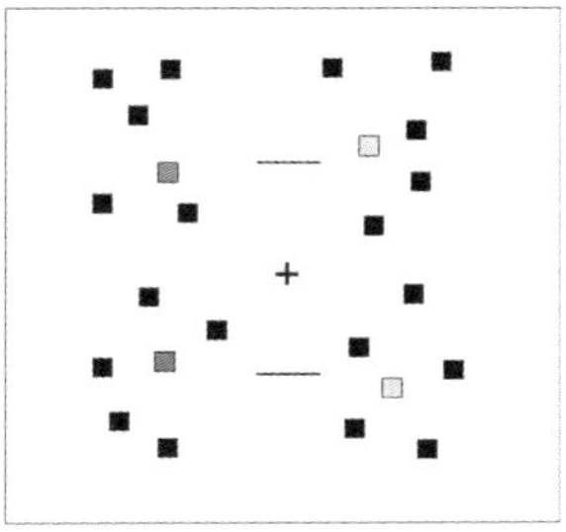

Figure 1. Example stimulus array. Squares filled with patterns represent the coloured items, and black squares represent the black distractor items. The stimuli were presented on a grey background.

their participation. All reported having normal or corrected-to-normal visual acuity and normal colour vision. Fourteen of the participants were female, and 16 were right-handed.

Stimuli

The stimuli were presented on a CRT at a viewing distance of 70 cm (see Figure 1). Stimulus chromaticity was measured with a Tektronix J17 LumaColour chromaticity meter using the 1931 CIE (Commission International d'Eclairage) coordinate system. A black fixation cross ($0.70^\circ \times 0.70^\circ$) and two black reference lines were continuously visible on a grey background (17.6 cd/m^2). The references lines were centred 3.6° above and below the fixation point and subtended 0.16° vertically and 1.64° horizontally.

The search arrays consisted of 20 black squares and four coloured squares, each subtending $0.46^\circ \times 0.46^\circ$. Five black squares and one coloured square were presented within each of the four quadrants of the display. The squares were randomly placed within a $6.54^\circ \times 5.23^\circ$ region in each quadrant, and this region was centred $3.89^\circ \times 3.23^\circ$ from the fixation point. The objects within a region were separated from each other by at least 0.65° (centre-to-centre) and were at least 2° from the fixation point. The coloured square was always centred 0.28° above or 0.28° below the nearest reference line, and was placed at one of three distances from the vertical meridian (2.3°, 2.8°, or 3.3°, selected at random).

Five colours were used for the coloured squares: red ($x = 0.647$, $y = 0.325$), blue ($x = 0.290$, $y = 0.133$), green ($x = 0.328$, $y = 0.555$), violet ($x = 0.296$, $y = 0.139$), and yellow ($x = 0.320$, $y = 0.545$). One of these colours was designated the target colour for a given block of trials, and one of the four coloured squares was the target colour on target-present trials. The colours of the nontarget coloured squares were selected at random (without replacement) from the four nontarget colours.

Procedure

Each search array was presented for 2000 ms, and successive arrays were separated by an intertrial interval that varied randomly between 800 and 1200 ms (rectangular distribution). The target colour was present on 50% of trials in all three conditions. When the target was present, it was equally likely to appear in the upper or lower field, and it was also equally (and independently) likely to appear slightly above or slightly below the nearby reference line.

In the detection condition, subjects were instructed to press one of two gamepad buttons on each trial to indicate whether the target was present or absent. In the coarse localization condition, subjects were instructed to press one of two buttons to indicate whether the target was in the upper or lower visual field and to press a third button if the target was absent. In the fine localization condition, subjects were instructed to press one of two buttons to indicate whether the target was above or below the nearest reference line and to press a third button if the target was absent. Subjects used their dominant hand for button pressing and were instructed to use the index finger to indicate target presence or relative location and the middle finger to indicate target absence. Speed and accuracy were equally emphasized.

The experiment consisted of 15 blocks of 64 trials. The target colour changed after every three blocks, and all five colours eventually served as target for each subject; the order of colours varied randomly across subjects. The three task conditions (detection, coarse localization, and fine localization) were tested in each set of three blocks in an order that varied randomly. At the beginning of each trial block, subjects were informed which one of the five colours would be the target for that block and whether they needed to detect it, localize it relative to the horizontal meridian, or localize it relative to the reference lines. Subjects were given 32 practice trials before the first time they experienced a particular task (i.e., before each of the first three blocks).

Recording and analysis

The electroencephalogram (EEG) was recorded using tin electrodes mounted in an elastic cap. Recordings were obtained from 10 standard scalp sites of the International 10/20 system (F3, F4, C3, C4, P3, P4, O1, O2, T5, and T6), two nonstandard sites (OL, halfway between O1 and T5, and OR, halfway between O2 and T6), and the left mastoid. All of these sites were referenced to an electrode on the right mastoid. The averaged ERP waveforms were algebraically rereferenced offline to the average of the activity at left and right mastoids (see Luck, 2005). The horizontal electrooculogram (HEOG) was recorded from electrodes placed lateral to the left and right eyes for monitoring horizontal eye movements. To monitor eye blinks, an electrode was placed below the left eye and referenced to the right mastoid. Electrode impedances were reduced to 5 KΩ or less. The EEG and EOG were amplified by an SA Instrumentation amplifier with a bandpass of 0.01–80 Hz and digitized at a rate of 250 Hz.

Trials with blinks or eye movements were automatically excluded from all behavioural and ERP analyses. Following our standard procedures, any subject with a rejection rate of 25% or higher was replaced; seven subjects were replaced for this reason. An average of 13.3% of trials per subject were rejected due to ocular artifacts in the remaining 20 subjects.

Averaged ERP waveforms were computed from target-present trials and collapsed across target colour conditions; after collapsing, there were 160 target-present trials in each condition. Target-absent waveforms were not relevant for the hypotheses being tested and will not be discussed further. N2pc amplitude was measured from the target-present waveforms as the mean voltage between 200 and 300 ms poststimulus relative to a 200 ms prestimulus baseline interval; measurements were obtained at the medial occipital, lateral occipital, and posterior temporal electrode sites (O1/2, OL/R, and T5/6). To isolate the N2pc component from other overlapping ERP components, we computed difference scores in which the voltage for trials with an ipsilateral target (with respect to the current electrode site) was subtracted from the voltage for trials with a contralateral target, averaged across the left and right hemisphere electrode sites; this difference represents the amplitude of the N2pc component. These difference scores were analysed in a two-way within-subjects analysis of variance (ANOVA). The ANOVA factors were task condition (detection vs. coarse localization vs. fine localization) and within-hemisphere electrode position (T5/6, OL/R, O1/2). All p-values reported here were corrected for nonsphericity using the Greenhouse-Geisser epsilon correction (Jennings & Wood, 1976).

RESULTS

Behavioural results

Mean reaction time (RT) from correct trials is shown in Figure 2A. Reaction times were computed separately for target-present and target-absent trials in each condition (collapsing across target locations in the localization conditions). RT for target-absent trials was largely constant across conditions, whereas RT for target-present trials was fastest for the detection condition, slowest for the fine localization condition, and intermediate for the coarse localization condition. In a two-way ANOVA with factors of condition and target presence, this pattern led to a significant interaction, $F(2, 38) = 194.31$, $p < .001$. In addition, the differences among conditions led to a significant main effect of condition, $F(2, 38) = 110.57$, $p < .001$, and the slower responses for target-present responses relative to target-absent responses led to a significant main effect of target presence, $F(1, 19) = 81.72$, $p < .001$. Planned pairwise comparisons of the three task conditions, conducted separately for target-present and target-absent trials, revealed significant differences between each pair of the conditions on target-present trials, $ps < .001$, but no significant differences on target-absent trials. The difference in target-present RTs between the coarse and fine localization conditions presumably reflects the greater

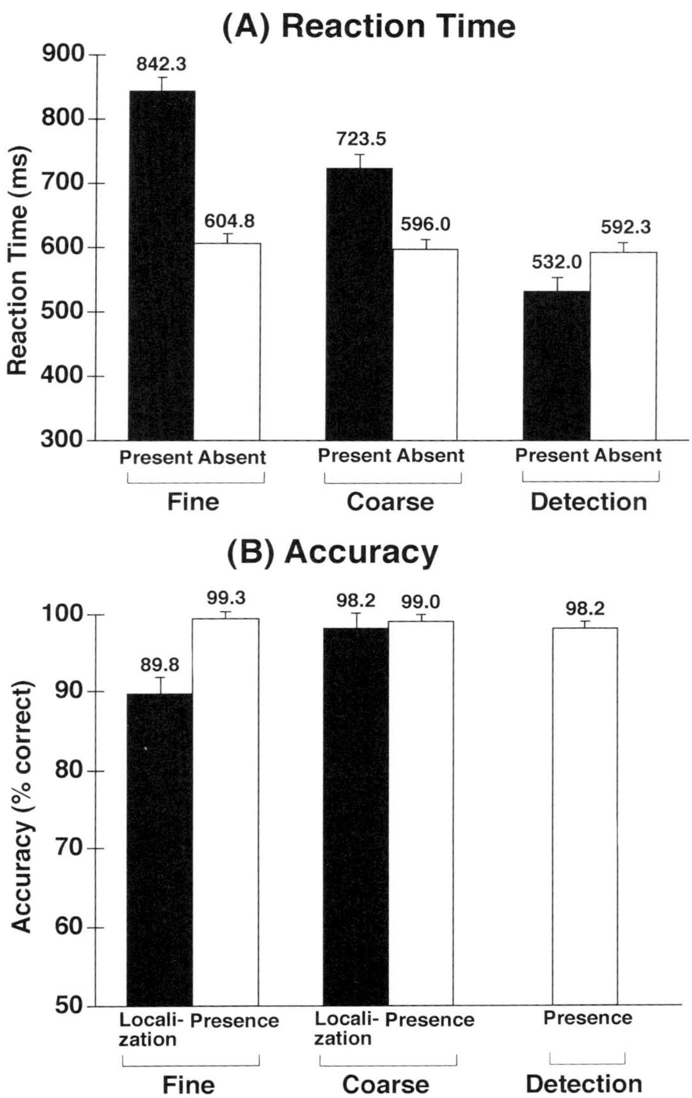

Figure 2. Reaction time (A) and accuracy (B) for the fine, coarse localization, and detection conditions. Reaction times were calculated separately for target-absent and target-present trials; for target-present trials in the localization conditions, reaction times were averaged over the two different spatial locations. Accuracy was calculated in two different ways. First, bars labelled "Presence" show the accuracy of determining whether a target was present (irrespective of whether it was correctly localized in the localization conditions). Second, bars labelled "Localization" show the accuracy of the localization response on target-present trials in the localization conditions. Error bars represent within-subjects 95% confidence intervals (Loftus & Masson, 1994).

difficulty of the fine discrimination task. Some of the difference between the detection and coarse localization conditions, however, almost certainly reflects the greater number of response alternatives in the coarse localization condition (RT typically increases as a function of the square root of the number of response alternatives; see Hick, 1952).

Accuracy, which is shown in Figure 2B, was computed in two ways. First, for all three conditions, we computed the percentage of trials for which subjects correctly indicated whether a target was present or absent (irrespective of whether the correct location was indicated; labelled "Presence" in Figure 2B). Second, for the two localization conditions, we computed the percentage of target-present trials for which the correct localization judgment was made (labelled "Localization" in Figure 2B). Accuracy for determining whether a target was present or absent was observed to be near ceiling for all three conditions; this observation was supported by a one-way ANOVA in which the effect of condition was not significant, $F(2, 38) = 2.42$, $p > .10$. In contrast, target localization on target-present trials was significantly less accurate in the fine localization condition than in the coarse localization condition, $F(1, 19) = 36.01$, $p < .001$.

Together, the RT and accuracy data indicate that the fine localization was, as intended, substantially more difficult than the coarse localization condition. In addition, the coarse localization and detection tasks yielded similar accuracy levels, but responses were slower in the coarse localization task (presumably due, in part, to the greater number of response alternatives).

Electrophysiological results

Figure 3 shows the grand-average ERPs recorded from a pair of lateral occipital electrode sites (OL and OR) in the detection, fine localization, and coarse localization conditions. These ERP waveforms compare activity elicited by targets that were ipsilateral versus contralateral to the electrode site, collapsed across the left and right hemispheres. That is, the contralateral waveform is the average of the left hemisphere waveform for right visual field targets and the right hemisphere waveform for left visual field targets, and the ipsilateral waveform is the average of the left hemisphere waveform for left visual field targets and the right hemisphere waveform for right visual field targets. The N2pc component was measured as the degree of difference in amplitude between the contralateral and ipsilateral waveforms between 200 and 300 ms poststimulus.

Consistent with previous studies, the N2pc component was largest at the lateral occipital sites (OL and OR), somewhat smaller at the posterior

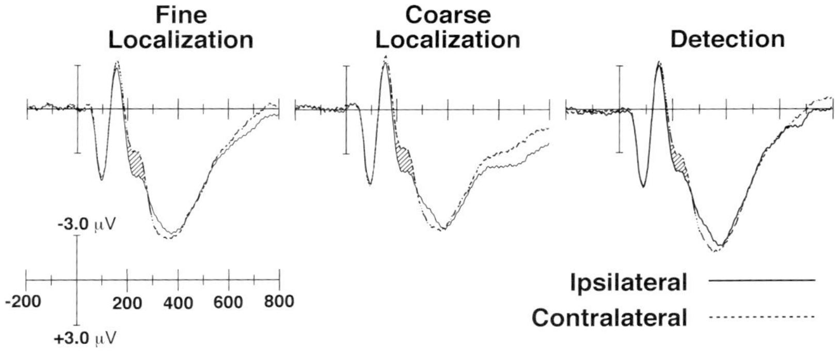

Figure 3. Event-related potential waveforms for correctly classified target-present trials in the three conditions, recorded from posterior temporal electrode sites (OL/OR) and averaged across subjects. The N2pc component is indicated by the hatched regions. Negative is plotted upward by convention, and time zero represents search array onset. For purposes of visual clarity, the waveforms were digitally filtered before plotting by convolving the original waveforms with a Gaussian impulse response function (standard deviation = 6 ms, 50% amplitude low-pass cutoff at approximately 35 Hz).

temporal sites (T5 and T6), and even smaller at the medial occipital sites (O1 and O2). This pattern led to a main effect of within-hemisphere electrode location in the omnibus ANOVA, $F(2, 38) = 3.74$, $p < .05$.

As can be seen in Figure 3, a clear N2pc component was present in all three conditions. The time course of the N2pc was similar across conditions, which is to be expected given that the stimuli and therefore the ease of finding the target should have been equivalent in all three conditions. N2pc amplitude was approximately equal in the two localization conditions (-0.74 μV for coarse localization and -0.70 μV for fine localization) but was smaller in the detection condition (-0.42 μV). The difference in N2pc amplitude across the three conditions led to a main effect of condition, $F(2, 38) = 4.01$, $p < .05$. In follow-up ANOVAs, a significant effect of condition was obtained when the detection and coarse localization conditions were compared, $F(1, 19) = 8.06$, $p < .05$, but not when the coarse and fine localization conditions were compared, $F < 1$. These analyses support the claim that the N2pc was larger in the localization conditions than in the detection condition but did not differ between the two localization conditions.

DISCUSSION

N2pc amplitude is a sensitive index of the degree to which perceptual-level attention is allocated to a target (Luck, Girelli, et al., 1997b; Luck & Hillyard, 1994a, 1994b). Consequently, the present results indicate that more attention was allocated to targets in the localization tasks than in the detection task, but attention was allocated approximately equally to targets in the coarse and fine localization tasks. That is, the observers had a greater need to orient attention to the target colour when they needed to report its location than when they merely needed to report its presence. This difference between the detection condition and the localization conditions supports for a key proposal in feature integration theory (Treisman, 1988; Treisman & Gelade, 1980; Treisman & Sato, 1990) and is consistent with other theories in which attention plays a key role in localizing features (Cohen & Ivry, 1989, 1991; Luck, Girelli, et al., 1997b; Luck & Hillyard, 1994a, 1994b, 1995; Prinzmetal et al., 1986).

Could these results be explained by differences in overall task difficulty rather than differences in the specific computations required for detection and localization? Not easily. Accuracy was at ceiling for the coarse localization and detection conditions, but N2pc amplitude differed. In contrast, accuracy was substantially impaired in the fine localization condition compared to the coarse localization condition, and yet there was no difference in N2pc amplitude between these conditions. RT was longer for the coarse localization condition than for the detection condition, but it was also longer for the fine localization condition than for the coarse localization condition. Thus, the difference in difficulty between the coarse and fine localization conditions appeared to be greater than the difference in difficulty between the detection and coarse localization conditions, and yet the N2pc differed only between the detection and coarse localization conditions. Moreover, previous studies have shown that that N2pc component is sometimes larger for easier targets than for more difficult targets (Luck & Hillyard, 1994a). In addition, the lack of an N2pc difference between the coarse and fine localization conditions does not a ceiling effect on N2pc amplitude, which is often twice as great as the amplitudes measured here (see, e.g., Luck, Girelli, et al., 1997b). Thus, although the coarse localization task presumably required additional processing relative to the detection task, the difference in N2pc amplitude between these conditions cannot easily be explained by overall differences in difficulty per se. Instead, the difference in N2pc amplitude reflects a specific difference in the computational requirements of the tasks, namely the increased need to use spatially focused attention when localizing a target.

We observed no difference in N2pc amplitude between the coarse and fine localization conditions. We cannot, of course, conclude from this null effect that coarse and fine localization have equivalent attentional demands. It is possible that, given a sufficiently large sample size, we would have observed significantly greater N2pc activity in the fine localization condition. However, we have conducted two additional experiments comparing coarse and fine localization tasks, and no tendency was observed toward larger

N2pc amplitudes in the fine localization conditions in either experiment. Thus, we are fairly confident that if there are any differences in N2pc amplitude between fine and coarse localization tasks, these differences are negligible. It is also possible that a significant effect would have been observed in the present experiment if we had employed a more extreme manipulation of the localization accuracy necessary for the coarse and fine location tasks. We cannot rule out this possibility, but it is reasonably safe to conclude that the fairly large differences in localization requirements tested in the present experiment—which led to more than a 10% difference in accuracy and more than a 100 ms difference in reaction time—do not elicit measurably different N2pc amplitudes.

In the decades since Treisman and Gelade (1980) first proposed that attention plays a special role in localizing and binding features, many studies have be published that either support or conflict with this proposal. Some studies conclude that attention is required for both detecting individual features and for binding multiple features together (e.g., Joseph, Chun, & Nakayama, 1997; Kim & Cave, 1995; Theeuwes, van der Burg, & Belopolsky, 2008), and others conclude that even bindings can be detected without attention (e.g., Eckstein, 1998; Mordkoff & Halterman, in press; Palmer, Verghese, & Pavel, 2000). How do the present findings fit within this large and contradictory set of studies? One possibility is that the discrepancies are a result of treating attention as a unitary mechanism that operates at a single locus, when in fact considerable evidence indicates that attention operates within different cognitive subsystems under different conditions (see Luck & Vecera, 2002; Vogel, Woodman, & Luck, 2005). Feature Integration Theory was intended to apply to the intermediate to high levels of visual perception, and the present findings support the idea that attention plays a special role in localizing and binding features within these levels. However, attention may not play any special role in feature binding at lower levels of perception (e.g., feature extraction) or at higher levels of cognition (e.g., working memory encoding and response selection). Because behavioural responses reflect contributions from both perceptual and postperceptual attention mechanisms, behavioural studies are usually unable to determine the system in which attention is operating. Consequently, it is likely that many of the apparent discrepancies about the role of attention in localizing and binding features are a result of the use of different experimental paradigms that emphasize different mechanisms of attention.

As an example, consider the study of Joseph et al. (1997), in which the second target was a masked visual search array. The size of the attentional blink effect was just as great for feature targets as for conjunction targets, leading to the conclusion that attention plays the same role for features and conjunctions. It has been well documented that the attentional blink reflects the operation of attention in working memory encoding rather than in perception (see, e.g., Giesbrecht & Di Lollo, 1998; Luck, Vogel, & Shapiro, 1996; Shapiro, Driver, Ward, & Sorensen, 1997; Vogel, Luck, & Shapiro, 1998), and it is also known that single-feature and multiple-feature objects require equivalent working memory capacity (Allen, Baddeley, & Hitch, 2006; Luck & Vogel, 1997; Vogel, Woodman, & Luck, 2001). Thus, the finding that the attentional blink is equivalent for features and conjunctions tells us nothing about the role of attention in feature binding during perception.

A significant advantage of neurophysiological measures of attention is that they can more easily isolate the operation of attention within a specific cognitive subsystem, making it possible to determine whether a given attention effect is perceptual or postperceptual and even subdividing perceptual processes (see reviews by Hillyard, Vogel, & Luck, 1998; Luck, 1995). In the present study, the N2pc results indicate that greater attentional resources are required to discriminate colour-location bindings than to detect individual colours, but this claim can be limited to the attentional mechanism indexed by the N2pc component. As reviewed in the introduction, we know that this mechanism operates after feature extraction but before object recognition is complete, and we know that it operates within intermediate and high levels of extrastriate visual cortex. This is exactly the level of processing that is the focus of Feature Integration Theory and related theories, and the present results thus provide support for this class of theories.

REFERENCES

Allen, R. J., Baddeley, A. D., & Hitch, G. J. (2006). Is the binding of visual features in working memory resource-demanding? *Journal of Experimental Psychology: General*, *135*, 298–313.

Chelazzi, L., & Desimone, R. (1994). Responses of V4 neurons during visual search. *Society for Neuroscience Abstracts*, *20*, 1054.

Chelazzi, L., Duncan, J., Miller, E. K., & Desimone, R. (1998). Responses of neurons in inferior temporal cortex during memory-guided visual search. *Journal of Neurophysiology*, *80*, 2918–2940.

Chelazzi, L., Miller, E. K., Duncan, J., & Desimone, R. (1993). A neural basis for visual search in inferior temporal cortex. *Nature*, *363*, 345–347.

Chelazzi, L., Miller, E. K., Duncan, J., & Desimone, R. (2001). Responses of neurons in macaque area V4 during memory-guided visual search. *Cerebral Cortex*, *11*, 761–772.

Cohen, A., & Ivry, R. (1989). Illusory conjunctions inside and outside the focus of attention. *Journal of Experimental Psychology: Human Perception and Performance*, *15*, 650–663.

Cohen, A., & Ivry, R. B. (1991). Density effects in conjunction search: Evidence for a coarse location mechanism of feature integration. *Journal of Experimental Psychology: Human Perception and Performance*, *17*, 891–901.

Eckstein, M. P. (1998). The lower visual search efficiency for conjunctions is due to noise and not serial attentional processing. *Psychological Science*, *9*(2), 111–118.

Eimer, M. (1996). The N2pc component as an indicator of attentional selectivity. *Electro-encephalography and Clinical Neurophysiology, 99*, 225–234.
Giesbrecht, B. L., & Di Lollo, V. (1998). Beyond the attentional blink: Visual masking by object substitution. *Journal of Experimental Psychology: Human Perception and Performance, 24*, 1454–1466.
Hick, W. E. (1952). On the rate of gain of information. *Quarterly Journal of Experimental Psychology, 4A*, 11–26.
Hillyard, S. A., Vogel, E. K., & Luck, S. J. (1998). Sensory gain control (amplification) as a mechanism of selective attention: Electrophysiological and neuroimaging evidence. *Philosophical Transactions of the Royal Society: Biological Sciences, 353*, 1257–1270.
Hopf, J.-M., Boehler, C. N., Luck, S. J., Tsotsos, J. K., Heinze, H. J., & Schoenfeld, M. A. (2006a). Direct neurophysiological evidence for spatial suppression surrounding the focus of atteniton in vision. *Proceedings of the National Academy of Sciences, 103*, 1053–1058.
Hopf, J.-M., Luck, S. J., Boelmans, K., Schoenfeld, M. A., Boehler, N., Rieger, J., et al. (2006b). The neural site of attention matches the spatial scale of perception. *Journal of Neuroscience, 26*, 3532–3540.
Hopf, J.-M., Luck, S. J., Girelli, M., Hagner, T., Mangun, G. R., Scheich, H., et al. (2000). Neural sources of focused attention in visual search. *Cerebral Cortex, 10*, 1233–1241.
Jennings, J. R., & Wood, C. C. (1976). The e-adjustment procedure for repeated-measures analyses of variance. *Psychophysiology, 13*, 277–278.
Johnston, J. C., & Pashler, H. (1990). Close binding of identity and location in visual feature perception. *Journal of Experimental Psychology: Human Perception and Performance, 16*, 843–856.
Joseph, J. S., Chun, M. M., & Nakayama, K. (1997). Attentional requirements in a "preattentive" feature search task. *Nature, 387*, 805–808.
Kim, M.-S., & Cave, K. R. (1995). Spatial attention in visual search for features and feature conjunctions. *Psychological Science, 6*, 376–380.
Loftus, G. R., & Masson, M. E. J. (1994). Using confidence intervals in within-subject designs. *Psychonomic Bulletin and Review, 1*(4), 476–490.
Luck, S. J. (1995). Multiple mechanisms of visual-spatial attention: Recent evidence from human electrophysiology. *Behavioural Brain Research, 71*, 113–123.
Luck, S. J. (2005). *An introduction to the event-related potential technique.* Cambridge, MA: MIT Press.
Luck, S. J., Chelazzi, L., Hillyard, S. A., & Desimone, R. (1997a). Neural mechanisms of spatial selective attention in areas V1, V2, and V4 of macaque visual cortex. *Journal of Neurophysiology, 77*, 24–42.
Luck, S. J., & Ford, M. A. (1998). On the role of selective attention in visual perception. *Proceedings of the National Academy of Sciences, USA, 95*, 825–830.
Luck, S. J., Girelli, M., McDermott, M. T., & Ford, M. A. (1997b). Bridging the gap between monkey neurophysiology and human perception: An ambiguity resolution theory of visual selective attention. *Cognitive Psychology, 33*, 64–87.
Luck, S. J., & Hillyard, S. A. (1994a). Electrophysiological correlates of feature analysis during visual search. *Psychophysiology, 31*, 291–308.
Luck, S. J., & Hillyard, S. A. (1994b). Spatial filtering during visual search: Evidence from human electrophysiology. *Journal of Experimental Psychology: Human Perception and Performance, 20*, 1000–1014.
Luck, S. J., & Hillyard, S. A. (1995). The role of attention in feature detection and conjunction discrimination: An electrophysiological analysis. *International Journal of Neuroscience, 80*, 281–297.
Luck, S. J., & Vecera, S. P. (2002). Attention. In S. Yantis (Ed.), *Stevens' handbook of experimental psychology: Vol. 1. Sensation and perception* (3rd ed., 235–286). New York: Wiley.

Luck, S. J., & Vogel, E. K. (1997). The capacity of visual working memory for features and conjunctions. *Nature, 390*, 279–281.

Luck, S. J., Vogel, E. K., & Shapiro, K. L. (1996). Word meanings can be accessed but not reported during the attentional blink. *Nature, 382*, 616–618.

Mordkoff, J. T., & Halterman, R. (in press). Feature integration without visual attention: Evidence from the correlated flankers task. *Psychonomic Bulletin and Review.*

Palmer, J., Verghese, P., & Pavel, M. (2000). The psychophysics of visual search. *Vision Research, 40*, 1227–1268.

Prinzmetal, W., Presti, D. E., & Posner, M. I. (1986). Does attention affect visual feature integration? *Journal of Experimental Psychology: Human Perception and Performance, 12*, 361–369.

Robertson, L., Treisman, A., Friedman-Hill, S., & Grabowecky, M. (1997). The interaction of spatial and object pathways: Evidence from Balint's syndrome. *Journal of Cognitive Neuroscience, 9*(3), 295–317.

Shapiro, K., Driver, J., Ward, R., & Sorensen, R. E. (1997). Priming from the attentional blink: A failure to extract visual tokens but not visual types. *Psychological Science, 8*, 95–100.

Theeuwes, J., van der Burg, I., & Belopolsky, A. (2008). Detecting the presence of a singleton involves focal attention. *Psychonomic Bulletin and Review, 15*, 555–560.

Treisman, A. (1988). Features and objects: The fourteenth Bartlett memorial lecture. *Quarterly Journal of Experimental Psychology, 40*, 201–237.

Treisman, A., & Sato, S. (1990). Conjunction search revisited. *Journal of Experimental Psychology: Human Perception and Performance, 16*, 459–478.

Treisman, A., & Schmidt, H. (1982). Illusory conjunctions in the perception of objects. *Cognitive Psychology, 14*, 107–141.

Treisman, A. M., & Gelade, G. (1980). A feature-integration theory of attention. *Cognitive Psychology, 12*, 97–136.

Vogel, E. K., Luck, S. J., & Shapiro, K. L. (1998). Electrophysiological evidence for a postperceptual locus of suppression during the attentional blink. *Journal of Experimental Psychology: Human Perception and Performance, 24*, 1656–1674.

Vogel, E. K., Woodman, G. F., & Luck, S. J. (2001). Storage of features, conjunctions, and objects in visual working memory. *Journal of Experimental Psychology: Human Perception and Performance, 27*, 92–114.

Vogel, E. K., Woodman, G. F., & Luck, S. J. (2005). Pushing around the locus of selection: Evidence for the flexible-selection hypothesis. *Journal of Cognitive Neuroscience, 17*, 1907–1922.

Woodman, G. F., Kang, M.-S., Rossi, A. F., & Schall, J. D. (2007). Nonhuman primate event-related potentials indexing covert shifts of attention. *Proceedings of the National Academy of Sciences, 104*, 15111–15116.

Woodman, G. F., & Luck, S. J. (1999). Electrophysiological measurement of rapid shifts of attention during visual search. *Nature, 400*, 867–869.

Woodman, G. F., & Luck, S. J. (2003). Serial deployment of attention during visual search. *Journal of Experimental Psychology: Human Perception and Performance, 29*, 121–138.

VISUAL COGNITION, 2009, 17 (1/2), 25–47

Psychology Press
Taylor & Francis Group

The role of reentrant processes in feature binding: Evidence from neuropsychology and TMS on late onset illusory conjunctions

Wouter Braet and Glyn W. Humphreys

Behavioural Brain Sciences Centre, School of Psychology, University of Birmingham, Birmingham, UK

We report data on illusory conjunctions (ICs) in a colour/letter identification task from a patient with simultanagnosia following bilateral parietal lesions and from a study using transcranial magnetic stimulation (TMS) with normal participants. We show that, even though target conjunctions were reported well above chance across a range of exposure durations, ICs were only generated at longer display exposures while feature errors decreased across time. With normal participants we found that TMS to the right posterior parietal cortex but not to occipital cortex increased the number of ICs. Moreover, ICs tended to occur after delayed stimulation, with the critical time window for stimulation being later for ICs than for feature errors. The data provide support for the critical role of posterior parietal cortex in a late process of feature binding.

Keywords: Attention; Illusory conjunction; Transcranial magnetic stimulation; Parietal cortex.

Visual illusions, where a person perceives an external object with attributes that do not correspond to external reality, have long been a topic of scientific and philosophical interest, with Plato's (c. 427–347 BC) division of illusions and ideas being one of the earliest known treaties on the subject. More recently, investigators have studied so-called "illusory conjunctions" (ICs), when people report two or more attributes from different objects as if they belong to a single object. ICs were first documented experimentally by Treisman and Schmidt (1982). They had participants pay attention to two external stimuli that flanked a set of central coloured letters. Subsequently, when reporting the coloured letters participants made errors by incorrectly

Please address all correspondence to Glyn Humphreys, Behavioural Brain Sciences, School of Psychology, University of Birmingham, Birmingham B15 2TT, UK. E-mail: g.w.humphreys@bham.ac.uk

This work was supported by grants from the BBSRC and MRC (UK).

© 2008 Psychology Press, an imprint of the Taylor & Francis Group, an Informa business
http://www.psypress.com/viscog DOI: 10.1080/13506280802193318

combining some of the colours with some of the shapes (IC errors).The probability of ICs was found to be greater than the probability of the participants reporting the feature of one object that was present and another that was not present (a so-called "feature error", FE). Treisman and Schmidt argued that ICs occurred when participants failed to pay full attention to the central items and that attention was required in order to correctly bind the features together (though see Donk, 1999, for an alternative view).

Treisman and Schmidt's (1982) data were interpreted in terms of Feature Integration Theory (FIT; Treisman & Gelade, 1980; Treisman & Kanwisher, 1998). According to FIT, individual visual features can be registered in parallel across a display without any attentional limitations on coding. However, in order to form correct conjunctions of features, attention is required to selectively highlight features in an attended region and to filter out competing features from other locations (Treisman, 1998). Treisman (1998) has further proposed that the neural locus controlling the focus of spatial attention is localized in the posterior parietal lobes (see Corbetta & Shulman, 2002, for a review of data from neuroimaging). Consistent with this, damage to posterior parietal cortex (PPC) is associated with patients making increased numbers of ICs (see Arguin, Cavanagh, & Joanette, 1994; Cohen & Rafal, 1991, for evidence from patients with unilateral lesions, and Friedman-Hill, Robertson, & Treisman, 1995; Humphreys, Cinel, Wolfe, Olson, & Klempen, 2000; McCrea, Buxbaum, & Coslett, 2006, for evidence from bilateral patients).

Other accounts of visual binding differ from FIT in proposing that forms of binding can take place preattentively (e.g., Humphreys, 2001). These accounts are supported by neuropsychological evidence on visual extinction. Extinction occurs when patients can report a single stimulus presented on the contralesional side of space, but fail to detect the same item when it appears simultaneously with a competing stimulus on the ipsilesional side (Karnath, 1988). Interestingly patients can show recovery from extinction if the contralesional stimulus groups with the stimulus in their ipsilesional field (e.g., if the two elements are collinear or are similar in shape and contrast polarity; Gilchrist, Humphreys & Riddoch, 1996; Humphreys, 1998; Mattingly, Davis, & Driver, 1997; Ward, Goodrich, & Driver, 1994). These data illustrate that visual elements can enter into grouping relationships prior to their being attended—indeed it is only when the items group that such patients are able to attend to both items present.

There is also evidence that ICs are influenced by grouping between visual elements. In both normal participants (Prinzmetal, 1981) and patients (Humphreys et al., 2000), ICs are greater between features that are part of a grouped set of forms than when the features are the same distance apart but belong to different perceptual groups. This suggests that an initial process of grouping between visual forms constrains the subsequent binding that might be required, for example, to report the colour of a given form. For example, surface colours tend to swap within the same object more than they do across different objects (Humphreys et al., 2000). To account for such results, Humphreys et al. (2000; see also Cinel & Humphreys, 2006; Humphreys, 2001) proposed a two-stage account of binding. At a first stage, visual elements are weakly bound but this process is noisy and binding may dissipate unless reinforced by top-down "attentional" feedback, which acts to consolidate a more stable, integrated perceptual representation of the stimulus (see Ahissar & Hochstein, 2004, and Rensink, 2000, for similar proposals). This feedback process is modulated by the PPC. Consequently, either limiting attention to the stimuli (in normal participants), or damage to the PPC, leads to a breakdown in this feedback process, enabling ICs to occur.

Evidence consistent with this two-stage view comes from data on implicit binding in patients with Balint's syndrome. Several investigators have now shown that these patients, who make frequent ICs in their explicit perceptual report, can nevertheless show evidence that visual elements have been bound—for example, the patients can be slower to detect a particular hue if it is is carried by an incongruent word corresponding to another colour (e.g., Cinel & Humphreys, 2006; Robertson, Treisman, Friedman-Hill, & Grabowecky, 1997; Wojciulik & Kanwisher, 1998). According to the two-stage account, the initial binding of visual elements may prime subsequent processes (e.g., an alternative name to that of the ink colour, in an incongruent Stroop word), even if this binding subsequently comes apart due to impaired feedback processes. Cinel and Humphreys (2006) further showed that implicit binding between elements was influenced by the same factors as explicit report. For example, the ability of their patient to explicitly report the hue and identity of a colour word increased when the spacing between this word and a distractor word increased. However, even on trials where the durations precluded explicit binding, evidence of implicit binding (evidenced by Stroop interference when the word and hue were incongruent) increased with wider spacing between the target and distractor words. Thus, explicit and implicit binding were affected in a similar way by target–distractor spacing. These qualitatively similar effects suggest that the binding processes reflect a common (two-stage) process rather than being qualitatively distinct.

The FIT and the two-stage model of binding both assume that attentional processes are critical for binding and that these processes are mediated by the PPC. However, the accounts differ in terms of the proposed timing of any attentional effects. According to FIT, attention can affect the initial coding of visual elements and the filtering out of irrelevant distractors (Treisman, 1998). Consequently, disrupting attention should have two effects: It should impair coding of the basic features of stimuli and so increase "feature errors" (where features not present in a display are reported), and it should also disrupt feature binding (increasing ICs). Feature errors should decrease across time, as feature information accumulates and as attention is applied to a stimulus. It is possible that ICs occur later in time than feature errors, since features have to be encoded first, before being bound together. However, provided the features of the stimuli are encoded well enough to support above-chance report of targets, the likelihood of ICs occurring should also decrease over time, as attention focuses more accurately on the target. That is, as soon as target features can be reported reliably, there should be a monotonic decrease if ICs across time.

In contrast, the two-stage account holds that attention acts to consolidate the features that are initially coded and bound together. This means that it is possible for there to be above-chance report of conjunctions of features prior to consolidation taking place. Disrupting attention (e.g., following a real or virtual lesion to posterior parietal cortex) should increase ICs but this could occur after a time when conjunctions can be reported reliably. Indeed, ICs may even increase across time as performance becomes more reliant on representations consolidated by reentrant feedback. This possibility was examined here using two sources of converging evidence: (1) Neuropsychological data from a "dorsal simultanagnosic" patient (with bilateral parietal lesions) who generates ICs with abnormally long display durations, and (2) data from transcranial magnetic stimulation (TMS) with normal participants. If the chronic lesion in the patient, and any "virtual lesion" induced by TMS to posterior parietal cortex (PPC), disrupts the reentrant processes necessary for robust binding, then ICs may increase across time even following a stage where conjunctive relations can be reported reliably. This was examined by varying the stimulus duration (in the patient) and the time at which TMS was delivered (in normal participants). We ask whether, for the patient, binding errors arise only when there is relatively prolonged exposure of the display, when reentrant feedback processes should (normally) help to consolidate binding. With normal participants we asked whether relatively late application of TMS led to ICs occurring. For both the patient and the TMS study, the report of target conjunctions was above chance even at the shorter durations/times of stimulation, indicating that there was sufficient time for feature coding largely to take place. The question then is whether ICs decrease monotonically, as durations/times to stimulation increase further. With the TMS study we also assessed whether binding was specifically linked to activation of the PPC, and not to the activation of primary occipital cortex, which could influence feature coding itself. To evaluate this, we initially examined the effects of TMS at three sites—PPC, occipital cortex, and over the vertex. If binding is specifically linked to attention operating through the PPC, TMS should increase ICs only following stimulation of that site.

In previous studies, TMS to the PPC has been shown to affect attention demanding processes in visual search (Ashbridge, Walsh, & Cowey, 1997; Walsh, Ashbridge, & Cowey, 1998a) and the attention blink (Cooper, Humphreys, Hulleman, Praamstra, & Georgeson, 2004). Recently, Esterman, Verstynen, and Robertson (2007) have also reported that offline TMS over the right intraparietal sulcus reduces ICs in perceptual report, relative to a pre-TMS test session and relative to a sham TMS condition (coil oriented away from the scalp).[1] This last result is consistent with there being a modulatory role of the PPC in coding visual conjunctions, if the TMS protocol led to enhanced activity in the intraparietal sulcus. Similar effects were not found after stimulation to other sites (TMS was also applied to the right angular gyrus at the junction of the occipital sulcus, and to the left intraparietal sulcus), suggesting that the benefit to report was not due to generally increased arousal. On the other hand, the benefit might reflect the role of the right intra-parietal sulcus in perceptual learning (Walsh, Ellison, Battelli, & Cowey, 1998b; Walsh, Ellison, Ashbridge, & Cowey, 1999), rather than in binding per se, given that offline TMS necessarily involves comparisons of a later test period (post TMS) with an earlier period (pre TMS). In addition, the offline TMS protocol did not enable Esterman et al. (2007) to study the time course of ICs or their relation to feature errors (FEs; reflecting poor encoding of features; FEs were close to floor in their study). In Experiments 2 and 3 here we examined effects with online TMS, where TMS is delivered on a trial-by-trial basis, to affect performance only during that trial. By varying the onset of the pulse in relation to when the stimuli were presented, we investigated the time course of parietal engagement in feature binding.

Three experiments are reported. In Experiment 1 we assessed ICs and FEs in a patient with simultanagnosia following bilateral parietal lesions. To assess if ICs arose only after processing had progressed sufficiently to engage PPC, we varied the exposure of the displays. Experiments 2 and 3 used TMS with normal participants. In Experiment 2 we established that TMS over the right parietal cortex, but not TMS over the occipital cortex or sham TMS, selectively increased conjunction errors but not feature errors or misses. In Experiment 3 we investigated the time course of parietal stimulation, and found a different "window" for the two types of errors, with ICs tending to

[1] In offline TMS a train of pulses is delivered to the region of interest at the start of the experiment, prior to a task being performed, with the aim being to affect cortical excitability for the duration of the task.

emerge only when TMS was applied relatively late (on average 150–200 ms after stimulus onset).

GENERAL METHOD

Participants

The neuropsychological patient, PF, was a right-handed female born in 1948. She suffered a first stroke at the age of 47. An MRI scan in autumn 2006 revealed bilateral lesions to the posterior parietal cortices including the superior parietal lobe and the intraparietal sulcus, extending more inferiorly in the left hemisphere (Figure 1). Subsequently she presented with a mild case of simultanagnosia. She found it difficult to assimilate the meaning of complex pictures. For example, she described the Boston Cookie Theft picture as "a boy getting some biscuits and there is a woman washing dishes and I think there is a girl playing too", failing to notice the water running out of the sink or the stool toppling over. She also required exposure durations of 200 ms to identify two letters each centred 3 degrees respectively in the left and right visual fields. This is over four times the slowest duration required across a small group of six age-matched controls. These characteristics, of impaired interpretation of complex scenes and poor assimilation of multi-item displays, are the hallmark of simultanagnosia (Kinsbourne & Warrington, 1962).

PF's performance was compared with that of two age-matched control participants, with no history of brain lesion.

Experiment 2 involved 10 normal participants (three males, seven females), aged between 23 and 49 years old. Experiment 3 had 10 participants, aged 22–49 years, of whom four were males. All participants gave written consent to participate, had normal or corrected-to-normal vision, and reported absence of epilepsy or any other neurological disorders in themselves and first degree relatives. For Experiments 1, 2, and 3, participants who had not previously participated in TMS studies were given an information leaflet on TMS prior to giving consent, and prior to the experiment taking place the procedures were explained and participants were given the opportunity to ask further questions. The study had approval of the local ethics committee, and conformed to the Declaration of Helsinki (1967) and safety procedures for TMS (Wasserman, 1998).

Apparatus and stimuli

For all experiments, the stimuli were presented on a 17-inch Gateway VX720 monitor at an approximate viewing distance of 100 cm, using E-Prime

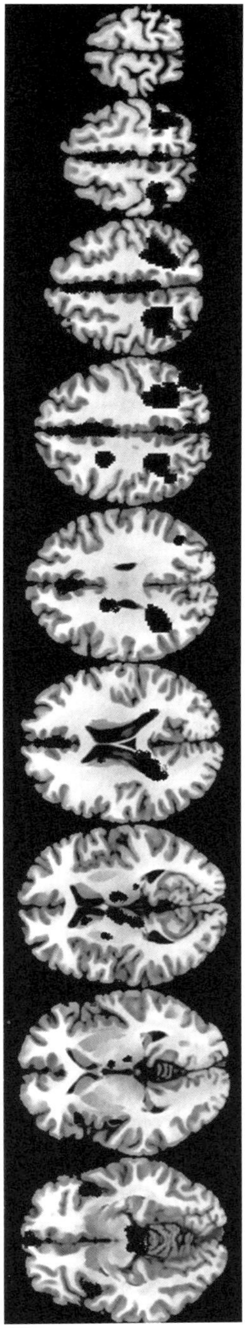

Figure 1. Lesion decomposition from MRI for PF (see Appendix).

software (Psychology Software Tools) run on a Pentium 4 (1.8 GHz). Responses were recorded on tape, for subsequent analysis for errors. Response latencies were not measured.

Stimulation

The stimulator used was a Magstim Rapid with two external boosters, in conjunction with a double circular 70 mm coil, which produces a maximum output of 2.2 T. With this coil configuration, the magnetic fields generated by both halves of the coil will add up, ensuring that the induced current is strongest in the region directly beneath the centre of the coil (Hovey, Houseman, & Jalinous, 2003).

Stimulation intensity was set at a fixed level of 60% of maximum stimulator output, for both Experiments 2 and 3. The stimulation during both experiments involved a train of two TMS pulses with an interpulse interval of 50 ms (double-pulse TMS, or dTMS). The onset of the first pulse was manipulated in both Experiments 2 and 3 (see Procedure). In Experiment 2, the total number of pulses was 576 (including 192 pulses of Sham TMS). Experiment 3 also had 576 pulses in total, all over the right parietal cortex (equivalent to the number of pulses in a 10 min train at 1Hz). To prevent overheating of the coil, and (in Experiment 2 only) to allow the coil to be placed over a different area within the experiment, both experiments consisted of three blocks of 96 trials each. The Intertrial interval was 1300 ms + the participant's RT.

In Experiment 2, three stimulation sites were used: Occipital, parietal, and sham over the vertex (e.g., see Cooper et al., 2004). For occipital stimulation, the centre of the coil was placed 3 cm above the inion, with the handle of the coil pointing upwards so that induced current would flow anterior-posterior. Stimulation of this region is assumed to affect area V1 in the primary visual cortex (see, e.g., Braet & Humphreys, 2006; Juan & Walsh, 2003; Lalli et al., 2006).

For parietal stimulation, the centre of the coil was placed over electrode site P4 in the 10–20 electrode system, overlying the PPC. MRI verification using our procedure suggests that this placement aligns stimulation at the border of the intraparietal sulcus and the angular gyrus (Mevorach, Humphreys, & Shalev, 2006). Induced current flow for this site was posterior–anterior and lateral–medial towards the vertex. In the sham condition, the coil was held over the vertex, but angled tangentially to the skull so that any cortical effects are unlikely to occur; this condition was included to control for nonspecific effects of TMS, such as caused by the sound (see Lisanby, Gutman, Luber, Schroeder, & Sackeim, 2001, for an evaluation of sham TMS). Both the parietal site and the vertex (Cz in the

10–20 electrode system) were marked on an electrode cap before the experiment taking place. The occipital site (3 cm anterior to the inion) was determined at the start of the experiment for each participant. Experiment 3 used only the parietal site (P4 in the 10–20 electrode system).

Procedure

All the experiments consisted of three blocks. In Experiment 1, the blocks were 192 trials long and were one of three different stimulus exposure durations: 100, 200, and 300 ms. In Experiment 2 the three blocks were each 96 trials long and represented the three different stimulation sites, and were counterbalanced across participants. In Experiment 3 there was no difference between the three blocks, and each comprised 96 trials.

The procedure was based on that of Cohen and Ivry (1989). In all the experiments, participants were asked to perform two consecutive tasks. First, they were asked to identify a one-digit number (ranging from 1 to 9), which appeared briefly (100 ms) at fixation. Immediately after the digit disappeared, two coloured letters appeared in the periphery (four possible locations: Top, bottom, left, and right; the distance between these locations and the centre of the screen was 8°). In Experiment 1 (for PF), the letters were exposed for either 100, 200, or 300 ms and they were not masked. In Experiment 2, the letters were visible for 100 ms, after which they were replaced by a 100 ms mask at the four different locations. The mask consisted of four white rectangles in Experiment 2, in addition to which a number of black letters (A, B, C, S, U, and Z) were added in Experiment 3 to increase the efficacy of the mask (see Figure 2). We used a black-and white mask to prevent additional (and irrelevant) colour features from the masks from being encoded along with the features of the stimuli.

For the letter identification task, participants had to identify the colour and identity of the target letter. Two letters appeared on every trial, a distractor letter (always O), and a target letter (either X or F, with equal probability). The letters were coloured red, green, blue, or yellow, with equal probability, and the target and distractor letters always differed in colour. The distance between the letters was 1.5° in Experiments 1 and 2, and 1.0° in Experiment 3 (this difference was introduced to increase the difficulty, and hence the number of errors, in the third experiment).

The identities of the target letters and the digit, as well as the colours and locations (up, down, left, or right) where the two letters (target and distractor) appeared, were randomized over trials.

In Experiment 2, the TMS pulses (two on each trial) were administered either at 50 and 100 ms after the onset of the letter-display (interval 50–100), or at 150 and 200 ms poststimulus onset (interval 150–200). In Experiment 2

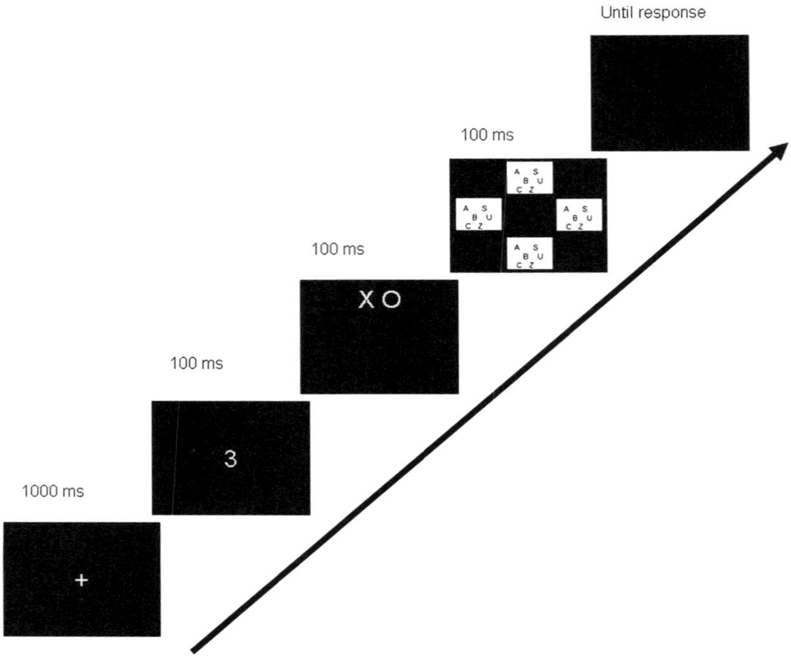

Figure 2. The sequence of visual events in a trial.

and 3, six different time points were used for the TMS: (1) 0 and 50 ms, (2) 50 and 100 ms, (3) 100 and 150 ms, (4) 150 and 200 ms, (5) 200 and 250 ms, and (6) 250 and 300 ms. This allowed for a more detailed investigation of the time course of the different error types.

Data analysis

Errors were analysed as one of three possible types: Feature errors (the participant named a colour or letter which was not present in the display), misses (when the digit was not correctly identified—this type of error may indicate that the participant was not fixating correctly at the beginning of the trial), and conjunction errors (where the participant correctly identified the target letter, but attributed the colour of the distractor letter to the target). This typology of feature and conjunction errors was originally used in a paper by Treisman and Schmidt (1982); miss errors were not included in the analyses presented here. Misses occurred in a very small proportion of the trials: 2.1% in Experiment 1,1.66% in Experiment 2, and 1.81% in Experiment 3.

EXPERIMENT 1: EFFECTS OF EXPOSURE DURATION ON ICS IN SIMULTANAGNOSIA

Previous research has demonstrated that simultanagnosic patients, with bilateral parietal lesions, make abnormally large numbers of ICs relative to normal participants (Friedman-Hill et al., 1995; Humphreys et al., 2000). We examined whether PF was prone to making ICs with relatively prolonged display durations (100 ms and above, with no mask), and whether the numbers of errors varied across the durations. This was assessed by comparing the number of observed ICs to the number of ICs expected from the total number of errors, using χ^2-tests.

Results

PF. PF made 126/192 (65.6%) correct letter–colour conjunction responses with stimuli exposed for 100 ms; 134/192 (69.8%) correct responses at an exposure duration of 200 ms, and 146/192 (76%) correct responses at an exposure duration of 300 ms. Chance report of the target conjunction was 12.5% (1/8). Performance was well above chance at each exposure duration. There was nevertheless a trend for identification to improve over time, $\chi^2(2) = 2.08$, $p > .05$. More crucially, relative to the total number of errors at each exposure, the number of conjunction errors increased as the exposure duration increased, $\chi^2(2) = 17.2$, $p < .001$, while the number of feature errors decreased, $\chi^2(2) = 15.93$, $p < .001$ (see Figure 3 for the percentages of each error type, relative to the total number of trials). There were more conjunction errors with a 200 ms exposure compared with a 100 ms exposure, $\chi^2(1) = 4.17$, $p < .05$, and more with a 300 ms exposure than with

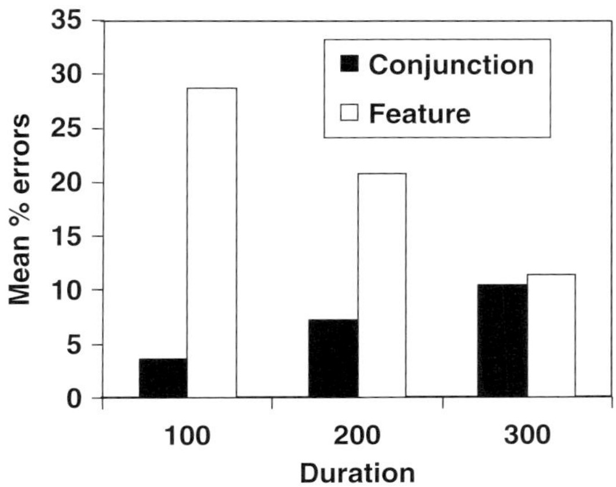

Figure 3. The percentage of conjunction and feature errors made by PF across three stimulus durations (Experiment 1).

both a 100 ms and a 200 ms exposure, $\chi^2(1) = 15.34$ and 4.86, $p < .001$ and .05, respectively. Relative to the total numbers of errors at each exposure, the number of conjunction errors at 100 ms did not differ from chance (for two letters and four colours, the expected proportions of CEs and FEs are 1/7 and 6/7 respectively, out of the total number of errors) at 100 ms, $\chi^2 < 1.0$, at 200 ms there was a trend for more conjunction errors than chance, $\chi^2(1) = 2.56$, $p > .05$, and at 300 ms conjunction errors were reliably greater than chance, $\chi^2(1) = 12.58$, $p < .001$.

Controls. The controls had a mean of 10% errors with stimuli exposed for 100 ms, with decreased to 2.6% errors at exposure durations 200 and 300 ms. At the shortest duration conjunctions errors occurred on 1.6% of the trials, which did not differ from chance, $t < 1.0$. There were too few data to analyse at the longer durations. PF's error rate was greater than that of the lowest control score, at each exposure duration, $\chi^2(1) = 31.71$, 53.34, and 38.01, all $ps < .001$, for durations 100, 200, and 300 ms, respectively.

Discussion

PF performed reliably worse than the controls. The controls never made conjunction errors at a rate greater than chance. At the short duration PF made feature errors while conjunction errors did not differ from chance. The report of target conjunctions, however, was well above chance, indicating that features were encoded sufficiently well to allow some conjunctive coding to take place. As the exposure duration increased, so there was a shift in error type; feature errors decreased and conjunction errors increased (and were greater than chance at the longest duration).

How can we account for this result? At the shortest duration PF's report of conjunctive targets was above chance, indicating that features were encoded to at least some degree, although it is clear that some FEs also occurred. As the exposure duration increased there was a decrease in FEs, consistent with attention gradually being focused on the target. According to FIT, this increased focusing on the target should also result in fewer distractor features being available and consequently a decrease in ICs. This was not the case, with ICs increasing rather than decreasing at longer exposure duration. Rather than this, we suggest a two-stage account of performance. At the short exposures, report was based on the initial encoding of features and feature bindings. The report of target conjunctions was above chance, but feature errors still occurred. As the exposure duration increased, feature coding improved and performance became more dependent on reentrant feedback from PPC. If this feedback is noisy in PF's case, due to her PPC lesion, then the feature bindings formed through this secondary process may be incorrect and "late" ICs emerge.

EXPERIMENT 2: TIME COURSE AND SITE OF STIMULATION IN NORMAL PARTICIPANTS

In Experiment 2, we investigated the types of errors made by normal participants following the application of TMS. TMS was applied over one of three possible sites: Parietal (P4), occipital, or sham TMS over the vertex (Cz). We also manipulated the onset of the stimulation (50–100 vs. 150–200 ms), to investigate possible differences in the time course of conjunction and feature errors.

Results

Overall accuracy, as well as the proportion of the errors that were conjunction errors,[2] are displayed in Table 1. The proportions of conjunction errors were also compared with those expected by chance (on 1/7 of the error trials). Conjunction errors were greater than chance only after P4 stimulation, but only at the longer stimulation time (150–200 ms). The data for conjunction and feature errors were analysed separately as they are not independent of one another. Each error type was subjected to a two-way repeated measures ANOVA, with time (early vs. late) and site (parietal, occipital, or sham) as the factors. For the ANOVAs, the data represent the overall percentage of errors, out of the total number of trials. There were no effects of stimulus location on the distribution of errors.

Conjunction errors. There was a significant main effect of site, $F(2, 18) = 10.27$, $p = .001$, but not of time ($F < 1$). The interaction between time and site was not significant, $F(2, 18) = 1.08$, $p = .362$. Participants made more conjunction errors when stimulation was applied to the parietal site, compared to either the occipital site or to when sham stimulation was given (both $ps = .014$, Bonferroni corrected). There was no difference in the number of conjunction errors between the occipital site and sham stimulation. The data are depicted in Figure 4.

[2] The scores for the percentage of conjunction errors here differ from those in Figure 4. The data in Table 1 show conjunction errors as a proportion of the total errors generated, needed to test performance relative to chance. Figure 4 shows conjunction errors as a percentage of the total numbers of trials in the experiment, to give an indication of errors relative to overall performance.

TABLE 1
The percentage correct responses, the percentage of the error responses that were conjunction errors, and the probability that the conjunction errors differed from chance (binomial test) (Experiment 2)

Site of stimulation	*TMS timing (ms)*	*% correct*	*% of errors that are conjunction errors*	*Probability of conjunction errors to chance*
P4	50–100	86.25%	18.75%	.1971
	150–200	89.58%	32.61%	.0013*
V1	50–100	89.17%	4.08%	.9952
	150–200	92.71%	14.29%	.5825
Vertex	50–100	90.63%	15.15%	.714
	150–200	92.50%	8.70%	.8908

Feature errors. The main effect of site was not significant, $F(2, 18) = 1.33$, $p = .298$, but there was a significant main effect of time, $F(1, 9) = 6.50$, $p = .031$, with participants making more FEs with early stimulation. The interaction between time and site was not significant, $F(2, 18) = 2.87$, $p = .083$ (see Figure 5).

Discussion

The data demonstrate that conjunction errors were observed only after stimulation of posterior parietal cortex (area P4). Overall conjunction errors only differed reliably from chance after P4 stimulation and only at the longer

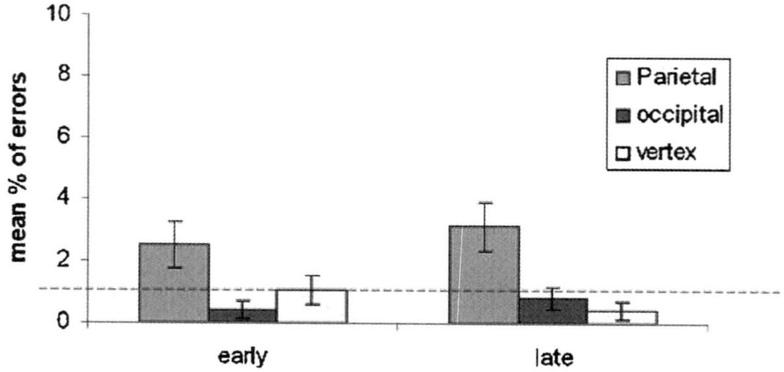

Figure 4. The mean percentage of conjunction errors (across all trials) made by controls as a function of the time at which TMS was applied and the site of stimulation. The dashed line represents the percentage of conjunction errors that would be expected by chance (Experiment 2).

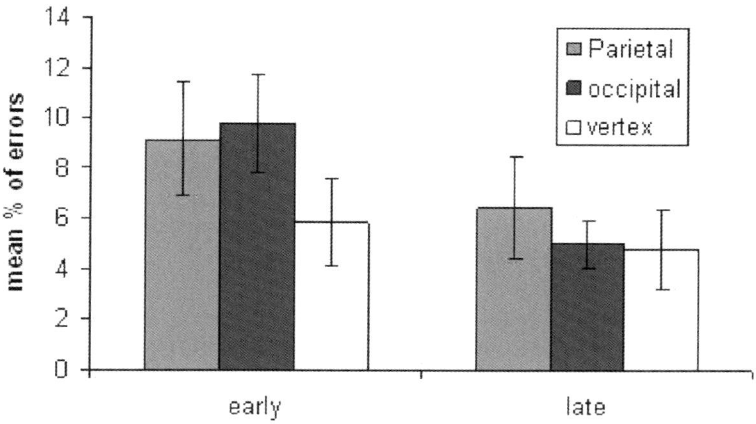

Figure 5. The mean percentage of feature errors (across all trials) made by controls as a function of the time of TMS and the site of stimulation (Experiment 2).

stimulation times (150–200 ms). Thus, neither occipital nor sham simulation was sufficient to induce conjunction errors. The overall ANOVA, however, only showed a trend for an interaction between stimulation time and conjunction errors after P4 stimulation. The time course of the effect will be explored further in Experiment 3. In contrast, feature errors showed a tendency to decrease as the time to stimulation increased, and these errors occurred with occipital as well as with parietal stimulation. The lack of any effects, with sham stimulation, counters an argument that the stimulation effects reflect nonspecific changes in arousal.

The failure to find conjunction errors at a level greater than chance after occipital stimulation is interesting and suggests that conjunction errors are not necessarily caused by impaired encoding of visual features, mediated by occipital cortex. The increase in feature errors found after both occipital and parietal stimulation, compared with sham stimulation, however, is consistent with stimulation disrupting feature encoding.

EXPERIMENT 3: A DETAILED ANALYSIS OF THE TIME COURSE OF PARIETAL STIMULATION

Experiment 3 was designed to investigate further the time course of conjunction errors following stimulation to the right PPC. Double-pulse stimulation was applied at six different points in time, always over the right parietal cortex (P4). Note that, in Experiment 2, there was no evidence for conjunction errors occurring at a level greater than chance after both occipital and sham stimulation. Hence, any evidence for the reliable generation of conjunction errors here is likely to be linked to the specific site of stimulation (PPC).

Results

The overall accuracy data, as well as the proportion of errors that were conjunction errors, are displayed in Table 2.

Conjunction errors. Conjunction errors occurred at a rate significantly greater than chance when stimulation was applied 150–200 ms after stimulus onset or later. Prior to this, conjunction errors did not differ from the levels expected by chance (Table 2). The effects of time were examined in a one-factor repeated measures ANOVA. There was a significant effect of time, $F(5, 45) = 4.48$, $p = .002$ (see Figure 6). Participants made the highest number of conjunction errors when stimulation was applied at 150–200 ms, compared to the two earliest windows of 0–50 ms ($p = .03$) and 50–100 ms ($p = .02$), but not when compared to 100–150 ms ($p \approx 1$), 200–250 ms ($p = .69$) or to 250–300 ms ($p = .15$) (pairwise comparisons, Bonferroni corrected).

Feature errors. The effect of time was also significant for feature errors, $F(5, 45) = 5.76$, $p < .001$ (see Figure 7). The highest number of feature errors was observed when stimulation was applied during the 100–150 ms window. This difference was significant compared to 50–100 ms ($p < .001$) and 200–250 ms ($p = .045$), but not compared to 0–50 ms ($p = .32$), 150–200 ms ($p = .34$), or to 250–300 ms ($p = .075$) (pairwise comparisons, Bonferroni corrected).

TABLE 2
The percentage of correct responses, the percentage of the total errors that were conjunction errors, and tests of whether the percentage of conjunctions errors were greater than chance (binomial test) (Experiment 3)

TMS timing (ms)	*% correct*	*% of errors that are conjunction errors*	*Probability of conjunction errors to chance*
0–50	81.46%	17.98%	.139
50–100	89.58%	8.00%	.881
100–150	73.54%	26.45%	.0003*
150–200	77.92%	35.85%	<.0001*
200–250	83.13%	29.63%	<.0001*
250–300	82.29%	30.59%	<.0001*

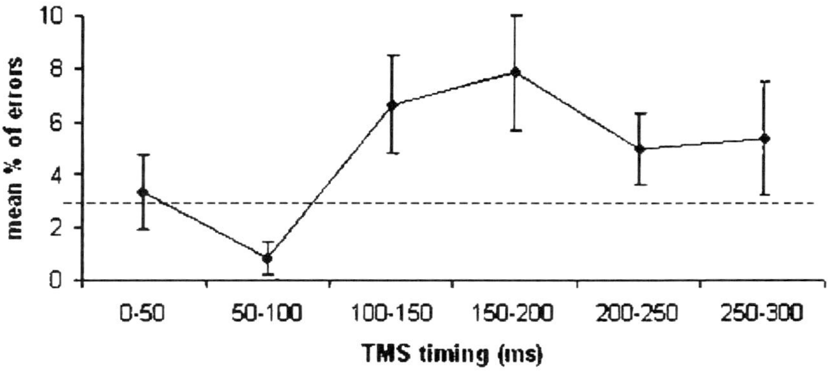

Figure 6. The mean percentage of conjunction errors (across all trials) made by controls as a function of the time TMS was applied to right PPC (Experiment 3). The dashed line represents the percentage of conjunction errors that would be expected by chance.

Conjunction errors versus feature errors. To evaluate the time course for these two types of errors, a sign test was carried out to compare the time points where the maximum number of each type of error was made. The test confirmed that, across participants, the point in time where TMS produced the most feature errors was earlier than that for producing the most conjunction errors ($p < .008$).

Discussion

The results reveal a distinct time course to conjunction errors in this paradigm, with the errors increasing when stimulation was applied at the

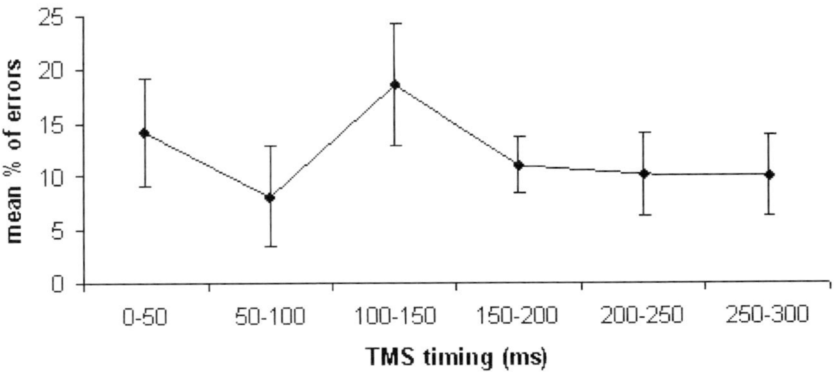

Figure 7. The mean percentage of FEs made as a function of when TMS was applied to right PPC (Experiment 2).

time interval of 150–200 ms onwards; prior to this conjunction errors did not occur at a rate greater than chance. This result replicates the data from Experiment 2, where again conjunction errors were only reliably greater than chance at the longer stimulation interval (though in that case there was a trend for an effect at the short stimulation interval; here there was no evidence for this). In contrast to this, there was evidence for feature errors occurring at an earlier stimulation interval, and, across participants, the peak of feature errors occurred at a stimulation time earlier than that found for the maximum conjunction errors. We suggest that early stimulation disrupts feature encoding while later stimulation disrupts feedback processes that are important for binding.

GENERAL DISCUSSION

We have used converging evidence from a patient with Balint's syndrome and from TMS studies with normal participants to examine the time course of conjunction errors in a task requiring the report of coloured letters. We found that the Balint patient, with bilateral parietal lesions, was generally worse at reporting targets than controls. In addition, while feature errors decreased as the exposure duration increased, conjunction errors increased. PF was more likely to make a conjunction error with display durations of 300 ms than with display durations of 100 ms. With control participants in Experiment 2 we found selective increases in conjunction errors when TMS was applied to the PPC, whereas conjunction errors were no greater than chance after occipital and sham stimulation. Also, with PPC stimulation conjunction errors only rose above chance with relatively late TMS (150–200 ms). Experiment 3 confirmed the increase in conjunction errors with late stimulation applied to the PPC. In addition, feature errors showed a peak at stimulation times less than those found to generate a peak of conjunction errors.

Both the data with PF and the TMS results are consistent with prior neuropsychological data (Friedman-Hill et al., 1995; Humphreys et al., 2000) and neuroimaging studies (Donner et al., 2002; Shafritz, Gore, & Marois, 2002, but see e.g., Nobre, Coull, Walsh, & Frith, 2003) linking structures in the parietal lobe to feature binding. In contrast, the present evidence indicates that stimulation of the occipital cortex was specifically linked to increases in feature errors. This fits with previous findings suggesting that the occipital cortex is critical for feature coding. In addition, the evidence indicates that feature coding can be temporarily isolated from binding, since (1) PF made feature rather than conjunction errors with short exposures of displays, (2) features errors tended to decrease while conjunction errors increased across time (PF, Experiments 2 and 3), and (3) feature errors peaked at durations and stimulation times shorter than those found for conjunction errors (PF, Experiments 2 and 3).

In addition to the "late" effects of parietal TMS on conjunction errors, there were earlier effects of parietal stimulation on feature errors. One possibility is that the two time windows reflect different processes in the parietal cortex, such as its role in directing eye movements and attention, and its role in feature binding. Leff, Scott, Rothwell, and Wise (2001), for example, have demonstrated that early but not late rTMS of the right parietal cortex disrupts the initiation and maintenance of a series of saccades (see also Yang & Kapoula, 2004). Given the close relations between saccadic programming and eye movements (see Schneider & Deubel, 2002, for a review), there is also likely to be disruption of the programming of attention. Hence, the early peak in feature errors here may reflect impaired programming of attention and saccades to the stimuli, resulting in poor feature coding. Interestingly, the time window for the peak of feature errors is similar to the timing of maximal TMS effects on conjunction search (Ashbridge et al., 1997; Walsh et al., 1998) and on generating contralateral neglect (Fierro et al., 2006). In both of these last cases, performance would be disrupted by impairing the process of shifting spatial attention.

The data on late conjunction errors, occurring even after conjunctive targets can be reported above chance, contradict the idea that conjunction errors reflect poor attentional allocation at early stages of visual processing (Treisman, 1998). Once features have been encoded to a level greater than chance, we would expect conjunction errors to decrease monotonically either as the stimulus exposure or the time to TMS increases, as attention is focused more accurately on the target. We did not find this. Instead there was an increase in conjunction errors either as the stimulus exposure increased (for PF) or as TMS was delayed, consistent with a second, reentrant binding process being disrupted by real and/or virtual lesioning of the PPC.

Our findings using TMS differ from those of Esterman and colleagues (2007), who observed a reduction of conjunction errors with right parietal stimulation. However, there are a number of methodological differences that may explain this difference between the two studies. In the present study we used two-pulse TMS while participants were engaged in the task, compared to 1 Hz stimulation prior to the task, which according to the authors may have facilitated, rather than inhibited, parietal processes (Esterman et al., 2007; though see, e.g., Mevorach et al., 2006). Our TMS experiments also used a higher stimulation intensity and were therefore more likely to disrupt underlying neural activity.

Like Esterman et al. (2007), we found that ICs were modulated by TMS applied to the right parietal lobe. Esterman et al. did not find the same result with stimulation of the left PPC, though we did not examine this. We did find, however, that the effect of TMS was not modulated by the stimulus field, suggesting that the right PPC may mediate binding across the visual field. On the other hand, studies with patients with unilateral PPC lesions have demonstrated problems primarily on the contralesional side of space (Cohen & Rafal, 1991), though it is possible that mild problems on the ipsilesional side may have gone undetected. However, marked deficits on both sides of space are usually associated with bilateral PPC damage (Friedman-Hill et al., 1995; Humphreys et al., 2000; this paper). From this we conclude that the left as well as the right PPC plays a role in feature binding, though the right PPC may be more dominant.

In conclusion, the data show that conjunction errors can be increased with either real or virtual lesioning of the PPC, with there being a relatively late critical time window to this effect. In contrast, feature errors are associated with shorter display durations and earlier stimulation, and with stimulation of occipital as well as parietal sites. The data therefore provide converging evidence that the PPC is critically involved in a relatively late process of feature binding.

REFERENCES

Ahissar, M., & Hochstein, S. (2004). The reverse hierarchy theory of visual perceptual learning. *Trends in Cognitive Sciences*, *8*, 457–464.

Arguin, M., Cavanagh, P., & Joanette, Y. (1994). Visual feature integration with an attention deficit. *Brain and Cognition*, *24*, 44–56.

Ashbridge, E., Walsh, V., & Cowey, A. (1997). Temporal aspects of visual search studied by transcranial magnetic stimulation. *Neuropsychologia*, *35*(8), 1121–1131.

Ashburner, J., & Friston, K. J. (2005). Unified segmentation. *Neuroimage*, *26*, 839–851.

Braet, W., & Humphreys, G. W. (2006). The "special effect" of case mixing on word identification: Neuropsychological and transcranial magnetic stimulation studies dissociating case mixing from contrast reduction. *Journal of Cognitive Neuroscience*, *18*, 1666–1675.

Cinel, C., & Humphreys, G. W. (2006). On the relations between implicit and explicit spatial binding: Evidence from Balint's syndrome. *Cognitive, Affective and Behavioral Neuroscience*, *6*, 127–140.

Cohen, A., & Ivry, R. (1989). Illusory conjunctions inside and outside the focus of attention. *Journal of Experimental Psychology: Human Perception and Performance*, *15*(4), 650–663.

Cohen, A., & Rafal, R. D. (1991). Attention and feature integration: Illusory conjunctions in a patient with a parietal lobe lesion. *Psychological Science*, *2*, 106–110.

Cooper, A. C. G., Humphreys, G. W., Hulleman, J., Praamstra, P., & Georgeson, M. A. (2004). Trans-cranial magnetic stimulation (TMS) to right parietal cortex modifies the attentional blink. *Experimental Brain Research*, *155*, 24–29.

Corbetta, M., & Shulman, G. L. (2002). Control of goal-directed and stimulus-driven attention in the brain. *Nature Reviews Neuroscience*, *3*, 201–215.

Crinion, J., Ashburner, J., Leff, A., Brett, M., Price, C., & Friston, K. (2007). Spatial normalization of lesioned brains: Performance evaluation and impact on fMRI analyses. *Neuroimage*, *37*, 866–875.

Donk, M. (1999). Illusory conjunctions are an illusion: The effects of target–nontarget similarity on conjunction and feature errors. *Journal of Experimental Psychology: Human Perception and Performance*, *25*, 1207–1253.

Donner, T. H., Kettermann, A., Diesch, E., Ostendorf, F., Villringer, A., & Brandt, S. A. (2002). Visual feature and conjunction searches of equal difficulty engage only partially overlapping frontoparietal networks. *Neuroimage*, *15*(1), 16–25.

Duvernoy, H. M. (1991). *The human brain: Surface, three-dimensional sectional anatomy and MRI*. Wien, Austria: Springer-Verlag.

Esterman, M., Verstynen, T., & Robertson, L. C. (2007). Attenuating illusory binding with TMS of the right parietal cortex. *Neuroimage*, *35*, 1247–1255.

Fierro, B., Brighina, F., Giglia, G., Palermo, A., Francolini, M., & Scalia, S. (2006). Paired pulse TMS over the right posterior parietal cortex modulates visuospatial perception. *Journal of the Neurological Sciences*, *247*(2), 144–148.

Friedman-Hill, S. R., Robertson, L. C., & Treisman, A. (1995). Parietal contributions to visual feature binding: Evidence from a patient with bilateral lesions. *Science*, *269*, 853–855.

Gilchrist, I., Humphreys, G. W., & Riddoch, M. J. (1996). Grouping and extinction: Evidence for low-level modulation of selection. *Cognitive Neuropsychology*, *13*, 1223–1256.

Hovey, C., Houseman, P., & Jalinous, R. (2003). *A guide to magnetic stimulation*. Whitland, UK: The Magstim Company.

Humphreys, G. W. (1998). Neural representations of objects in space: A dual coding account. *Philosophical Transaction of the Royal Society, Series B*, *353*, 1341–1351.

Humphreys, G. W. (2001). A multi-stage account of binding in vision: Neuropsychological evidence. *Visual Cognition*, *8*, 381–410.

Humphreys, G. W., Cinel, C., Wolfe, J., Olson, A., & Klempen, N. (2000). Fractionating the binding process: Neuropsychological evidence distinguishing binding of form from binding of surface features. *Vision Research*, *40*(10–12), 1569–1596.

Juan, C. H., & Walsh, V. (2003). Feedback to V1: A reverse hierarchy in vision. *Experimental Brain Research*, *150*(2), 259–263.

Karnath, H. O. (1988). Deficits of attention in acute and recovered visual hemi-neglect. *Neuropsychologia*, *26*, 27–43.

Kinsbourne, M., & Warrington, E. K. (1962). A disorder of simultaneous form perception. *Brain*, *85*, 461–486.

Lalli, S., Hussain, Z., Ayub, A., Cracco, R. Q., Bodis-Wollner, I., & Amassian, V. E. (2006). Role of the calcarine cortex (V1) in perception of visual cues for saccades. *Clinical Neurophysiology*, *117*(9), 2030–2038.

Leff, A. P., Scott, S. K., Rothwell, J. C., & &Wise, R. J. S. (2001). The planning and guiding of saccades: A repetitive transcranial magnetic stimulation study. *Cerebral Cortex*, *11*, 918–923.

Lisanby, S. H., Gutman, D., Luber, B., Schroeder, C., & Sackeim, H. A. (2001). Sham TMS: Intracerebral measurement of the induced electrical field and the induction of motor-evoked potentials. *Biological Psychiatry*, *49*, 460–463.

Mattingly, J. B., Davis, G., & Driver, J. (1997). Pre-attentive filling in of visual surfaces in parietal extinction. *Science*, *275*, 671–674.

McCrea, S. M., Buxbaum, L. J., & Coslett, H. B. (2006). Illusory conjunctions in simultanagnosia: Coarse coding of visual feature location? *Neuropsychologia*, *44*, 1724–1736.

Mechelli, A., Price, C. J., Friston, K. J., & Ashburner, J. (2005). Voxel-based morphometry of the human brain: Methods and applications. *Current Medical Imaging Reviews*, *1*, 105–113.

Mevorach, C., Humphreys, G. W., & Shalev, L. (2006). Opposite biases in salience-based selection for the left and right posterior parietal cortex. *Nature Neuroscience*, *9*, 740–742.

Nobre, A. C., Coull, J. T., Walsh, V., & Frith, C. D. (2003). Brain activations during visual search: Contributions of search efficiency versus feature binding. *Neuroimage*, *18*(1), 91–103.

Penny, W., Holmes, A., & Friston, K. (2003). Random effects analysis. In R. S. J. Frackowiak, K. J. Friston, C. Frith, R. Dolan, C. J. Price, S. Zeki, et al. (Eds.), *Human brain function* (2nd ed., pp. 843–850). Oxford, UK: Academic Press.

Prinzmetal, W. (1981). Principles of feature integration. *Perception and Psychophysics, 30*, 330–340.

Rensink, R. A. (2000). The dynamic representation of scenes. *Visual Cognition, 7*, 17–42.

Robertson, L. C., Treisman, A., Friedman-Hill, S., & Grabowecky, M. (1997). The interaction of spatial and object pathways: Evidence from Balint's syndrome. *Journal of Cognitive Neuroscience, 9*, 295–317.

Rorden, C. (2007). MRIcron [Computer software]. http://www.sph.sc.edu/comd/rorden/mricron/.

Schneider, W. X., & Deubel, H. (2002). Selection-for-perception and selection-for-spatial-motor-action are coupled by visual attention: A review of recent findings and new evidence from stimulus-driven saccade control. In W. Prinz & B. Hommel (Eds.), *Attention and performance XIX: Common mechanisms in perception and action* (pp. 609–627). Oxford, UK: Oxford University Press.

Shafritz, K. M., Gore, J. C., & Marois, R. (2002). The role of the parietal cortex in visual feature binding. *Proceedings of the National Academy of Science USA, 99*(16), 10917–10922.

Talairach, J., & Tournoux, P. (1988). *Co-planar stereotactic atlas of the human brain*. Stuttgart, Austria: Thieme-Verlag.

Treisman, A. (1998). Feature binding, perception and object perception. *Philosophical Transaction of the Royal Society, 353*, 1295–1306.

Treisman, A. M., & Gelade, G. (1980). A feature-integration theory of attention. *Cognitive Psychology, 12*(1), 97–136.

Treisman, A. M., & Kanwisher, N. G. (1998). Perceiving visually presented objects: Recognition, awareness, and modularity. *Current Opinion in Neurobiology, 8*, 218–226.

Treisman, A. M., & Schmidt, H. (1982). Illusory conjunctions in the perception of objects. *Cognitive Psychology, 14*, 107–141.

Walsh, V., Ashbridge, E., & Cowey, A. (1998a). Cortical plasticity in perceptual learning demonstrated by transcranial magnetic stimulation. *Neuropsychologia, 36*(1), 45–49.

Walsh, V., Ellison, A., Ashbridge, E., & Cowey, A. (1999). The role of the parietal cortex in visual attention-hemispheric asymmetries and the effects of learning: A magnetic stimulation study. *Neuropsychologia, 37*, 245–251.

Walsh, V., Ellison, A., Battelli, L., & Cowey, A. (1998b). Task-specific impairments and enhancements induced by magnetic stimulation of human visual area V5. *Proceedings of the Royal Society London, Series B, 265*, 537–543.

Ward, R., Goodrich, S., & Driver, J. (1994). Grouping reduces visual extinction: Neuropsychological evidence for weight-linkage in visual selection. *Visual Cognition, 1*, 101–130.

Wasserman, E. M. (1998). Risk and safety of repetitive transcranial magnetic stimulation: Report and suggested guidelines from the International Workshop on the Safety of Transcranial Magnetic Stimulation, June 5–7, 1996. *Electroencephalography and Clinical Neurophysiology/Evoked Potentials Section, 107*, 1–16.

Wojciulik, E., & Kanwisher, N. (1998). Implicit but not explicit feature binding in a Balint's patient. *Visual Cognition, 5*, 157–181.

Worsley, K. J. (2003). Developments in random field theory. In R. S. J. Frackowiak, K. J. Friston, C. Frith, R. Dolan, C. J. Price, S. Zeki, et al. (Eds.), *Human brain function* (2nd ed) (pp. 881–886). Oxford, UK: Academic Press.

Yang, Q., & Kapoula, Z. (2004). TMS over the left posterior parietal cortex prolongs latency of contralateral saccades and convergence. *Investigative Ophthalmology and Visual Science, 45*, 2231–2239.

APPENDIX: LESION RECONSTRUCTION

High resolution ($1 \times 1 \times 1$ mm) T1 weighted images (of the healthy controls and patients) were used for the lesion reconstruction. Image preprocessing and statistical analysis were done using SPM5 (Wellcome Department of Imaging Neuroscience, London). The images were transformed into the standard MNI space using the advanced segment-normalize procedure (Ashburner & Friston, 2005). Note that this procedure has been shown to be optimal for normalization of abnormal brain tissues (Crinion et al., 2007). In brief, the segment-normalize procedure uses the intensity signal in each voxel as well as a priori knowledge of the expected localization of grey matter (GM), white matter (WM), and cerebral blood fluid (CSF) in the brains, and iteratively segments the tissues and warps them onto standard space. Abnormal tissue intensity (i.e., a lesion) in regions that normally present GM intensity tissue for example, will be classified as less likely to be GM (see Figure 1). To ensure that abnormal GM/WM tissue intensities will not be classified as normal we restricted the number of Gaussians per class to 1 for GM and WM tissues. Finally, the segmented images were smoothed to accommodate the assumption of the random field theory used in the statistical analysis (Worsley, 2003).

In order to objectively determine the significance of tissue abnormality, we performed Voxel-Based Morphometry (VBM) analysis (Mechelli, Price, Friston, & Ashburner, 2005). We used general linear model with subjects as random variable (Penny, Holmes, & Friston, 2003) to compare the segmented GM of each patient to the segmented GM images of the 140 healthy controls (see earlier). In the statistical model we also included age and gender as covariates of no interest. Finally, we used a threshold of $p < .05$ corrected for family-wise error (height threshold, $t[137] = 5.1359$) with an extended cluster of at least 150 voxels (larger than ~ 350 mm^3). Finally we used *The Human Brain* atlas by (Duvernoy, 1991) and the *Co-Planer Stereotaxis Atlas of the Human Brain* (Talairach & Tournoux, 1988) for the anatomical labels of the lesion site. Lesions were confirmed by visual analysis.

For presentation, clusters that were classified significantly as abnormal were overlayed on a T1-weighted image (Ch2bet) using MRIcron (Rorden, 2007). Ch2bet is a scalp-stripped version of the average of 27 T1-weighted scans from the same individual (displayed at www.bic.mni.mcgill.ca/cgi/icbm_view). The whole brain on the right shows the slices used. Left of the slice represents the left hemisphere.

VISUAL COGNITION, 2009, 17 (1/2), 48–66

Psychology Press
Taylor & Francis Group

Attentive tracking disrupts feature binding in visual working memory

Daryl Fougnie and René Marois
Vanderbilt University, Nashville, TN, USA

One of the most influential theories in visual cognition proposes that attention is necessary to bind different visual features into coherent object percepts (Treisman & Gelade, 1980). Although considerable evidence supports a role for attention in perceptual feature binding, whether attention plays a similar function in visual working memory (VWM) remains controversial. To test the attentional requirements of VWM feature binding, here we gave participants an attention-demanding multiple object tracking task during the retention interval of a VWM task. Results show that the tracking task disrupted memory for colour-shape conjunctions above and beyond any impairment to working memory for object features, and that this impairment was larger when the VWM stimuli were presented at different spatial locations. These results demonstrate that the role of visuospatial attention in feature binding is not unique to perception, but extends to the working memory of these perceptual representations as well.

Keywords: Visual working memory; Attention; Binding.

Visual scenes regularly contain multiple objects, each defined by its unique featural properties such as its colour, shape, and motion. The richness of this visual information presents a "binding" problem to the visual system: How does our brain correctly associate features with their proper objects, especially considering that these features are processed in distinct and highly specialized cortical regions (DeYoe & van Essen, 1988)? It is not yet fully understood how features become conjoined into objects during visual perception, but one influential proposal is that visuospatial attention may assist in the binding process by selecting an object's location and linking all features at that location to the object (Treisman, 1998, 2006; Treisman & Gelade, 1980). The finding that subjects may incorrectly bind features of objects together if attention is diverted provides converging evidence for a role of attention in perceiving an

Please address all correspondence to Daryl Fougnie, Department of Psychology, Wilson Hall, 111 21st Avenue South, Vanderbilt University, Nashville, TN 37240-1103, USA. E-mail: d.fougnie@vanderbilt.edu

This work was supported by NIMH grant (R01-MH70776) to RM.

© 2008 Psychology Press, an imprint of the Taylor & Francis Group, an Informa business
http://www.psypress.com/viscog DOI: 10.1080/13506280802281337

integrated visual world (Briand & Klein, 1987; Prinzmetal, Presti, & Posner, 1986; Treisman & Schmidt, 1982; but see Donk, 1999; Navon & Ehrlich, 1995).

A considerable amount of work has illuminated the function of attention in visual perception, but its role in visual working memory (VWM) is much less understood. Dual-task studies have shown that shifts of attention can interfere with VWM (Awh & Jonides, 2001; Awh, Jonides, & Reuter-Lorenz, 1998; Fougnie & Marois, 2006; Oh & Kim, 2004; Woodman & Luck, 2004; but see Woodman, Vogel, & Luck, 2001), clearly highlighting a role for attention in VWM maintenance. Wheeler and Treisman (2002) have proposed that the role of attention in VWM is not in the storage of object features, but rather in the maintenance of proper bindings between these features. According to this view, visuospatial attention plays a similar role in visual perception and VWM—the formation and maintenance of feature bindings. This theory is supported by work suggesting that attention is involved in creating a representational format, termed "object files", which maintain an object's identity in both perception and working memory (Irwin, 1992, 1996; Irwin & Andrews, 1996; Irwin & Zelinsky, 2002; Kahneman & Treisman, 1984; Kahneman, Treisman, & Gibbs, 1992; Treisman, 2006; Treisman & Zhang, 2006). In contrast to the view that attention is necessary to maintain feature bindings in VWM, it has been suggested that features are automatically conjoined in VWM. According to this hypothesis, participants can store the same number of items in VWM regardless of whether the items are defined by a single feature, or by a conjunction of features (Luck & Vogel, 1997; Vogel, Woodman, & Luck, 2001). Thus, theories of VWM differ on the purported role of attention in maintaining bound features.

If attention is required to keep features bound together in VWM, then diverting attention during a VWM retention interval should result in impaired memory for feature bindings. Indeed, the importance of attention in perceptual feature binding is often demonstrated by the improper feature conjunctions that result when attention is diverted from the primary perceptual task (Treisman & Schmidt, 1982). When this approach has been used to investigate the role of attention in working memory, the results have generally failed to demonstrate that attention is specifically involved in VWM feature binding (Allen, Baddeley, & Hitch, 2006; Gajewski & Brockmole, 2006; Yeh, Yang, & Chiu, 2005). One study disrupted attention by requiring subjects to identify letters that were briefly presented at various positions during the retention interval of a VWM task (Yeh et al., 2005); another used a briefly presented exogenous cue to draw attention during the VWM retention interval (Gajewski & Brockmole, 2006). Although both studies showed that the withdrawal of attention affected VWM performance, neither found that it specifically disrupted VWM feature bindings. However, considering that attention may not need to be continuously applied to maintain object representations in VWM (Hollingworth, 2004; Hollingworth, Williams, & Henderson, 2001; Irwin, 1992, 1996; Schneider, 1999), transient shifts of attention may be insufficient to impair VWM feature binding. In contrast to the two aforementioned studies, Allen and colleagues (Allen et al., 2006) used a continuously demanding attention task during the VWM retention interval, but nevertheless still failed to show specific disruptions of VWM feature bindings. However, that study's attention-demanding secondary task—which consisted in either backward counting or supraspan digit recall—may not have tapped onto the type of attention that is required for binding. Backward counting and digit recall tasks are considered to load on central attention (Han & Kim, 2004), whereas visuospatial attention is believed to be involved in feature binding during perception (Treisman & Gelade, 1980), and these two types of attention have been proposed to be distinct (Johnston, McCann, & Remington, 1995; Pashler 1991, 1993; Posner & Petersen, 1990; Vogel, Woodman, & Luck, 2005).

Thus, the goal of the present study was to reexamine the role of attention in VWM feature binding. Specifically, we tested the hypothesis that a secondary attention task, which is both visuospatial and continuously demanding, could disrupt feature bindings in VWM.

EXPERIMENT 1

To test whether a continuously demanding attention task would disrupt feature binding in VWM, we required subjects to perform a multiple object tracking (MOT) task (Cavanagh & Alvarez, 2005; Pylyshyn & Storm, 1988) during the retention interval of a VWM task (Figure 1). The MOT task involved attentively tracking moving targets among distractors. The VWM task involved holding in working memory, over a brief retention interval, just the colour, just the shape, the colour and the shape, or the specific conjunctions of colour and shape of the objects in the memory display. Based on previous work (Fougnie & Marois, 2006), we predicted that the MOT task would disrupt VWM performance. More importantly, we predicted that the MOT task would be most disruptive for VWM in the conjunction condition because this condition should specifically rely on the type of attention taxed by MOT.

Methods

Participants

Twenty young adults (eight males) participated for course credit or monetary reward. One participant's data was discarded because VWM

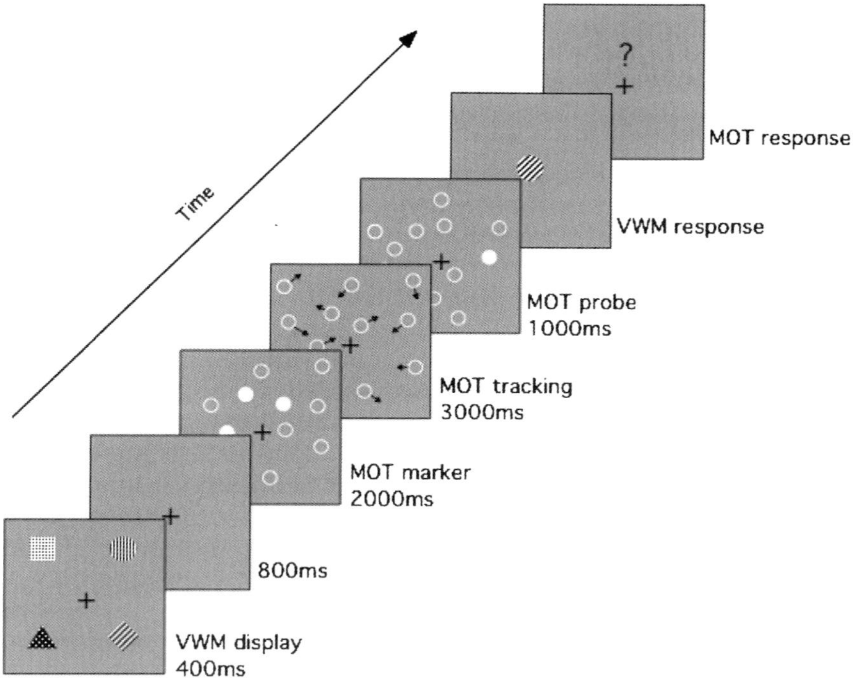

Figure 1. Trial design for Experiment 1. Different fill patterns represent different solid colours.

performance did not meet our a priori criterion of above chance VWM performance in all conditions. This criterion prevented the inclusion of participants who would not show an effect of tracking on VWM performance because of chance VWM performance even without the tracking task.

Procedure

VWM task. This task was based on a change detection procedure (Vogel et al., 2001) in which a memory display of three objects was first briefly presented, followed by a retention interval, and by a single probe item that required a same–different judgement on the task-relevant feature(s). The relevant features differed across four VWM conditions (colour-only, shape-only, either, binding). In the colour-only condition, participants memorized the colour of the stimuli, whereas they memorized the shape in the shape-only condition. In the either and binding conditions, participants were required to memorize both the colour and shape of the stimuli, but only the binding condition required participants to remember the specific colour–shape pairings of the objects in the memory display.

The memory display consisted of three coloured shapes (0.78° × 0.78°). Stimuli were spaced evenly apart and appeared along an imaginary circle (2.5° radius) around a centrally presented fixation cross. There were six possible colours (green, brown, blue, yellow, purple, or red) and six possible shapes (circle, square, octagon, cross, diamond, or triangle). Task-relevant features did not repeat in a display. In the colour-only condition, the stimuli all shared the same shape, selected randomly every trial. Similarly, the stimuli all shared the same randomly selected colour in the shape-only condition.

The memory display was presented for 400 ms and, after a 6800 ms retention interval, a probe display appeared containing one coloured shape (0.78° × 0.78°) at fixation. The probe display remained until participants made an unspeeded response (accuracy stressed) by pressing one of two keys on a keyboard with their right hand to indicate whether the task-relevant features matched an item from the memory display (50% match trials). In the colour-only and shape-only conditions, the probe either matched one of the memory items, or differed in the task-relevant feature. In the either condition, the probe display tested shape or colour memory (randomly determined). To minimize confusion in this condition, the untested feature property was a colour (black) or shape (bar) that would never appear in the memory display (see Figure 2). In the binding condition, the probe was either a correct or incorrect pairing of shape and colour from the memory display.

MOT task. The MOT task occurred during the VWM retention interval beginning 800 ms after memory display offset to allow sufficient time to fully encode the VWM display. MOT stimuli were hollow white discs (0.50°) moving about within an 8.5° × 8.5° area centred around fixation. Each 6000 ms MOT movie had three phases: Marker, tracking, and probe, lasting

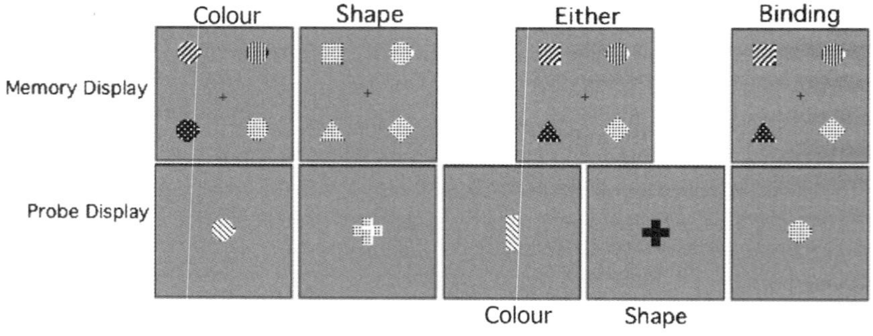

Figure 2. Examples of memory and probe displays in the four VWM conditions (colour, shape, either, and binding). Different fill patterns represent different solid colours.

2000, 3000, and 1000 ms, respectively. During the *marker* phase, the three target discs (among nine distractors) were filled white. During the *tracking* phase, the target indicators disappeared and both targets and distractors began to move in a random direction. The speed of each disc varied from 0.00215°/ms to 0.0195°/ms, and disc direction had a 10% chance to change at every refresh (13.3 ms). The discs bounced off the boundaries of the MOT display, other MOT discs, and the three VWM stimuli locations. During the *probe* phase, a single disc was marked. Half of the time the probe disc corresponded to a target.

Participants responded to the tracking task after responding to the VWM task. A question mark appeared above fixation, notifying participants to make a left-handed button press to indicate whether the MOT probe item corresponded to a target. Responses were not speeded and accuracy was stressed.

Control condition. Performance in the VWM task during concurrent MOT was contrasted with VWM performance during a control condition in which a stimulus display similar to that of the MOT task was presented but no accompanying task was required. The control condition included a MOT display during the VWM retention interval, as in the MOT task, except that no targets were highlighted in the marker phase and all discs were highlighted during the probe phase. In the control condition, only the VWM response was collected.

Articulatory suppression. To minimize contamination form verbal working memory, participants performed an articulatory suppression task (repeating the word "the" at a 2 Hz rate) beginning 1 s prior to the memory display and continuing until responses for both tasks had been collected. Articulatory suppression was monitored by an experimenter.

Design

Participants performed eight blocks of 24 trials. Half of the trials in each block required tracking, with the tracking and control trials randomly intermixed. VWM conditions were blocked, and participants were assigned to one of four possible orderings, with each ordering differing by the starting condition. For each ordering, the four conditions were first presented sequentially for the first four blocks, and this sequence was reversed for the last four blocks (for example, a participant might receive either-binding-colour-shape–shape-colour-binding-either blocks of trials). In all experiments, there was no effect of VWM condition order on either VWM or MOT performance (*ps* > .5); thus, this factor is not discussed any further. At the beginning of the experiment participants completed a practice block consisting of 12 trials of each VWM type. Participants were instructed to maintain fixation on the central cross throughout the trial and to emphasize the two tasks equally.

Results

VWM task. VWM accuracy is plotted in Figure 3A. Following prior convention, we separately analysed colour and shape probes in the either condition (labelled either-colour and either-shape, respectively; see also Allen et al., 2006; Wheeler & Treisman, 2002). Importantly, the results of this experiment (and Experiment 2) are statistically equivalent if the analyses are performed on the combined either condition data. We performed a two-way within-subject ANOVA as a function of tracking condition (tracking, control) and VWM condition (colour-only, shape-only, either-colour, either-shape, binding) on the VWM accuracy data. There were main effects of VWM condition, $F(4, 72) = 31.3$, $p < .0001$, and tracking condition, $F(1, 18) = 13.9$, $p < .005$. The interaction between tracking and VWM condition was also significant, $F(4, 72) = 5.3$, $p < .01$. To measure the effect of tracking in each VWM condition, VWM accuracy during no tracking (control condition) was subtracted from VWM accuracy during tracking. Two-tailed t-tests revealed an effect of tracking in the binding ($p < .001$) and shape-only conditions ($p = .02$), but not in any other VWM conditions (all, $ps > .05$). Most importantly, two-tailed paired t-tests demonstrated that the effect of tracking was significantly larger in the binding condition than in any other VWM condition, all $ps < .05$.

MOT task. MOT accuracy is illustrated in Figure 3B. A one way within-subject ANOVA, with a factor of VWM condition (colour-only, shape-only, either-colour, either-shape, binding), revealed that VWM condition had no affect on MOT performance, $F(4, 72) = 1.02$, $p = .41$.

Discussion

An attention-demanding tracking task performed during the retention interval of a VWM task specifically disrupted feature bindings in VWM. That the effect of tracking was largest in the binding condition cannot be explained by an unequal allocation of resources to tracking between VWM conditions, since performance on the tracking task was comparable across these conditions. This result also cannot be explained by the fact that tracking can additively impair VWM performance of two features in the binding condition compared to a single feature in the colour-only and shape-only conditions because the costs of tracking in the binding condition are larger than the sum of the costs of tracking in the colour-only and

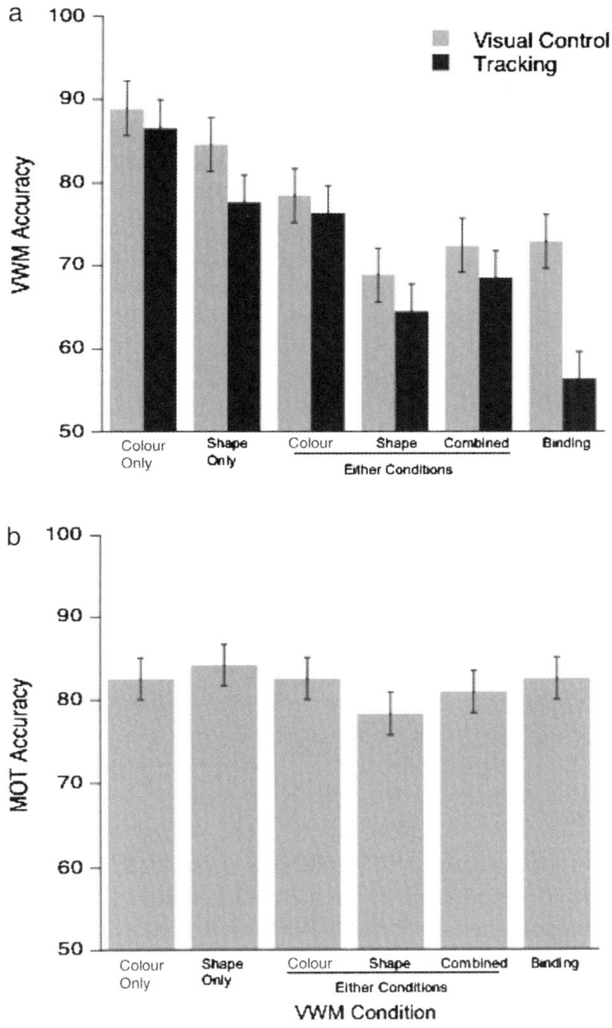

Figure 3. Accuracy in Experiment 1 for the VWM task (a) and the MOT task (b) by VWM condition. In the either condition, in addition to combined performance, scores are separately given for colour and shape memory probes. VWM accuracy (a) is black for the tracking condition and grey for the control condition. Error bars represent within-subject errors of the mean.

shape-only conditions ($p < .05$, one tailed). It is also unlikely that the larger binding interference occurred because that condition was more difficult than the other conditions. VWM performance in the absence of tracking was worse in the binding condition than either the colour-only or shape-only conditions ($ps < .001$), but it was equivalent in the binding and either conditions ($p = .88$). The latter results accord well with those of Allen and colleagues (2006), demonstrating that general secondary task difficulty does not affect VWM binding.

Taken together, the findings of Experiment 1 are consistent with Wheeler and Treisman's (2002) suggestion that disruptions of visuospatial attention impair VWM binding. However, in addition to attentive tracking, the MOT task involves other cognitive processes, including encoding and retrieval of target identity. In order to demonstrate that the interference of MOT on VWM feature binding results from attentional demands, nonattentional factors need to be ruled out. Experiment 2 accomplished this by replacing the control task of Experiment 1 with a static task. The static task was identical to the tracking task during the marker and probe phases, but the tracking phase differed in that the stimuli remained stationary instead of moving about throughout that phase. Although the static condition still necessitated the encoding and retrieval of targets, the requirement to attentively track stimuli was virtually eliminated. If the impairment in Experiment 1 was due to the demands of tracking, then binding should still be impaired during tracking relative to the static condition.

EXPERIMENT 2

Method

Participants

Twenty-five young adults (11 males) participated for course credit or monetary reward. Data from three participants were discarded because of chance performance in one of the VWM conditions.

Procedure

The procedure for Experiment 2 was identical to Experiment 1 except for the following differences.

VWM task. The colour (green, brown, red, yellow, and blue) and shape (triangle, octagon, cross, diamond, and square) sets were altered to further minimize potential confusion between tasks.

Static memory task. The static task had three phases: Marker (2 s), memory (3 s), and probe (1 s). The memory phase was identical to the tracking phase of the MOT task, except that the disks remained stationary.

A total of 256 trials were included with 32 trials in each block. The type of probe in the either condition was counterbalanced across conditions.

Results and discussion

VWM task. VWM accuracy is plotted in Figure 4A. We performed a two-way within-subject ANOVA as a function of tracking condition (tracking, static) and VWM condition (colour-only, shape-only, either-colour, either-shape, binding) on VWM accuracy. There was a main effect of VWM condition, $F(4, 84) = 71.9$, $p < .0001$, and tracking condition, $F(1, 21) = 6.6$, $p < .05$, as well as an interaction between tracking and VWM condition, $F(4, 84) = 2.4$, $p < .05$. Two-tailed t-tests showed an effect of tracking (VWM accuracy during the static condition subtracted from VWM accuracy during tracking) in the binding condition ($p < .001$) but not in any other VWM condition ($ps > .05$). Additionally, two-tailed, paired t-tests revealed that the effect of tracking was larger in the binding condition than in all other conditions (colour-only, shape-only, either-colour, either-shape), all $ps < .05$. Furthermore, costs due to tracking were larger in the binding condition than the added costs of tracking in the colour-only and shape-only conditions ($p = .01$). The observed impairment in VWM performance with concurrent tracking, which was largest in the binding condition, replicates Experiment 1's findings while ruling out the possibility that nonattentional components of the MOT task (i.e., encoding and retrieval) caused the binding impairment.

Secondary task. Secondary task accuracy is plotted in Figure 4B. We performed a two-way within-subject ANOVA as a function of tracking condition (tracking, static) and VWM condition (colour-only, shape-only, either-colour, either-shape, binding) on secondary task accuracy. There was a main effect of VWM condition, $F(4, 84) = 2.9, p < .05$, and tracking condition, $F(1, 21) = 89.3$, $p < .001$ (tracking worse than static), but no interaction between tracking and VWM condition, $F(4, 84) = 0.7, p = .6$. Consistent with the failure to find an interaction between tracking and VWM condition, paired t-tests revealed that the difference in secondary task accuracy (tracking minus static) in the binding condition was similar to the other VWM conditions ($ps >$ .2). Thus, the large interference of tracking on VWM performance in the binding condition cannot be explained by participants differentially allocating resources to the VWM and secondary tasks across conditions.

EXPERIMENT 3

It has been suggested that visuospatial attention promotes feature binding during visual perception by disambiguating the relationship between

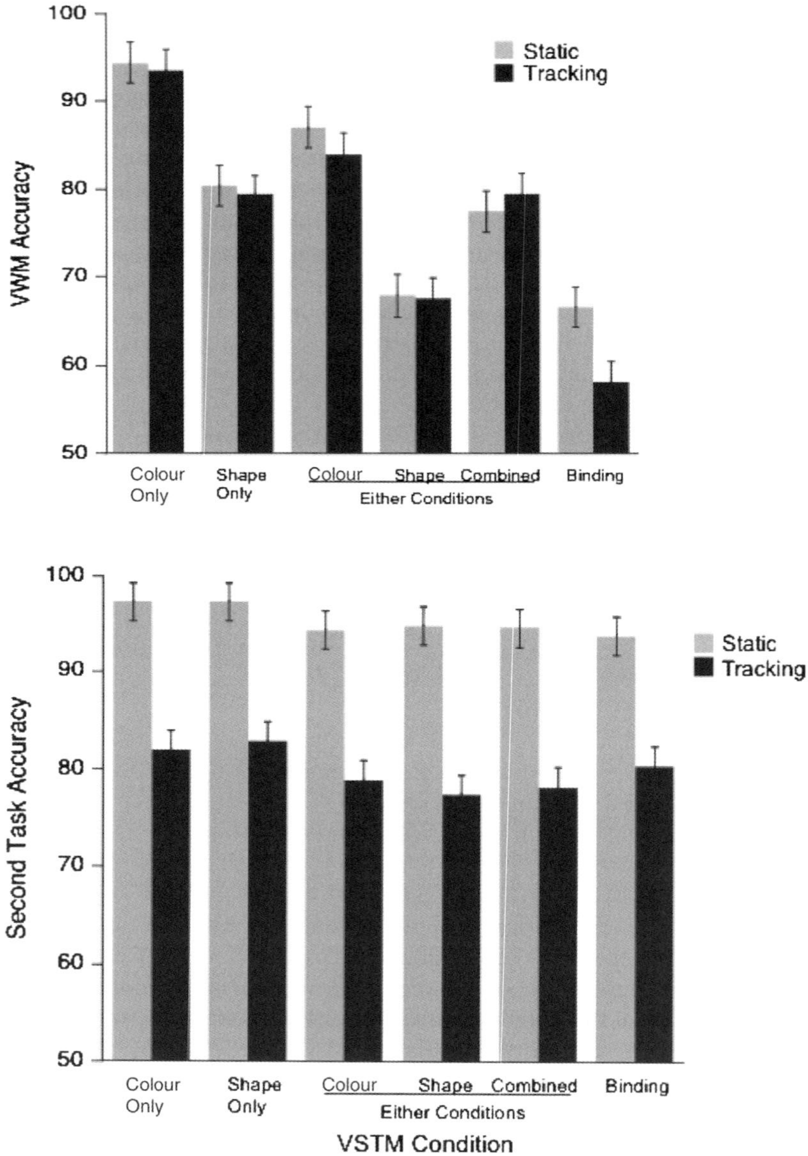

Figure 4. Accuracy in Experiment 2 for the VWM task (a) and the MOT task (b) by VWM condition. VWM accuracy (a) is black for the tracking condition and grey during the static condition. MOT accuracy (b) is black for the tracking condition and grey for the static condition. Error bars represent within-subject errors of the mean.

features and objects in a visual scene containing multiple objects (Desimone & Duncan, 1995; Luck & Ford, 1998; Luck, Girelli, McDermott, & Ford, 1997; Treisman, 1998, 2006). According to this proposal, attention selects an object location and filters out all other unattended objects, allowing the attended features to be bound together into an object representation (Treisman, 1998, 2006). Consistent with this disambiguation theory, there is both neurological (Friedman-Hill, Robertson, & Treisman, 1995) and neuroimaging (Shafritz, Gore, & Marois, 2002) evidence that the posterior parietal cortex—a brain region critical for visuospatial attention (Kastner & Ungerleider, 2000; Shafritz et al., 2002)—promotes feature binding chiefly when there is potential for confusion about the relationship between each object and their constituent features. Specifically, the posterior parietal cortex was found to be preferentially involved in feature integration when multiple objects were presented simultaneously in a visual display, but not when they were presented sequentially at the same location (Friedman-Hill et al., 2005; Shafritz et al., 2002). Following on these findings, we tested in the present experiment whether the role of visuospatial attention in maintaining feature bindings would be reduced if the VWM stimuli were presented sequentially at fixation. If so, this would suggest that one role of attention in VWM is the maintenance of location-specific object representations formed during visual perception (Treisman & Zhang, 2006).

Method

Participants

Twenty-five young adults (11 males) participated for course credit or monetary reward. One participant's data was removed from all analyses because she was not engaging in articulatory suppression.

Procedure

The procedure for Experiment 3 was identical to Experiment 2 except that the VWM stimuli were presented sequentially at fixation. Each stimulus was presented for 400 ms with a 400 ms interstimulus interval. The colour and shape conditions were not included since the principal comparison is between the binding and either conditions.

Results and discussion

VWM task. VWM accuracy is plotted in Figure 5A. We performed a two-way within-subject ANOVA as a function of tracking condition

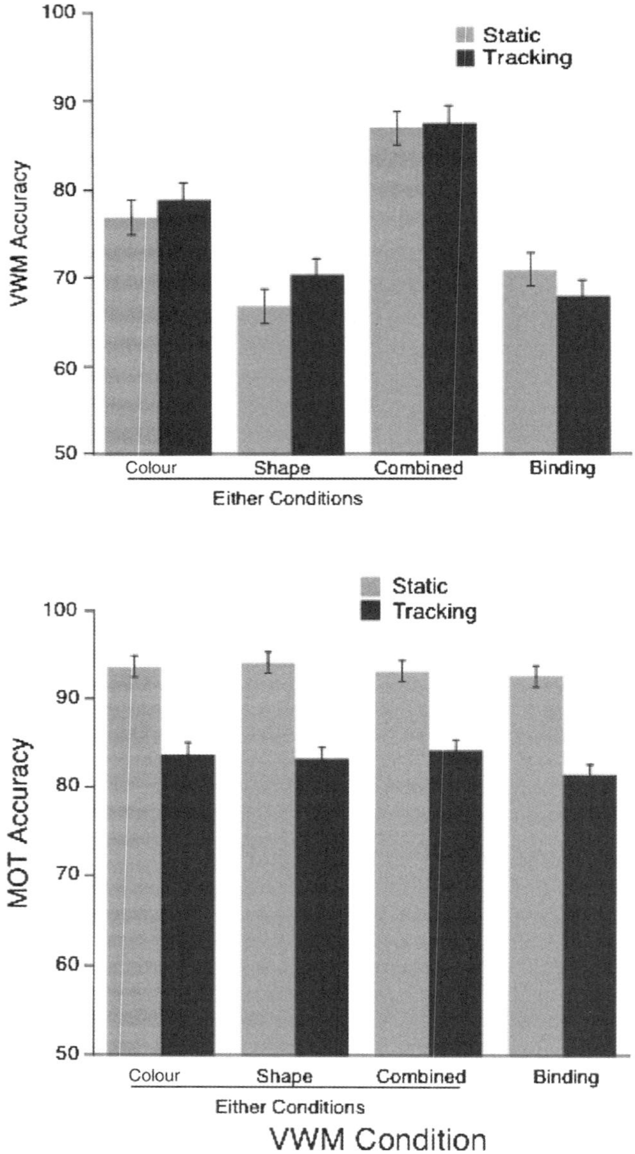

Figure 5. Accuracy in Experiment 3 for the VWM task (a) and the MOT task (b) by VWM condition. VWM accuracy (a) is black for the tracking condition and grey during the static condition. MOT accuracy (b) is black for the tracking condition and grey for the static condition. Error bars represent within-subject errors of the mean.

(tracking, static) and VWM condition (either-colour, either-shape, binding) on the VWM accuracy data. There was a main effect of VWM condition, $F(2, 46) = 53.78$, $p < .0001$, but there was no effect of tracking condition, $F(1, 23) = 0.04$, $p = .84$, and a marginal interaction between tracking and VWM condition, $F(2, 36) = 2.94$, $p = .06$. A two-tailed *t*-test revealed a marginal effect of tracking in the binding condition (VWM performance during the static condition subtracted from VWM performance during the tracking condition, $p = .07$). The effect of tracking in the binding condition was similar to the one observed in the either-colour or either-shape conditions (two-tailed paired *t*-tests, both $ps > .15$). However, we did observe a difference in the effect of tracking between the binding and the combined either condition ($p = .04$), suggesting that tracking might still impair feature binding in VWM even when VWM stimuli are presented sequentially at fixation. Importantly, this effect is much reduced compared to when VWM stimuli were presented at distinct locations in Experiment 2 (two-sample *t*-test of the tracking effect in the binding condition between Experiments 2 and 3, $p < .05$; Figures 4 and 5).

Previous studies have found that visuospatial attention is primarily involved in perceptual feature binding when objects are presented at distinct spatial locations (Friedman-Hill et al., 1995; Shafritz et al., 2002). Correspondingly, here we show that the amount of impairment produced by a secondary tracking task on VWM feature binding was significantly reduced when the VWM stimuli were presented sequentially at the same location. However, although the tracking effect was attenuated it was not altogether eliminated with foveal stimulus presentation. These results suggest that multiple object tracking may disrupt VWM feature binding by affecting both spatial and nonspatial attentional components of working memory.

Secondary task. We performed a two-way within-subject ANOVA as a function of tracking condition (tracking, static) and VWM condition (either-colour, either-shape, binding) on secondary task accuracy (Figure 5B). The main effect of tracking condition was significant, $F(1, 23) = 16.5$, $p < .001$, but there was no main effect of VWM condition, $F(2, 46) = 2.25$, $p = .12$, and no interaction between tracking and VWM condition, $F(2, 46) = 0.99$, $p = .38$. Paired *t*-tests revealed that the difference in secondary task accuracy (tracking minus static) in the binding condition was similar to the other VWM conditions ($ps > .2$), suggesting that the failure to observe significant effects of tracking on VWM performance cannot be explained by participants differentially allocating resources to the VWM and secondary tasks across conditions.

GENERAL DISCUSSION

In the present study, we carried out three experiments to test the hypothesis that visuospatial attention supports feature binding in visual working memory. In Experiment 1 we found that a secondary tracking task impaired memory for colour–shape bindings to a larger degree than memory for single features such as colour or shape. Experiment 2 showed that the effect is due to the attentive tracking component of the tracking task, and Experiment 3 demonstrated that the interference of the MOT task on VWM feature binding performance largely depends on the VWM stimuli occupying distinct spatial locations. Taken together, the results of these three experiments support the hypothesis that visuospatial attention plays an important role in storing bound representations in VWM (Delvenne & Bruyer, 2004; Wheeler & Treisman, 2002). These findings are consistent with a study suggesting that VWM feature binding is vulnerable to the spatial configuration of objects in a visual display (Treisman & Zhang, 2006), and with neuroimaging studies showing that brain regions involved in visuospatial attention and VWM—particularly the parietal cortex—also support visual feature binding (Corbetta, Kincade, Ollinger, McAvoy, & Shulman, 2000; Corbetta, Shulman, Miezin, & Petersen, 1995; Culham, Cavanagh, & Kanwisher, 2001; Jovicich et al., 2001; Shafritz et al., 2002; Todd & Marois, 2004).

Our results are at variance with previous studies that did not observe an effect of a secondary task on VWM feature binding (Allen et al., 2006; Gajewski & Brockmole, 2006; Yeh et al., 2005). This difference may be attributed to the fact that some of these studies used secondary tasks that loaded on central attention rather than on visuospatial attention. Central attention may not contribute to VWM binding, even when the secondary central tasks (e.g., digit recall) are just as difficult as ours (Allen et al., 2006). Consistent with this notion, we found in Experiment 3 that a secondary task that puts heavy demands on spatial attention barely affected VWM feature binding when spatial information could no longer be used for disambiguating the relationship between objects and features in VWM. Additionally, studies that did not use continuously demanding secondary tasks may not have observed VWM binding-specific deficits because the secondary task may not have sufficiently taxed attention (Gajewski & Brockmole, 2006; Yeh et al., 2005). A similar argument may also account for the difference between our results and those of a recent study (Johnson, Hollingworth, & Luck, 2008) reporting that a visual search task does not disrupt feature bindings in VWM. Because the visual search task demanded attention for a shorter duration (≈ 1 s) than our MOT task (6 s) and may only have required few shifts of visuospatial attention (two on average for set sizes of four), that task may have insufficiently taxed attentional resources to specifically impair feature bindings in VWM.

Previous work (Desimone & Duncan, 1995; Friedman-Hill et al., 1995; Shafritz et al., 2002) has suggested that visuospatial attention can be used to create bound object representations if objects occur at distinct spatial locations. Our dual-task study demonstrates that visuospatial attention also appears critical for the continued maintenance of these representations. In conjunction with previous findings, this may suggest that attention plays a critical role in VWM when spatial information is important for the VWM task (Awh & Jonides, 2001; Awh et al., 1998; Oh & Kim, 2004; Treisman & Zhang, 2006; Woodman & Luck, 2004; Woodman et al., 2001). In analogy to the proposed role of visuospatial attention in spatial working memory (Awh & Jonides, 2001; Awh et al., 1998; Awh, Vogel, & Oh, 2006; Postle, Awh, Jonides, Smith, & D'Esposito, 2004; Smith & Jonides, 1998; Smyth & Scholey, 1994), visuospatial attention may assist VWM by scanning the objects' locations during the retention interval as a means of refreshing the features that are bound to that location. If the role of attention in VWM primarily consists in iteratively refreshing stored representations, it could also explain why bound VWM representations may only be impaired by a secondary task that strongly and continuously withdraws attention away from working memory.

Although the present results suggest a role for visuospatial attention in feature binding in VWM, they do not imply that such binding is solely dependent on visuospatial attention. Indeed, it is interesting to note that, even with a concurrent difficult tracking task, participants' VWM performance was nevertheless above chance in the binding condition (50% being chance performance in Figures 3–5). These results are consistent with the notion that some binding can occur in the absence of visuospatial attention (Holcombe & Cavanagh, 2001). It is also consistent with the recent finding that VWM capacity, including the capacity for colour–location bindings, is not solely based on visuospatial attention, but is also constrained by central attention and VWM-specific sources of processing (Fougnie & Marois, 2006). But, irrespective of the extent to which other factors may contribute to feature binding in VWM, the present results suggest that visual features are not automatically integrated in VWM. Instead, working memory of feature bindings, just as their perceptual representations, is seemingly vulnerable to the withdrawal of visuospatial attention.

REFERENCES

Allen, R. J., Baddeley, A. D., & Hitch, G. J. (2006). Is the binding of visual features in working memory resource-demanding? *Journal of Experimental Psychology: General*, *135*(2), 298–313.

Awh, E., & Jonides, J. (2001). Overlapping mechanisms of attention and spatial working memory. *Trends in Cognitive Sciences*, *5*, 119–126.

Awh, E., Jonides, J., & Reuter Lorenz, P. A. (1998). Rehearsal in spatial working memory. *Journal of Experimental Psychology: Human Perception and Performance, 24*, 780–790.

Awh, E., Vogel, E. K., & Oh, S. H. (2006). Interactions between attention and working memory. *Neuroscience, 139*(1), 201–208.

Briand, K. A., & Klein, R. M. (1987). Is Posner's "beam" the same as Treisman's "glue?" On the relation between visual orienting and feature integration theory. *Journal of Experimental Psychology: Human Perception and Performance, 13*(2), 228–241.

Cavanagh, P., & Alvarez, G. A. (2005). Tracking multiple targets with multifocal attention. *Trends in Cognitive Sciences, 9*(7), 349–354.

Corbetta, M., Kincade, J. M., Ollinger, J. M., McAvoy, M. P., & Shulman, G. L. (2000). Voluntary orienting is dissociated from target detection in human posterior parietal cortex. *Nature Neuroscience, 3*(3), 292–297.

Corbetta, M., Shulman, G. L., Miezin, F. M., & Petersen, S. E. (1995). Superior parietal cortex activation during spatial attention shifts and visual feature conjunction. *Science, 270*(5237), 802–805.

Culham, J. C., Cavanagh, P., & Kanwisher, N. G. (2001). Attention response functions: Characterizing brain areas using fmri activation during parametric variations of attentional load. *Neuron, 32*(4), 737–745.

Delvenne, J. F., & Bruyer, R. (2004). Does visual short-term memory store bound features? *Visual Cognition, 11*(1), 1–27.

Desimone, R., & Duncan, J. (1995). Neural mechanisms of selective visual attention. *Annual Review of Neuroscience, 18*, 193–222.

DeYoe, E. A., & van Essen, D. C. (1988). Concurrent processing streams in monkey visual cortex. *Trends in Neurosciences, 11*(5), 219–226.

Donk, M. (1999). Illusory conjunctions are an illusion: The effects of target–nontarget similarity on conjunction and feature errors. *Journal of Experimental Psychology: Human Perception and Performance, 25*(5), 1207–1233.

Fougnie, D., & Marois, R. (2006). Distinct capacity limits for attention and working memory: Evidence from attentive tracking and visual working memory paradigms. *Psychological Science, 17*(6), 526–534.

Friedman-Hill, S. R., Robertson, L. C., & Treisman, A. (1995). Parietal contributions to visual feature binding: Evidence from a patient with bilateral lesions. *Science, 269*(5225), 853–855.

Gajewski, D. A., & Brockmole, J. R. (2006). Feature bindings endure without attention: Evidence from an explicit recall task. *Psychonomic Bulletin and Review, 13*(4), 581–587.

Han, S. H., & Kim, M. S. (2004). Visual search does not remain efficient when executive working memory is working. *Psychological Science, 15*(9), 623–628.

Holcombe, A. O., & Cavanagh, P. (2001). Early binding of feature pairs for visual perception. *Nature Neuroscience, 4*(2), 127–128.

Hollingworth, A. (2004). Constructing visual representations of natural scenes: The roles of short- and long-term visual memory. *Journal of Experimental Psychology: Human Perception and Performance, 30*(3), 519–537.

Hollingworth, A., Williams, C. C., & Henderson, J. M. (2001). To see and remember: Visually specific information is retained in memory from previously attended objects in natural scenes. *Psychonomic Bulletin and Review, 8*(4), 761–768.

Irwin, D. E. (1992). Memory for position and identity across eye movements. *Journal of Experimental Psychology: Learning, Memory, and Cognition, 18*(2), 307–317.

Irwin, D. E. (1996). Integrating information across saccadic eye movements. *Current Directions in Psychological Science, 5*(3), 94–100.

Irwin, D. E., & Andrews, R. V. (Eds.). (1996). *Integration and accumulation of information across saccadic eye movements.* Cambridge, MA: MIT Press.

Irwin, D. E., & Zelinsky, G. J. (2002). Eye movements and scene perception: Memory for things observed. *Perception and Psychophysics, 64*(6), 882–895.

Johnson, J. S., Hollingworth, A., & Luck, S. J. (2008). The role of attention in the maintenance of feature bindings in visual short-term memory. *Journal of Experimental Psychology: Human Perception and Performance, 4*(1), 41–55.

Johnston, J. C., McCann, R. S., & Remington, R. W. (1995). Chronometric evidence for two types of attention. *Psychological Science, 6*(6), 365–369.

Jovicich, J., Peters, R. J., Koch, C., Braun, J., Chang, L., & Ernst, T. (2001). Brain areas specific for attentional load in a motion-tracking task. *Journal of Cognitive Neuroscience, 13*(8), 1048–1058.

Kahneman, D., & Treisman, A. (1984). Changing views of attention and automaticity. In R. Parasuraman & D. R. Davies (Eds.), *Varieties of attention* (pp. 29–61). Orlando, FA: Academic Press.

Kahneman, D., Treisman, A., & Gibbs, B. J. (1992). The reviewing of object files: Object-specific integration of information. *Cognitive Psychology, 24*, 175–219.

Kastner, S., & Ungerleider, L. G. (2000). Mechanisms of visual attention in the human cortex. *Annual Review of Neuroscience, 23*, 315–341.

Luck, S. J., & Ford, M. A. (1998). On the role of selective attention in visual perception. *Proceedings of the National Academy of Sciences, USA, 95*(3), 825–830.

Luck, S. J., Girelli, M., McDermott, M. T., & Ford, M. A. (1997). Bridging the gap between monkey neurophysiology and human perception: An ambiguity resolution theory of visual selective attention. *Cognitive Psychology, 33*(1), 64–87.

Luck, S. J., & Vogel, E. K. (1997). The capacity of visual working memory for features and conjunctions. *Nature, 390*(6657), 279–281.

Navon, D., & Ehrlich, B. (1995). Illusory conjunctions: Does inattention really matter? *Cognitive Psychology, 29*(1), 59–83.

Oh, S. H., & Kim, M. S. (2004). The role of spatial working memory in visual search efficiency. *Psychonomic Bulletin and Review, 11*(2), 275–281.

Pashler, H. (1991). Shifting visual attention and selecting motor responses: Distinct attentional mechanisms. *Journal of Experimental Psychology: Human Perception and Performance, 17*(4), 1023–1040.

Pashler, H. (Ed.). (1993). *Dual-task interference and elementary mental mechanisms.* Cambridge, MA: MIT Press.

Posner, M. I., & Petersen, S. E. (1990). The attention system of the human brain. *Annual Review of Neuroscience, 13*, 25–42.

Postle, B. R., Awh, E., Jonides, J., Smith, E. E., & D'Esposito, M. (2004). The where and how of attention-based rehearsal in spatial working memory. *Cognitive Brain Research, 20*(2), 194–205.

Prinzmetal, W., Presti, D. E., & Posner, M. I. (1986). Does attention affect visual feature integration? *Journal of Experimental Psychology: Human Perception and Performance, 12*(3), 361–369.

Pylyshyn, Z. W., & Storm, R. W. (1988). Tracking multiple independent targets: Evidence for a parallel tracking mechanism. *Spatial Vision, 3*(3), 179–197.

Schneider, W. X. (1999). Visual-spatial working memory, attention, and scene representation: A neuro-cognitive theory. *Psychological Research, 62*(2–3), 220–236.

Shafritz, K. M., Gore, J. C., & Marois, R. (2002). The role of the parietal cortex in visual feature binding. *Proceedings of the National Academy of Sciences, USA, 99*, 10917–10922.

Smith, E. E., & Jonides, J. (1998). Neuroimaging analyses of human working memory. *Proceedings of the National Academy of Sciences, USA, 95*(20), 12061–12068.

Smyth, M. M., & Scholey, K. A. (1994). Interference in immediate spatial memory. *Memory and Cognition, 22*(1), 1–13.

Todd, J. J., & Marois, R. (2004). Capacity limit of visual short-term memory in human posterior parietal cortex. *Nature*, *428*, 751–754.

Treisman, A. (1998). Feature binding, attention and object perception. *Philosophical Transactions of the Royal Society of London, Series B: Biological Sciences*, *353*(1373), 1295–1306.

Treisman, A. (2006). How the deployment of attention determines what we see. *Visual Cognition*, *14*(4–8), 411–443.

Treisman, A., & Gelade, G. (1980). A feature-integration theory of attention. *Cognitive Psychology*, *12*(1), 97–136.

Treisman, A., & Schmidt, H. (1982). Illusory conjunctions in the perception of objects. *Cognitive Psychology*, *14*(1), 107–141.

Treisman, A., & Zhang, W. (2006). Location and binding in visual working memory. *Memory and Cognition*, *34*(8), 1704–1719.

Vogel, E. K., Woodman, G. F., & Luck, S. J. (2001). Storage of features, conjunctions, and objects in visual working memory. *Journal of Experimental Psychology: Human Perception and Performance*, *27*(1), 92–114.

Vogel, E. K., Woodman, G. F., & Luck, S. J. (2005). Pushing around the locus of selection: Evidence for the flexible-selection hypothesis. *Journal of Cognitive Neuroscience*, *17*(12), 1907–1922.

Wheeler, M. E., & Treisman, A. M. (2002). Binding in short-term visual memory. *Journal of Experimental Psychology: General*, *131*(1), 48–64.

Woodman, G. F., & Luck, S. J. (2004). Visual search is slowed when visuospatial working memory is occupied. *Psychonomic Bulletin and Review*, *11*(2), 269–274.

Woodman, G. F., Vogel, E. K., & Luck, S. J. (2001). Visual search remains efficient when visual working memory is full. *Psychological Science*, *12*(3), 219–224.

Yeh, Y. Y., Yang, C. T., & Chiu, Y. C. (2005). Binding or prioritization: The role of selective attention in visual short-term memory. *Visual Cognition*, *12*(5), 759–799.

VISUAL COGNITION, 2009, 17 (1/2), 67–82

Psychology Press
Taylor & Francis Group

New evidence for rapid development of colour–location binding in infants' visual short-term memory

Lisa M. Oakes and Ian M. Messenger
University of California, Davis, CA, USA

Shannon Ross-Sheehy
University of Iowa, Iowa City, IA, USA

Steven J. Luck
University of California, Davis, CA, USA

Change-detection tasks reveal that infants' ability to bind colour to location in visual short-term memory (VSTM) develops rapidly: Seven-month-old infants, but not six-month-old infants, detect that successive arrays of three objects are different if they contain the same colours in different locations (Oakes et al., 2006). Here we test a counterintuitive consequence of the hypothesis that 6-month-old infants are unable to bind colours to locations: When comparing two successive stimulus arrays, these infants will often compare noncorresponding items, making it impossible for them to distinguish between identical arrays and nonidentical arrays. As a result, they will not show a preference for changing arrays over nonchanging arrays even when all of the items change. We tested this prediction by presenting 6- and 7-month-old infants ($N = 36$) with nonchanging displays of three items and changing displays in which all three items simultaneously changed colours. As predicted, 7-month-old infants, but not 6-month-old infants, responded to the difference between these changing and nonchanging displays, providing additional evidence that the ability to bind colours to locations develops rapidly across this age range.

Keywords: Infancy; Visual short-term memory; Binding.

Please address all correspondence to Lisa M. Oakes, Center for Mind and Brain, 267 Cousteau Pl., University of California, Davis, CA 95618, USA. E-mail: lmoakes@ucdavis.edu

This research and preparation of this manuscript were made possible by NIH grant HD49840 awarded to LMO; SRS was funded by predoctoral and postdoctoral NRSAs (HD055040, MH068934). We thank Shaena Stille, Kristine Kovack-Lesh, and the undergraduate students in the Infant Perception and Cognition Laboratory at the University of Iowa for their help with this project.

© 2008 Psychology Press, an imprint of the Taylor & Francis Group, an Informa business
http://www.psypress.com/viscog DOI: 10.1080/13506280802151480

Understanding the early development of visual short-term memory (VSTM) is important for several reasons. For example, infants must encode and maintain information in VSTM for daily tasks such as comparing objects located on opposite sides of a room or recognizing the continuity of objects that go in and out of view. In addition, experimental procedures used to assess infants' visual cognition often involve momentarily occluding some or all of the objects in the display (e.g., Baillargeon & Graber, 1988; Wilcox & Chapa, 2004; Xu, 2003). Therefore, we can best understand infants' performance on such tasks by considering their emerging abilities to store and maintain information in short-term memory. Finally, studies documenting developmental changes in memory abilities can constrain theories about the neural and cognitive systems underlying visual short-term memory. For example, if the ability to store bound features in visual short-term memory has the same developmental time course as the ability to store unbound features, then this will suggest that both involve the same mechanism (see Vogel, Woodman, & Luck, 2001).

We use the phrase *short-term memory* rather than *working memory* because our experiments involve infant subjects, making it difficult to determine whether the memory system we are studying is used in the service of other tasks, which is the defining feature of a *working* memory system (Baddeley, 1986). However, the memory system we study is almost certainly a short-term memory system because our experimental paradigm uses conditions that are known to promote the use of short-term memory and to minimize the use of long-term memory (e.g., short encoding durations, brief retention intervals, and high levels of proactive interference). Moreover, this paradigm is quite similar to the change detection paradigm that has been used extensively to study VSTM in adults (Vogel et al., 2001).

Using the paradigm illustrated in Figure 1, we have documented clear developmental changes in VSTM over the first 12 months. In this paradigm, infants are simultaneously presented with two stimulus streams and their looking at each one is recorded. Each stream contains a specific number of objects, which cycle on and off over a period of many seconds (as in the flicker version of the change detection paradigm—see Simons & Rensink, 2005). In our streams, the array of objects is on for 500 ms, off for 250–300 ms, on for 500 ms, and so on. On one monitor infants see a *changing* stream, in which some aspect of the array changes from cycle to cycle; for example, a randomly chosen item might change colour between cycle N and cycle $N+1$ (as in Figure 1C). On another monitor, infants see a *nonchanging* stream in which the arrays are identical from cycle to cycle (as in Figure 1A). Using this general paradigm, we can determine the conditions under which infants prefer to look at a changing stream more than to a simultaneously presented nonchanging stream. It is well established that infants prefer (i.e., look longer at) visual arrays that are more complex, or contain more elements

(Cohen, 1991), and that they prefer dynamic stimuli to static ones (Shaddy & Colombo, 2004). Consequently, they will prefer a changing stream to a nonchanging stream if they can detect that the changing stream is changing and that the nonchanging stream is not. Given that a gap of 250–300 ms separates consecutive arrays within a stream, the infants will be able to distinguish between the changing and nonchanging streams only if they are able to store some of the information from a given array in VSTM and compare it with the corresponding information from the subsequent array. The combination of the 250–300 ms gap and the large transient caused by the onset of each array make it impossible to use iconic memory to solve this task. That is, even though the iconic memory of a given array will not have completely faded after 250–300 ms, the transient caused by the next array will eliminate this iconic memory so that it cannot be used to detect changes. Indeed, Rensink, O'Regan, and Clark (1997) found that iconic memory could not be used to perform change detection even when the delay was only 80 ms (see also Becker, Pashler, & Anstis, 2000). In addition, because the stimuli are brief and change frequently, infants cannot easily use long-term memory representations to detect the changes in the changing stream (see Ross-Sheehy, Oakes, & Luck, 2003).

Using this procedure, Ross-Sheehy et al. (2003) found that 6-month-old infants detected a change (as evidenced by a preference for changing streams) when there was one item in each array (Figure 1B), but they did not detect a change (i.e., they showed no preference for the changing stream) when there were 2 or more items on each array (Figure 1C). Thus, although these infants exhibited the ability to remember the colour of a single item in VSTM, they appeared to be unable to remember the colours of multiple objects. Ten-month-old infants, in contrast, significantly preferred the streams in which one randomly chosen item changed colour to nonchanging streams when there were one, two, three, or four items in each stream (Figure 1B, C; Ross-Sheehy et al., 2003), but they showed no significant preference at set size 6. Thus, VSTM abilities appear to undergo dramatic change in the first year of life—infants' ability to detect changes in multiobject arrays develops between 6- and 10-months of age, perhaps reaching adult-like level of three to four objects by 10 months of age (other work has lead to similar estimates of the number of objects infants at this age can store, e.g. Cheries, Wynn, & Scholl, 2006; Feigenson, 2007), although it is difficult to determine their precise capacity with confidence using our procedure (see Cowan et al., 2005, for an extensive discussion of the development of VSTM capacity across development).

The failure of the 6-month-old infants to detect change in multiobject arrays is particularly noteworthy because infants could, in principle, notice changes in an array of two or more objects even if they stored only one of the objects in VSTM. That is, if they remembered one of the N items in the

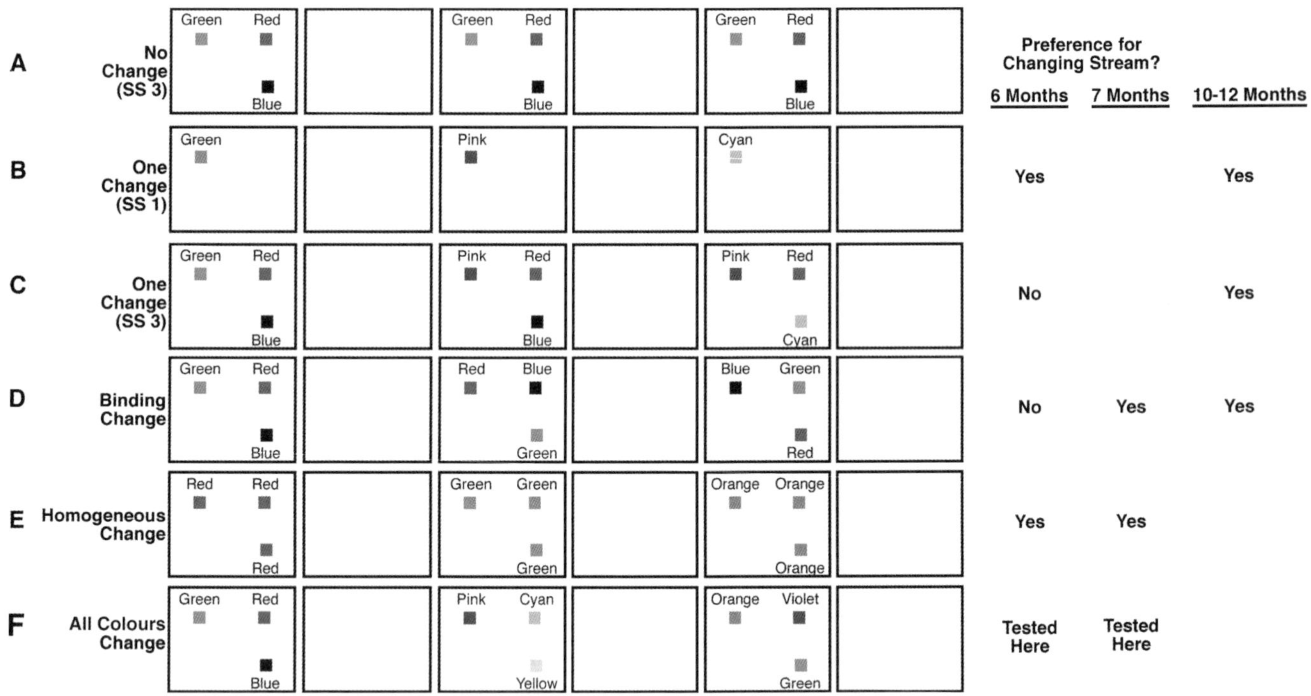

Figure 1 (*Continued*)

array, and if the colour of one randomly chosen item changes on each cycle, they should be able to detect $1/N$ of the changes in the changing stream. If infants did adopt this strategy, however, their preference would be small at set size 3 because they would detect only one out of three changes, and their preference may not be statistically significant. The 6-month-old infants observed by Ross-Sheehy et al. (2003) did not show a gradually decreasing preference as a function of set size (as predicted by their having detected $1/N$ changes); rather their preference was robust at set size one and near chance for both set sizes 2 and 3. Thus, 6-month-old infants' failure to show a significant preference for changing arrays containing two or more objects may not solely reflect a limited storage capacity, but rather may reflect some other difficulty that arises when multiple objects are present. In particular, infants may have difficulty binding object features to specific locations in the array. That is, they may represent the object features and the object locations, but without any link between the features and their locations.

A failure of object-location binding would make it difficult for infants to differentiate between changing and nonchanging streams of multielement stimulus arrays because of the *correspondence problem* that must be solved in this task. Specifically, determining whether or not a given item changed between array N and array $N+1$ requires that the infant is able to determine which objects in array N correspond to which objects in array $N+1$ so that the corresponding objects can be compared. If infants are unable to bind colour and location they may compare noncorresponding objects and perceive a change even when no change occurred.

Consider, for example, the nonchanging stream in Figure 1A. An infant who remembers the red item from cycle N–1 but does not remember the location of this item may compare the remembered red colour with the visible blue item in cycle N (i.e., comparing noncorresponding objects), thus perceiving a change when there was no change. Thus, infants who are unable

Figure 1 (previous page). Sequence of events in several different types of stimulus streams: (A) Nonchanging streams in which the array is identical from cycle to cycle. (B) One-change streams at set size 1, in which the arrays contain only one object and that one object changes colour from cycle to cycle (Ross-Sheehy et al., 2003). (C) One-change streams at set size 3, in which arrays contain three differently coloured objects, and the colour of a different randomly chosen object changes on each cycle (Ross-Sheehy et al., 2003). (D) Binding change streams, in which arrays contain three differently coloured objects, and the colour-location bindings (but not the particular colours or the particular locations) change from cycle to cycle (Oakes et al., 2006). (E) Homogeneous change cycles, in which arrays contain three identically coloured objects, and the colours of all the objects change from cycle to cycles (Oakes et al., 2006). (F) All colours change streams, in which arrays contain three differently coloured objects, and the colours of all the objects change from cycle to cycle. In addition, to the right of each cycle, we present what we know about whether infants prefer each type of changing stream when it is paired with a nonchanging stream (illustrated in A for each of the comparisons except for the homogeneous change streams in which were paired with corresponding homogeneous no-change streams).

to bind object identity to location will have difficulty differentiating changing from nonchanging arrays at set sizes of 2 or greater, even if they could in principle store multiple object identities in VSTM.

Oakes, Ross-Sheehy, and Luck (2006) demonstrated rapid developmental changes in infants' ability to bind information in VSTM. In this study, the changing stream contained the same colours and same locations on each cycle, but the locations of the colours swapped from cycle to cycle (Figure 1D). Six-month-old infants failed to differentiate changing from non-changing streams in this experiment, whereas 7-month-old infants strongly preferred the changing side. Kaldy and Leslie (2003)Kaldy and Leslie (2005) reported converging results for developmental changes in binding in this same age range. Thus the ability to bind colour and location in VSTM develops rapidly around 7 months of age. One might be concerned that in our procedure the 6-month-olds could detect the colour-location binding changes but that these changes were too subtle to have an impact on looking time. However, in this experiment all three items in the changing stream swapped locations on every cycle, and the changes should have been very salient if the colours were bound to the locations. Thus, the 6-month-old infants showed no preference for changing streams even though *every location in the changing stream changed colour each time the array reappeared.* If the infants had been able to remember just one colour at one location, they would have been able to detect the change on every cycle. These results indicate that the 6-month-old infants' lack of preference for the changing side was not solely a result of limited VSTM storage capacity. Instead, they were unable to bind the colour of an object to its location in VSTM. In contrast, 7-month-old and 12-month-old infants showed a significant preference for the changing arrays, indicating that they were able to bind colour and location in VSTM.

Two control experiments demonstrated that 6-month-old infants are not simply overwhelmed by the presence of multiple items. In one experiment, all the items in a given array of three items were the same colour, but the colour of these three items changed from cycle to cycle in the changing stream (Figure 1E). Six-month-old infants showed a strong preference for the changing side in this experiment, demonstrating that they can use VSTM in the face of multiple-object stimulus arrays when no colour-location binding is required to detect a change. In a second control experiment, each array in one stream contained three identical colours and each array in the other stream contained three different colours. Six-month-old infants preferred the arrays containing three different colours, demonstrating that they could discriminate the colour differences. Moreover, in tasks with exposure times of tens of seconds (or more), by 6 months infants can recognize colour–location bindings (e.g., Catherwood, Skoien, Green, & Holt, 1996), suggesting that they both can perceive such relations and that they can store them in long-term memory. Thus, the failure of 6-month-old infants to show a preference for streams in which all colour–location bindings are swapped on every trial is best explained by an inability to bind colour and location together in VSTM, and the success of 7-month-old infants in this task indicates that the ability to bind colour and location develops rapidly between 6 and 8 months of age.

The present study was designed to extend these previous findings and test a counterintuitive prediction that arises from our hypothesis that the ability to bind objects to locations develops over this period. Specifically, we hypothesized that an inability to bind colour and location would lead to an inability to differentiate between changing and nonchanging streams even if every item in the changing stream changed to a completely new colour on each cycle (see Figure 1F). This prediction is counterintuitive because 6-month-old infants have a VSTM capacity of at least one item, which should make it trivial to detect a change when every item changes to a colour that was absent in the previous cycle. Such a failure would be remarkable given that memory for a single item should be sufficient to perform this task. However, memory for a single item will be useful only if it contains location information so that this memory can be compared to the appropriate item. Without the ability to bind colour and location, infants will be unable to determine which item in the currently visible array should be compared with any items they have stored in VSTM from the previous array. As a result, even if infants retain one colour in VSTM they are likely to see changes even in the nonchanging stream and it should be extremely difficult for them to distinguish between changing and nonchanging arrays containing multiple items, even if all the feature values vary from cycle to cycle in the changing stream.

Because 7-month-old infants, in contrast, can bind colour and location, they should be able to determine that the nonchanging arrays are in fact nonchanging, and they should find it trivial to determine that the changing arrays are changing given that every item changes to a new colour on every cycle. Thus, we predicted that 7-month-olds would prefer the changing stream but 6-month-old infants would not. Such a finding would provide converging evidence for rapid developmental change in VSTM binding, which would suggest that changes in neural structures in this period underlie the ability to form colour-location bindings in VSTM.

METHOD

Participants

Thirty-six healthy infants with no history of birth complications, vision problems, or risk of colourblindness were tested. They included eighteen

6.5-month-old infants ($M = 193$ days, $SD = 5.43$) and eighteen 7.5-month-olds ($M = 231$ days, $SD = 3.93$) (19 boys and 17 girls). The majority of the infants were from White, middle-class families and were recruited using our usual procedures (Ross-Sheehy et al., 2003). An additional four infants were tested but were excluded from the final analysis because of experimenter error (one 7.5-month-old), equipment failure (one 6.5-month-old), or extreme side bias (one 6.5-month-old, one 7.5-month-old).

Apparatus

A Macintosh G3 computer was used to present the stimuli on two 17-inch ViewSonic monitors, each with viewable surface of 18.26 degrees (width) × 13.5 degrees (height) at a distance of 100 cm. The two monitors were positioned side by side with a 24 cm (13.5 degrees) gap between them. The total width of the two displays and gap was approximately 88 cm (47.5 degrees). With this setup, infants could detect that there was a stimulus on the nonfixated display while attending to a fixated monitor, but they could not perceive the details of the nonfixated display due to the $> 30°$ distance between the centres of the monitors, which would have led to extensive crowding within the nonfixated display (Pelli, Palomares, & Majaj, 2004). Thus, when performing this task, the infants are focused on one monitor at any given moment rather than attending to both stimulus streams at the same time.

Stimuli

Each array contained three coloured squares (2.9 × 2.9 degrees) on a grey background. Each of the three squares was a different colour, selected from a set of eight highly discriminable values (red, green, cyan, white, yellow, black, brown, and blue). The colours within a display were always different from each other. During each 20 s trial, the array of coloured squares on each monitor continually appeared and disappeared (visible for 500 ms, off for 300 ms, visible for 500 ms, etc.). For the changing stream, the colours of all three squares changed between disappearing and reappearing; the new values were selected at random on each cycle from the colours that were not present in the previous cycle. For the nonchanging stream, the colours of all three squares remained the same.

Procedure

Infants sat on a parent's lap 100 cm in front of a large black curtain that obscured their view of the experimental apparatus. Holes were cut in the curtain for the two computer monitors, a small black box positioned between the monitors, and the lens of a video camera below the black box. To direct infants' attention between the two monitors at the start of each trial, and thereby reduce side bias, the black box produced a flashing light and beeping tone between trials.

Infants received six 20 s trials in which a *changing stream* was presented on one monitor and a *nonchanging stream* was presented on the other. The left/right position of the changing stream was counterbalanced across trials (i.e., all infants received three trials with the changing stream on the right and three trials with the changing stream on the left). A trained observer, unaware of the location of the changing stream, recorded the looking time to each monitor online, and a second trained observer recoded the looking time offline for a randomly chosen 25% of the infants. The average correlation between the two observers' looking times was high ($r = .98$), with an average difference of 0.42 s.

RESULTS

Our main dependent variable was the *change-preference score*, which was calculated by dividing the duration of looking to the changing stream by the total time spent looking at either of the two streams for a given trial (i.e., excluding time spent looking somewhere other than the two streams). The mean scores, and the mean looking scores used to derive them, are presented in Table 1.

To determine whether infants discriminate the changing and nonchanging streams, we compared the change-preference score at each age to chance (.50) with a two-tailed t-test. If infants can determine that only the changing stream involves a change, they should prefer it and their change-preference score should be greater than chance. If infants are unable to determine that only the changing stream involves a change, they should look equivalently at the changing and nonchanging streams and their change-preference score should not be different from chance. The mean novelty preference score (with 95% confidence intervals) and individual scores for each infant are presented in Figure 2. It is clear that 7-month-old infants, but not 6-month-old infants, differentiated the two types of streams. Indeed, 7-month-old

TABLE 1

Average looking times and change preference scores in s (*SD* in parentheses) by age

Age	*Changing streams*	*Nonchanging streams*	*Change preference*
6 months	4.72 (2.38)	4.46 (1.70)	.50 (.09)
7 months	6.30 (1.87)	4.81 (1.36)	.57 (.05)

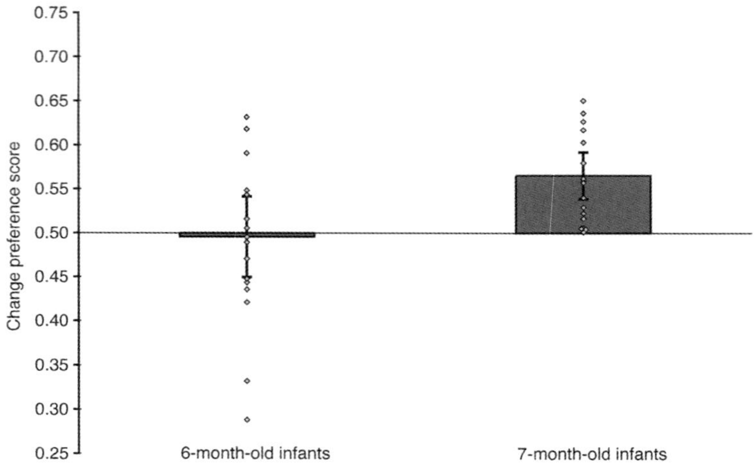

Figure 2. Mean change preference score (error bars represent 95% confidence intervals) and individual infants' change preference scores by age.

infants' change-preference score was significantly greater than chance, $t(17) = 3.37$, $p = .004$, whereas 6-month-old infants' change-preference score did not differ from chance, $t(17) = -0.17$, $p = .87$.[1]

To determine whether the preference score of the 7-month-old infants was significantly greater than that of the 6-month-old infants, we compared the preference scores across age. This comparison also was significant, $t(34) = 2.15$, $p = .039$, confirming that not only did 7-month-old infants have a preference score that was greater than chance, but they also preferred the changing side more than did the 6-month-old infants.

Finally, we compared the proportion of 6-month-old infants whose preference score was greater than .50 (9 out of 18) to the proportion of 7-month-old infants whose preference score was greater than .50 (18 out of 18). There was a significantly higher number of 7-month-old infants than 6-month-old infants who had scores greater than .50, $\chi^2(df = 1) = 12.00$, $p = .001$.

[1] One might expect that the individual 6-month-old infants would all have preference scores approximating .50. However, although most infants had scores near .50, a few had substantially higher or lower scores (see Figure 2). We examined the data of these infants carefully to see if we could find a clear explanation for their divergent scores, but we found no obvious differences between these infants and the infants whose scores were nearer to chance (e.g., they did not differ in age from the other infants and they generally looked at both streams on each trial). It is therefore likely that their divergent scores reflect measurement noise rather than true preferences for the changing or nonchanging streams.

DISCUSSION

This experiment reveals a striking pattern of findings: 6-month-old infants, but not 7-month-old infants, failed to prefer a changing stream at set size 3 even though all the items changed to a new colour on every cycle. This is a remarkable failure, especially given that 6-month-old infants show a robust and replicable preference for changing streams that consist of a single object or three identically coloured objects. Together, this work reveals that at 6 months infants can represent a single object—or a single object feature—but are unable to detect changes when multiple object identities must be stored and compared. After only one more month of development, however, infants could detect the changes with ease. The mean change preference score of the 7-month-old infants in the present experiment was .57, which means that they spent 33% more time looking towards the changing stream than towards the nonchanging stream, even though they were provided with no external incentives for doing so. This preference was highly significantly greater than what would be expected by chance, and it was also significantly greater than the preference exhibited by the 6-month-old infants, which was not significantly greater than what would be expected by chance. The timing of this difference in performance is precisely the timing of the dramatic change we previously observed in a different test of VSTM binding (Oakes et al., 2006), providing converging evidence for a key developmental change in this age range.

Detecting changes in the present paradigm seems trivially easy—infants need only remember a single object and compare it to the corresponding object in the next array to detect the change. However, this comparison requires that infants can determine which items correspond across the arrays, a process that requires binding. That is, recognizing that the red object has become green or remained red requires that the observer can remember which object was the red one, which in turn requires remembering where it was located. The inability of 6-month-old infants to prefer the changing stream in the present study therefore indicates that they either lacked information about the colour–location bindings or were unable to use this information. Infants at this age do show a preference when each stream contains a single item or three identical items, ruling out a lack of storage capacity or an inability to process multielement arrays as explanations for this result.

It should be noted that colour–location bindings are not strictly necessary, in a formal sense, to perform the present task. An observer who could remember only the colours could, in principle, determine whether a change is present or absent by comparing a representation of the statistical properties of one array (e.g., the mean colour of the entire array) with those of the next array. Indeed, adult observers can extract and compare some statistical properties, such as size (Chong & Treisman, 2003, 2005), and this ability may influence VSTM performance (Johnson, Hollingworth, & Luck, 2008). There were large changes in the statistical properties of the arrays in the changing streams of the present experiment on every cycle, giving the 6-month-old infants every opportunity to use representations of these statistical properties and show a preference for the changing streams. Their failure to do so indicates that they either do not form these representations or do not use them to control their looking behaviour. Moreover, 7-month-old infants do not solely rely on statistical properties because they prefer changing arrays both when they involve large changes in statistical properties (as in the present experiment) and when they involve no changes in statistical properties (as in the binding-changing experiment illustrated in Figure 1D; Oakes et al., 2006). Further research is necessary to determine whether observers of any age can use statistical information to perform tasks such as this.

One might also suppose that 6-month-old infants—who appear to be able to store a single item in VSTM—would be able to detect changes in the present paradigm by simply focusing attention onto a single location, storing this item in VSTM, and comparing it with the next item that appears at that location. Their lack of a preference for the changing stream therefore might reflect a problem with attention rather than a problem with binding, per se. However, by 6 months of age, attention can effectively perform simple stimulus selection operations such as this, and there is no evidence of a rapid transition in attentional selection between 6 and 8 months (Colombo, 2001). Thus, although we cannot completely rule out an attentional explanation of our findings, it is unlikely. Moreover, the binding of features to locations appears to require attention (Hyun, Woodman, & Luck, 2009 this issue), so a failure of attention may be viewed as a failure of one major component of binding.

Kaldy and Leslie (2003, 2005) also observed that the ability to bind object location to identity changes in the second half of the first year. However, Kaldy and Leslie argue that at 6 months infants can bind, but they have a limited capacity to do so—specifically, they can bind only a single object and location. Thus, for Kaldy and Leslie, binding and capacity develop somewhat independently. We argue, in contrast, that infants' ability to detect changes in multiobject arrays emerges from their ability to bind; that is, binding *allows* infants to compare the corresponding items in multiobject arrays, which is a necessary prerequisite for detecting changes, and thus the ability to bind features and to represent multiple objects are intertwined whenever the task requires comparing arrays separated by a gap.

These two different explanations have different implications for the brain mechanisms involved in binding. That is, although solving Kaldy and Leslie's (2003, 2005) task may involve working memory (i.e., infants must update and maintain a representation of an object on each trial), the encoding and retention periods may be sufficiently long to engage long-term memory representations.[2] Indeed, they argued that their results reflected maturation of the medial temporal lobes, which appear to play a role in binding only with delays that exceed 1 s (Olson, Page, Moore, Chatterjee, & Verfaellie, 2006). This system may be able to bind objects to locations by 6 months of age given a sufficiently long encoding period.[3]

In contrast, binding in our task requires rapid encoding, and infants must retain information over a very short period of time. Recent evidence suggests that VSTM representations are maintained by means of interactions between the intraparietal sulcus (IPS) and inferotemporal cortex (ITC). Both of these regions exhibit sustained activity during the delay period of change-detection tasks, but IPS activity seems to be more closely tied to storage capacity and to location binding (Todd & Marois, 2004; Vogel & Machizawa, 2004; Xu & Chun, 2006). The parietal cortex has also been linked to the binding of objects and locations in multielement stimulus arrays in other contexts. For example, an fMRI study by Shafritz, Gore, and Marois (2002) found that parietal regions were activated when subjects were required to bind the features of multiple objects presented simultaneously. In addition, Balint's syndrome patients, who have bilateral parietal damage, are unable to bind object identity to location (Robertson, 2003). Thus, the kind of binding required in our task seems to be more closely related to the kind of binding that engages parietal cortex.

Indeed, consistent with our behavioural findings, several studies using a variety of methods suggest increases in connectivity and activity in parietal regions until 3 months after birth, and a gradual decrease approaching asymptotic change by approximately 6 months (e.g., Chugani, 1998; Johnson, Mareschal, & Csibra, 2001). These data are obviously suggestive and should be considered with caution—establishing the developmental time course of changes in neuroanatomy in infancy is extremely difficult. Nevertheless, these conclusions are supported by behavioural findings such as those presented here that infants 6 months and younger have difficulty with tasks that appear to involve parietal cortex in adults. Thus, the developmental changes of changes in infants' ability to bind features in

[2] Substantial evidence supports the existence of separable short-term and long-term visual memory systems, which differ in terms of both their functional characteristics and their neural implementation (reviewed in Luck & Hollingworth, 2008). These systems may operate concurrently in many tasks that use relatively short retention intervals (< 10 s) but also use relatively long encoding periods (> 500 ms).

[3] It should also be noted that the pattern of performance exhibited by the 6-month-old infants in the experiments of Kaldy and Leslie (2003, 2005) is also consistent with infants simply remembering the identity of the last item shown, with no binding of identity and location.

VSTM before 6 months may be related to the immaturity of parietal structures that support these abilities in adults.

In summary, we argue that infants' inability to bind colour to location makes it difficult—if not impossible—to make use of VSTM representations in the context of multielement stimulus arrays. In particular, an inability to bind colour and location will make it difficult to determine which representation(s) should be compared with the current sensory input. Thus, even though they have the ability to store one object in VSTM, infants in the first year of life will be able to use VSTM only when the visual input contains a single salient object (e.g., a single toy, a parent's face, etc.), and the resolution of their VSTM representations may be highly limited. This may have a significant impact on their ability to integrate visual information across eye blinks and eye movements (see Currie, McConkie, Carlson-Radvansky, & Irwin, 2000; Hollingworth, Richard, & Luck, 2008) and their ability to compare objects during categorization (Kovack-Lesh & Oakes, 2007; Oakes & Ribar, 2005). The present results also support the hypothesis that VSTM develops rapidly from 6 to 8 months, and they suggest that binding is necessary for representing multiple objects in VSTM. Moreover, this developmental change occurs just after a period of rapid maturation in parietal cortex, providing support for the hypothesis that parietal cortex plays a key role in binding and in representing multiple objects in VSTM.

REFERENCES

Baddeley, A. D. (1986). *Working memory.* Oxford, UK: Clarendon.

Baillargeon, R., & Graber, M. (1988). Evidence of location memory in 8-month-old infants in a nonsearch AB task. *Developmental Psychology, 24*, 502–511.

Becker, M. W., Pashler, H., & Anstis, S. M. (2000). The role of iconic memory in change-detection tasks. *Perception, 29*, 273–286.

Catherwood, D., Skoien, P., Green, V., & Holt, C. (1996). Assessing the primary moments of infant encoding of compound visual stimuli. *Infant Behavior and Development, 19*, 1–11.

Cheries, E. W., Wynn, K., & Scholl, B. J. (2006). Interrupting infants' persisting object representations: An object-based limit? *Developmental Science, 9*, F50–F58.

Chong, S. C., & Treisman, A. (2003). Representation of statistical properties. *Vision Research, 43*, 393–404.

Chong, S. C., & Treisman, A. (2005). Statistical processing: Computing the average size in perceptual groups. *Vision Research, 45*, 891–900.

Chugani, H. T. (1998). A critical period of brain development: Studies of cerebral glucose utilization with PET. *Preventative Medicine, 27*, 184–188.

Cohen, L. B. (1991). Infant attention: An information processing approach. In M. J. Weiss & P. R. Zelazo (Eds.), *Newborn attention: Biological constraints and the influence of experience* (pp. 1–21). Norwood, NJ: Ablex.

Colombo, J. (2001). The development of visual attention in infancy. *Annual Review of Psychology, 52*, 337–367.

Cowan, N., Elliott, E. M., Saults, J. S., Morey, C. C., Mattox, S., Hismjatullina, A., et al. (2005). On the capacity of attention: Its estimation and its role in working memory and cognitive aptitudes. *Cognitive Psychology, 51*, 42–100.

Currie, C., McConkie, G., Carlson-Radvansky, L. A., & Irwin, D. E. (2000). The role of the saccade target object in the perception of a visual stable world. *Perception and Psychophysics, 62*, 673–683.

Feigenson, L. (2007). Continuity of format and computation in short-term memory development. In L. M. Oakes & P. J. Bauer (Eds.), *Short- and long-term memory in infancy: Taking the first steps toward remembering* (pp. 51–74). New York: Oxford University Press.

Hollingworth, A., Richard, A. M., & Luck, S. J. (2008). Understanding the function of visual short-term memory: Transsaccadic memory, object correspondence, and gaze correction. *Journal of Experimental Psychology: General, 137*, 163–181.

Hyun, J.-S., Woodman, G. F., & Luck, S. J. (2009). The role of attention in the binding of surface features to locations. *Visual Cognition, 17*, 10–24.

Johnson, J. S., Hollingworth, A., & Luck, S. J. (2008). The role of attention in the maintenance of feature bindings in visual short-term memory. *Journal of Experimental Psychology: Human Perception and Performance, 34*, 41–55.

Johnson, M. H., Mareschal, D., & Csibra, G. (2001). The functional development and integration of the dorsal and ventral visual pathways: A neurocomputational approach. In C. A. Nelson & M. Luciana (Eds.), *The handbook of developmental cognitive neuroscience* (pp. 339–351). Cambridge, MA: MIT Press.

Kaldy, Z., & Leslie, A. M. (2003). Identification of objects in 9-month-old infants: Integrating "what" and "where" information. *Developmental Science, 6*, 360–373.

Kaldy, Z., & Leslie, A. M. (2005). A memory span of one? Object identification in 6.5-month-old infants. *Cognition, 97*, 153–177.

Kovack-Lesh, K. A., & Oakes, L. M. (2007). Hold your horses: How exposure to different items influences infant categorization. *Journal of Experimental Psychology, 2*, 69–93.

Luck, S. J., & Hollingworth, A. (Eds.). (2008). *Visual memory*. New York: Oxford University Press.

Oakes, L. M., & Ribar, R. J. (2005). A comparison of infants' categorization in paired and successive presentation familiarization tasks. *Infancy, 7*, 85–98.

Oakes, L. M., Ross-Sheehy, S., & Luck, S. J. (2006). Rapid development of binding in visual short-term memory. *Psychological Science, 17*, 781–787.

Olson, I. R., Page, K., Moore, K. S., Chatterjee, A., & Verfaellie, M. (2006). Working memory for conjunctions relies on the medial temporal lobe. *Journal of Neuroscience, 26*, 4596–4601.

Pelli, D. G., Palomares, M., & Majaj, N. (2004). Crowding is unlike ordinary masking: Distinguishing feature integration from detection. *Journal of Vision, 4*, 1136–1169.

Rensink, R. A., O'Regan, J., & Clark, J. J. (1997). To see or not to see: The need for attention to perceive changes in scenes. *Psychological Science, 8*, 368–373.

Robertson, L. C. (2003). Binding, spatial attention and perceptual awareness. *Nature Reviews Neuroscience, 4*, 93–102.

Ross-Sheehy, S., Oakes, L. M., & Luck, S. J. (2003). The development of visual short-term memory capacity in infants. *Child Development, 74*, 1807–1822.

Shaddy, D. J., & Colombo, J. (2004). Developmental changes in infant attention to dynamic and static stimuli. *Infancy, 5*, 355–365.

Shafritz, K. M., Gore, J. C., & Marois, R. (2002). The role of the parietal cortex in visual feature binding. *Proceedings of the National Academy of Science, 99*, 10917–10922.

Simons, D. J., & Rensink, R. A. (2005). Change blindness: Past, present, and future. *Trends in Cognitive Sciences, 9*, 16–20.

Todd, J. J., & Marois, R. (2004). Capacity limit of visual short-term memory in human posterior parietal cortex. *Nature, 428*, 751–754.

Vogel, E. K., & Machizawa, M. G. (2004). Neural activity predicts individual differences in visual working memory capacity. *Nature*, *428*, 748–751.

Vogel, E. K., Woodman, G. F., & Luck, S. J. (2001). Storage of features, conjunctions, and objects in visual working memory. *Journal of Experimental Psychology*, *27*, 92–114.

Wilcox, T., & Chapa, C. (2004). Priming infants to attend to color and pattern information in an individuation task. *Cognition*, *90*, 265–302.

Xu, F. (2003). The development of object individuation in infancy. In H. Hayne & J. W. Fagen (Eds.), *Progress in infancy research* (Vol. 3, pp. 159–192). Mahwah, NJ: Lawrence Erlbaum Associates, Inc.

Xu, Y., & Chun, M. M. (2006). Dissociable neural mechanisms supporting visual short-term memory for objects. *Nature, 440*, 91–95.

VISUAL COGNITION, 2009, 17 (1/2), 83–102

Psychology Press
Taylor & Francis Group

Cross-modal binding and working memory

Richard J. Allen

Institute of Psychological Sciences, University of Leeds, Leeds, UK

Graham J. Hitch and Alan D. Baddeley

Department of Psychology, University of York, York, UK

We examine the role of general attention in the binding of colour and shape across the visual and verbal modalities. Three experiments studied the effects of concurrent tasks on the binding and retention of either unified visual stimuli, namely coloured shapes, or cross-modal stimuli in which one feature involved visual and the other auditory presentation. Performance accuracy was broadly equivalent across conditions, and was unimpaired by spatial tapping but impaired by backward counting. The decrement was however, no greater for the cross-modal binding conditions, suggesting that the act of binding is not itself attention demanding. Implications for this unexpected finding are discussed.

Keywords: Binding; Attention; Working memory; Colour; Shape.

The original Baddeley and Hitch (1974) model of working memory had three components comprising visuospatial and phonological temporary storage systems controlled by a limited capacity executive which was by implication capable of both storage and attentionally based control. In attempting to specify this central executive system in more detail, Baddeley (1986) adapted the model of attentional control proposed by Norman and Shallice (1986). The emphasis on attention rather than storage was further emphasized in an attempt to constrain the model, which could otherwise be regarded as hardly more testable than an all-powerful homunculus (Baddeley, 1996; Baddeley & Logie, 1999). However, having abandoned the assumption that the central executive had a storage function, it became clear that the model encountered some major limitations.

Please address all correspondence to Graham J. Hitch, Department of Psychology, University of York, Heslington, York YO10 5DD, UK. E-mail: gjh3@york.ac.uk

This research was supported by MRC grant G9423916. We thank Robert Logie and Daniel Gajewski for their useful comments on an earlier version of this paper.

© 2008 Psychology Press, an imprint of the Taylor & Francis Group, an Informa business
http://www.psypress.com/viscog DOI: 10.1080/13506280802281386

These limitations fell into two broad categories. The first comprised problems in explaining how information from the separate phonological and visuospatial subsystems could be combined given their mutually exclusive basic coding systems. The second concerned the question of how working memory could interface with long-term memory. In an attempt to solve these problems, Baddeley (2000) proposed a fourth working memory component, the episodic buffer.

The episodic buffer is assumed to comprise a storage system based on a multidimensional code, that is able to hold a limited number of episodes or chunks. Although its capacity in chunks is limited, its informational content can be increased by binding additional information into each chunk (Miller, 1956). The system was furthermore assumed to be accessible through conscious awareness, a process that allows information from a range of sensory channels to be combined into perceptual objects and scenes (Baddeley, 2000).

This version of the model is shown in Figure 1, from which it can be seen that access to the episodic buffer is assumed to depend crucially on the central executive. In this respect, it resembles the initial 1974 model in which control and storage were assumed to be closely linked. Direct links between the visuospatial and phonological subsystems were explicitly excluded. This was for reasons of parsimony. Given the central role assumed for the episodic buffer within the model, a link with the central executive would clearly be necessary, and it seemed entirely possible that all information in the buffer was routed through the executive, rather than having direct access from the visual and verbal subsystems. Furthermore, it seemed possible to test this assumption by using dual task methodology to block the normal operation of each of the three components of the initial working memory

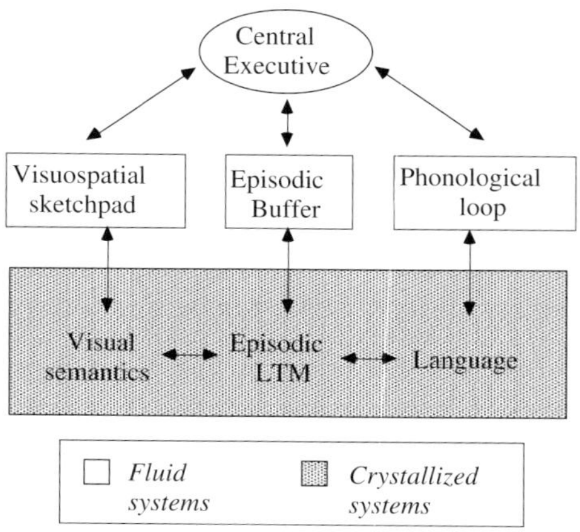

Figure 1. Model of working memory (Baddeley, 2000).

model. This has been the focus of our subsequent work. Given that a crucial feature of the buffer is its assumed capacity to bind information from a number of sources, binding seemed to be an obvious target for our research.

Our initial conceptualization of binding was influenced by research on visual imagery, whereby a pair of words such as "elephant" and "umbrella" could readily be associated by forming an interactive image of the elephant holding the umbrella over its head, whereas imagining the two side by side failed to enhance learning (Bower, 1970). We assumed that the process of manipulating the material so as to create the binding was intrinsically attentionally demanding. We went on to test this in two contrasting fields, one concerned with the binding of words within sentences, and the other concerned with the binding of colour and shape into perceived and remembered objects in visual cognition. In both cases, we have used dual task methodology to study the role of the phonological loop, the visuospatial sketchpad and the central executive in encoding the material in separate or bound form. According to the model outlined in Figure 1, memory for separate features reflects storage in the phonological or visuospatial subsystems and is less attention demanding than memory for bound chunks, which depends critically on accessing the episodic buffer. It follows that disrupting the operation of the central executive should differentially interfere with the capacity to bind features into chunks. In the case of sentences, our research is still incomplete, but suggests that with auditory presentation at least, a demanding concurrent executive task influences overall performance, but does not appear to interfere differentially with the process of binding (Allen & Baddeley, 2008; Baddeley, Allen, & Hitch, 2008). Interpretation, however, awaits subsequent experimentation. Of more direct relevance to the present study is a range of recent experimental work on the binding of visual features such as colour and shape into perceived objects.

In a series of experiments, Vogel, Woodman, and Luck (2001; see also Luck & Vogel, 1997) estimated the capacity of visual short-term memory at around three to four objects, with this limit constrained by the number of objects in memory, rather than the number of visual features, as change detection was as accurate for a set of four single-feature objects as for four objects each varying on four feature dimensions (e.g., colour, size, orientation, gap presence/absence). Based on these and previous findings (e.g., Duncan, 1984; Egly, Driver, & Rafal, 1994), Vogel et al. argued that integrated object representations are first created by perceptual processes before subsequently being stored in visual working memory.

Treisman and Gelade (1980) proposed that selective attention to the location of each object plays a crucial role in the process of feature integration. One possibility is that selective attention to location enables visual features to be bound together through the synchronous firing of neurons that code the individual features (e.g., Raffone & Wolters, 2001; Vogel et al., 2001). Alternatively, O'Reilly, Busby, and Soto (2003) describe a binding process based within multiple, distributed units that specifically code feature conjunctions. The coarse-coded nature of these units, and the distributed nature of the representations avoids the problem of a possible "combinatorial explosion" that undermines localist descriptions of conjunctive units.

Using a more direct test of binding memory than those implemented by Vogel et al. (2001), Wheeler and Treisman (2002) observed that accuracy for feature combinations was equivalent to single feature conditions only when a single test probe was used. When the standard change detection paradigm was implemented (with a full display of all items at test), binding memory was less accurate than feature memory. Wheeler and Treisman suggested that the onset of the multi-item test display disrupts attention more than a single-item test probe and concluded that attention plays a critical role in maintaining bound object representations in memory. Gajewski and Brockmole (2006) tested this idea through the use of an exogenous spatial cue placed between visual presentation and subsequent verbal recall of shape, colour, or both shape and colour. Although the cue did influence performance, indicating the role of attention generally in maintaining object representations, Gajewski and Brockmole observed a pattern of "all or none" forgetting. This suggests that multifeature objects are processed as single units, rather than falling apart into individual features when attention is withdrawn as claimed by Wheeler and Treisman (2002).

Our own visual binding studies combined the paradigm developed by Wheeler and Treisman (2002) with the dual-task methodology that we have used extensively in developing the working memory model (Allen, Baddeley, & Hitch, 2006). When attention-demanding concurrent tasks were performed during presentation and a short retention interval, we found a major overall effect of disrupting the central executive, in line with other findings indicating a role for the executive in encoding and maintaining visual items in working memory (e.g., Dell'Acqua & Jolicoeur, 2000; Morey & Cowan, 2004). However, we found that this effect was not substantially greater in tasks requiring the binding of features than it was on retention of single features. In a subsequent series of experiments (Karlsen, Allen, Baddeley, & Hitch, 2008) we increased the difficulty of binding by presenting each colour and its corresponding shape in different though adjacent locations. This manipulation did indeed reduce accuracy and performance was impaired by a concurrent executive task. However, once again, performance on the binding condition was not differentially impaired by placing a concurrent load on the central executive.

Our observation that a demanding executive load impaired overall performance but did not differentially disrupt the process of binding (Allen et al., 2006) was initially surprising, but in retrospect consistent both with the earlier work of Vogel et al. (2001), and with the observation that Gestalt factors such as pattern symmetry also influence performance regardless of an attentionally demanding task (Rossi-Arnaud, Pieroni, & Baddeley, 2006). It seems reasonable to assume a degree of perceptual processing that occurs prior to working memory, with the result that a task that impairs overall working memory does not necessarily prevent perceptual binding. We were somewhat more surprised however, to find that this was also the case when the colour and shape features were presented in physically separate locations (Karlsen et al., 2008), since this would appear to involve combining what were perceptually two separate objects. In this respect the task could be seen as a similar to the imagery task of combining two objects into an integrated whole (Bower, 1970), something that we would assume to be quite attentionally demanding. It is plausible to suggest that the binding of a colour and shape is automatic, but a visual system that automatically bound features that were separately located would seem likely to lead to perceptual chaos. However, it could be argued that when both visual features are relevant and presented in an uncluttered field, this produces conditions where binding might be facilitated. The purpose of the present study is to extend this situation further by presenting one feature visually and the second auditorily. These conditions might be regarded as involving the integration of two separate objects, one visual the other auditory, and thus more likely to be attentionally demanding.

Experiment 1 studied the effect of presenting features cross-modally on recognition memory performance, and included a spatial separation condition, as used by Karlsen et al. (2008), in order to gauge the relative difficulty of our cross-modal task. As is customary with this paradigm, presentation was always accompanied by articulatory suppression to discourage verbally based strategies, although the evidence suggests that such strategies are rare (Allen et al., 2006; Vogel et al., 2001).

EXPERIMENT 1

Method

Participants. Sixteen undergraduate and postgraduate students from the University of York took part, receiving course credit or payment. There were seven males and eleven females, with an age range of 18–37 years.

Materials. Visual stimuli utilised a set of eight shapes (circle, cross, diamond, star, arch, chevron, flag, triangle) and eight colours (green, red, blue, yellow, black, grey, purple, turquoise), taken from Allen et al. (2006). In addition, in the relevant spatially separated and cross-modal conditions, we used a neutral formless shape (a "blob") to present any of the eight colours, and a set of unfilled shapes with three-point black outlines to present any of the eight shapes. All stimuli subtended a visual angle of approximately 0.95°, presented on a white background. A male English speaker digitally recorded the names of each of the test features. Testing was controlled on a Macintosh iMac with a 17-inch inch screen, using a SuperCard program.

Design and procedure. All participants performed each of four binding conditions in a counterbalanced order. In the visually unitized condition, each shape–colour combination was presented as a single integrated object, whereas in the spatially separated condition the colours and shapes were presented as visually separate entities. In addition, there were two cross-modal conditions: Auditory colour and auditory shape. In the auditory colour condition (XM colour), shapes were visually presented in synchrony with colour names, while the reverse was true for the auditory shape condition (XM shape). Examples of the stimuli presented in each condition are provided in Figure 2. Each block consisted of 10 practice trials and 60 test trials, with three colour–shape combinations presented in each trial.

At the start of the session, the set of eight shapes and eight colours were displayed on screen, along with the names associated with each, to ensure that participants knew which verbal label applied to which feature (for the purposes of the cross-modal conditions). The first block of practice and test trials then followed.

Each trial commenced with a fixation cross at screen centre for 500 ms, followed by a 250 ms blank screen delay. Each of the three visual stimuli in each trial was then serially presented at screen centre for 1000 ms, with interstimulus intervals of 250 ms. In the visually unitized condition, each stimulus consisted of a single coloured shape, whereas spatially separated stimuli consisted of a shape outline just above centre screen, vertically adjacent to a colour blob presented approximately 0.38° visual angle below. In each of the two cross-modal conditions, one feature dimension (e.g., shape) was presented in the visual modality, and the other (e.g., colour) in the auditory modality. Visual features were displayed one at a time at screen centre, for 1 s each. For the cross-modal auditory–colour condition, shapes were visually presented as black outlines; colour blobs were used in the auditory–shape condition. In synchrony with each visual stimulus presentation, participants heard a feature name from the other dimension (e.g., colour) through headphones.

A 900 ms blank screen delay followed presentation of the three feature pairs. The test probe, consisting of a single visually unitized shape–colour combination, was then presented just below screen centre. On half the trials, this was a target probe, with the feature combination having initially been

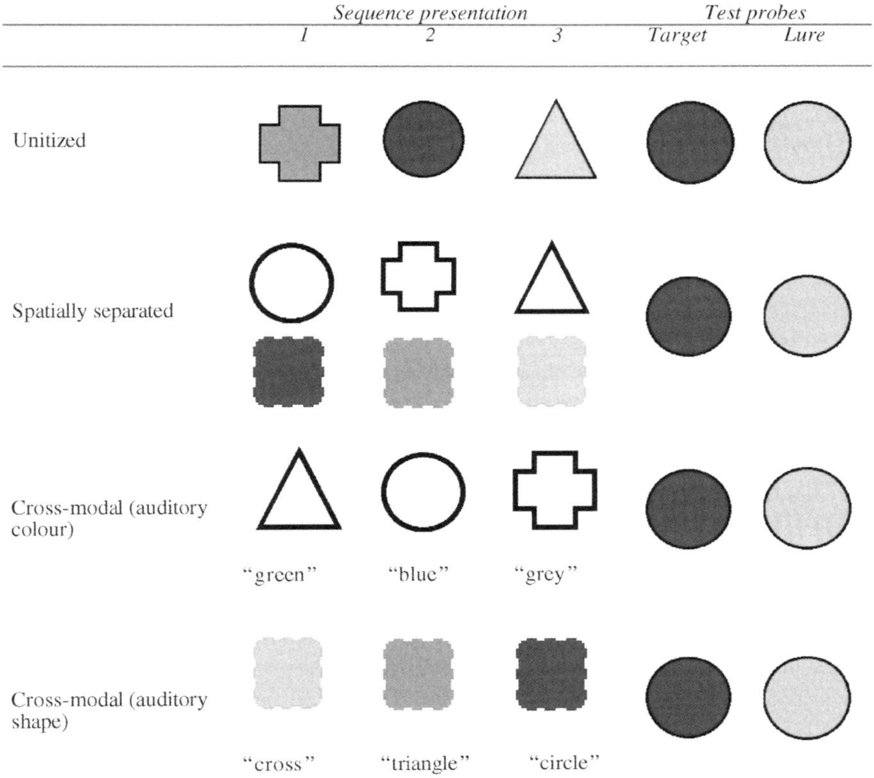

Figure 2. Examples of presentation and test stimuli in each condition.

presented as one of the three to-be-remembered combinations, with each of the serial positions probed an equal number of times across the trial block. The remaining trials involved lure probes, in which shape and colour were drawn from two different feature combinations (as illustrated in Figure 2). Participants were instructed to respond by pressing the "z" key if they thought the test probe combination was present and the "/" key if they thought the test features were not presented together in the original sequence. Reaction times were recorded, but response accuracy was emphasized over speed. Feedback was not given in any of the reported experiments.

It is possible that the lure probe methodology just described enables a "shortcut" strategy to be applied in judging that the test feature combination was not initially presented. As described by Allen et al. (2006), memory for a single combination of features (e.g., "red diamond") may enable participants to decide that the test probe (e.g., "red circle") was not part of the sequence. To prevent the effective application of this strategy, a subset of trials were included in which two features were repeated. For example, remembering that a red diamond was part of the sequence would not necessarily mean that the red circle test probe was not also present. Four of the ten practice trials involved a feature repetition (in either dimension), as did 12 of the 60 test trials, and participants were alerted to the possible presence of such repetitions at the start of each block. Repetition trials were randomly interspersed throughout the block, and performance on these trials was removed from analysis.

Finally, in order to prevent verbal recoding of the visually presented stimuli, articulatory suppression (repeating the sequence "one-two-three-four" at approximately two digits a second) was performed from the fixation cue to the test probe in each trial.

Results

Overall performance in each of the binding conditions is reported as A' (Grier, 1971; Pollack & Norman, 1964). Mean accuracy was $A' = .80$ in the visually unitized condition, .77 in the spatially separated condition, .81 for cross-modal (auditory colour), and .80 for cross-modal auditory shape. An ANOVA revealed that the effect of binding condition was not significant, $F(3, 45) = 1.21$, $MSE = 0.01$, $p = .319$, $\eta_p^2 = .08$. It appears that accuracy was generally equivalent across the four binding conditions.[1] An analysis of response bias (B'') indicated no significant differences in bias across the conditions.

Discussion

Unlike the studies reported by Karlsen et al. (2008), unitized presentation did not lead to significantly better memory than spatially separated feature presentation, though there was a trend in this direction. Perhaps more surprisingly, separating features by modality had no adverse effect on recall as compared with unitized presentation. Despite the lack of any effect on recall, cross-modal binding may nevertheless involve different resources. The next experiment omitted the visually separated condition and used dual-task

[1] Serial position curves showed clear recency effects in all three experiments, in agreement with previous data on memory for feature binding for sequentially presented stimuli (see, e.g., Allen et al., 2006). However, serial position effects were not very informative over and above this, as they did not show any consistent interactions with experimental conditions.

methodology to investigate the resources required to support memory for cross-modal feature bindings.

EXPERIMENT 2

Having established that participants were able to bind features presented cross-modally, we moved on to study the effects on performance of concurrent tasks designed to differentially disrupt specific components of working memory. Experiment 1 had used articulatory suppression during presentation, as is typical in this area of research, thereby limiting any use of the phonological loop. In Experiment 2, we attempted to look at the role of the visuospatial sketchpad in binding. Operation of the sketchpad can be separated into visual and spatial components (Baddeley, 2007; (Logie, 1995), and it seemed likely that our memory task involved both, since the visual features of shape and colour were defined by their spatial location within a complex visual array. We employed as our visual-spatial concurrent task, tapping keys in a figure-of-eight pattern. The keys were masked, but it is certainly conceivable that maintaining the figure-of-eight path also involved a degree of visual pattern coding. It could be argued that we should have also used a task that was more clearly visual, such as presentation of visual noise (Quinn & McConnell, 1996). However, the effect of presenting visual noise is not always readily detectable (Andrade, Werniers, May, & Szmalek, 2002) and, given that our main task involved visual stimuli, any effect might be due to disrupting perception. We accept, however, that although our concurrent task will disrupt spatial processing, its impact on visual processing is uncertain.

Experiment 2 therefore examined whether memory for cross-modal feature bindings would be more sensitive to disruption from concurrent spatial tapping than bindings for visually unitized stimuli. Such a result would imply that cross-modal binding places greater demands on working memory, though without specifying whether these demands are located on the subsystems themselves (loaded by tapping and by articulatory suppression) or by the central executive (loaded by performing these two concurrent tasks at the same time).

Method

Participants. Twenty-four undergraduate and postgraduate students from the University of York took part, receiving course credit or payment. There were 7 males and 17 females, with an age range of 18–39 years.

Materials. All visual and auditory stimuli were taken from Experiment 1.

Design and procedure. This experiment followed a 3×2 repeated measures design, with binding condition (visually unitized, cross-modal auditory–colour, cross-modal auditory–shape) and concurrent task (no task; spatial tapping) as factors. Each condition was implemented in a trial block containing eight practice trials (including four repetitions) and 30 test trials (six repetitions). Condition order was counterbalanced across participants, with conditions blocked by concurrent task.

Spatial tapping practice and baseline measure. The session began with a 30 s spatial tapping practice block in order to demonstrate the pace at which tapping responses were to be made. A tone was played through the computer's speakers every 500 ms, with participants required to respond with a keypress on each tone. If timing was deemed by the experimenter to be too slow or too fast, the practice session was repeated. Tapping responses were recorded using the keyboard's numerical keypad, on which a "figure-of-eight" pattern was repeatedly tapped out using the right hand (following the sequence 1-2-3-6-5-4-7-8-9-6-5-4-1-2-3 . . .). The keypad was hidden from view by a metal screen, placed over the right side of the keyboard to enable free hand movement while preventing participants from visually guiding their responses.

Following the tapping practice session, a set of five tapping trials was performed, to obtain a pretest baseline measure of tapping performance. In line with the timing schedule of the primary memory trials, each baseline tapping trial commenced with the phrase "Start tapping" displayed on screen for 1 s, followed by a blank screen for 5150 ms. The figure-of-eight pattern was tapped out on the keypad during this period, with participants instructed to aim both for pattern accuracy and the steady rhythm established in the preceding practice block (rather than speed). This procedure was repeated at the end of the session to obtain a posttest measure, again containing five trials. In order to provide a close match with the concurrent task conditions, articulatory suppression (repeatedly articulating the sequence "1-2-3-4") was performed in the tapping baseline trials.

Visual and cross-modal memory. The stimulus presentation conditions and test procedure from Experiment 1 were implemented again in this study (though the visually separated binding condition was omitted). In the spatial tapping conditions, the fixation cue was preceded by presentation of the "Start tapping" command, on screen for 1 s. Tapping responses were made from this point through to test probe presentation. At this point, tapping ceased and a response was made to the probe using the left hand, either "z" if the feature combination was judged to be part of the test sequence, or "x" if it was deemed to be an incorrect combination. The articulatory suppression task was also performed in all conditions, from fixation cue to test probe presentation, to prevent verbal recoding of visual stimuli.

Results

Accuracy in each condition was scored as A', with the results illustrated in Figure 3. A 3×2 ANOVA revealed no significant effects of stimulus condition, $F(2, 46) = 0.46$, $MSE = 0.01$, spatial tapping, $F(1, 23) = 0.01$, $MSE = 0.01$, or the interaction, $F(2, 46) = 0.70$, $MSE = 0.01$. It is therefore apparent that cross-modal binding accuracy was as accurate as visually unitized binding, and that performing spatial tapping as a concurrent task did not have a significant effect on any of the memory conditions.

Analysis of response bias (B'') in each of the no tapping conditions yielded values of .17, .19, and .17, for the unitized, cross-modal (colour), and cross-modal (shape) conditions respectively. For the spatial tapping conditions, $B'' = .20$, .17, and .22 for each of the stimulus conditions in turn. Analysis of variance revealed no significant effects of stimulus condition, $F(2, 46) = 0.28$, $MSE = 0.01$, or spatial tapping, $F(1, 23) = 2.28$, $MSE = 0.01$, $p = .145$, $\eta_p^2 = .09$. However, the interaction was significant, $F(2, 46) = 3.90$, $MSE = 0.01$, $p < .05$, $\eta_p^2 = .15$. This indicates that the tapping task produced a somewhat more negative response bias in the visually unitized and cross-modal (shape) conditions, relative to cross-modal (colour).

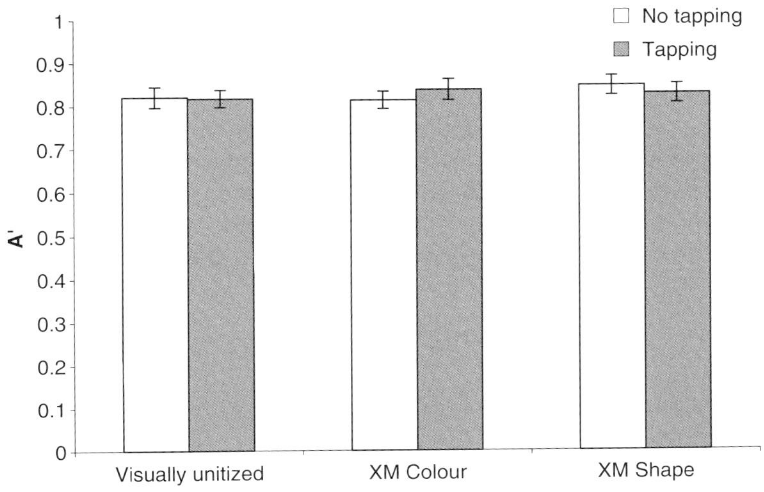

Figure 3. Mean accuracy (A') in each condition in Experiment 2 (with standard error).

Spatial tapping. Pre- and posttest baseline measures were collapsed to provide a mean baseline measure of tapping performance. In the concurrent task conditions, only those responses made during visual and cross-modal stimulus presentation and the subsequent 900 ms delay were included in subsequent analysis. Mean reaction time and variability (standard deviation) in spatial tapping latency for the baseline and concurrent task conditions are reported in Table 1. The main measure of interest in this task was reaction time variability, with lower variability indicating better performance. An ANOVA on baseline and concurrent task conditions revealed a significant effect of condition, $F(3, 69) = 2.89$, $MSE = 1091$, $p < .05$, $\eta_p^2 = .11$, indicating that a more accurate response rhythm was maintained in the baseline than the concurrent task tapping conditions, which themselves did not differ, $F(2, 46) = 0.13$, $MSE = 924$. Errors in tapping (i.e., keypress responses in the wrong order) were infrequent, at less than 0.02 of responses in all conditions, and so were not analysed.

Discussion

The absence of any detrimental effect of presenting colour and shape in different modalities confirms the result obtained in Experiment 1. The amount of dual-task interference observed was generally rather small with an effect on the variability of tapping but not on performance of the memory task. Neither measure gave any indication of greater dual-task interference in the cross-modal condition. These observations indicate that binding the features of visual objects places the same load on working memory regardless of whether features are presented in the same or different modalities. The relatively small amount of dual-task interference observed suggests that the spatial component of the sketchpad is relatively unimportant in the memory task. However, since combining tapping with articulatory suppression probably does not place a particularly onerous load on the central executive, the experiment was not a strong test of the hypothesis that cross-modal binding depends on the executive. The next experiment turned to examine the effect of loading the central executive more substantially, using backwards counting in decrements of three as an

TABLE 1
Mean reaction times and standard deviations for baseline and concurrent task spatial tapping conditions (standard errors in parentheses)

	Baseline	*Visual*	*XM colour*	*XM shape*
RT (ms)	458 (15)	426.23 (19.46)	421.23 (20.03)	422.33 (18.27)
Variability (*SD*)	61.90 (6.58)	84.66 (9.99)	86.70 (10.57)	82.25 (9.58)

attentionally demanding concurrent verbal task. The substantial load that this task places on executive resources has already been shown to disrupt the encoding of visual features and their conjunctions (Allen et al., 2006).

EXPERIMENT 3

Method

Participants. Twenty-four undergraduate and postgraduate students from the University of York took part, receiving course credit or payment. There were nine males and fifteen females, with an age range of 18–40 years.

Materials. All visual and auditory stimuli were taken from the previous experiments.

Design and procedure. As in Experiment 2, there were three binding conditions (visually unitized, cross-modal auditory–colour, cross-modal auditory–shape) and two concurrent task conditions in this study. However, spatial tapping was replaced with backwards counting in decrements of three. Each condition was implemented in a trial block containing six practice trials (including three repetitions) and 30 test trials (six repetitions). Condition order was counterbalanced across participants, with conditions blocked by concurrent task.

Articulatory suppression and backward counting. A new version of the suppression task was used in this study, in order to match its output demands with those of backward counting and to provide a comparable measure of performance in each. Each trial commenced with a three-digit number (e.g., 362) presented at the top of screen centre. In the simple suppression condition, this number string was repeatedly articulated (e.g., "three six two, three six two, . . ."). In the backward counting condition, participants were instructed to count backwards in decrements of three (e.g., "three six two, three five nine, three five six, . . .").

Each session commenced with five pretest trials of backward counting and five of suppression, in order to obtain baseline measures of performance in these tasks. This procedure was repeated at the end of the session to obtain a posttest measure.

When performed as a concurrent task alongside the primary memory task, verbal responses were made from the point of number presentation, through to presentation of the recognition test probe. Total trial duration in both baseline and concurrent task versions of the number tasks was 5150 ms.

Visual and cross-modal memory. In both concurrent task conditions, the three-digit start number was presented above screen centre for 1 s, followed by a 500 ms delay and then the fixation cue. The remainder of each trial featured the same procedure as that reported in the previous experiments.

Results

Accuracy (A') for each condition is illustrated in Figure 4. A 2 × 3 ANOVA revealed a significant effect of backward counting, $F(1, 23) = 31.09$, $MSE = 0.02$, $p < .001$, $\eta_p^2 = .58$, but no effect of binding condition, $F(2, 46) = 2.17$, $MSE = 0.01$, $p = .126$, $\eta_p^2 = .09$. The task by condition interaction was not significant, $F(2, 46) = 1.61$, $MSE = 0.03$, $p = .210$, $\eta_p^2 = .07$. Backward counting had a large effect on memory performance that was equivalent in size across the different binding conditions.

Response bias (B'') analysis of the simple suppression conditions revealed values of .20, .20, and .18, for visually unitized, cross-modal (colour), and cross-modal (shape), respectively. For the backward counting conditions the corresponding values of B'' were .26, .23, and .24. Analysis of variance revealed a significant effect of backward counting, $F(1, 23) = 15.89$, $MSE = 0.01$, $p < .01$, $\eta_p^2 = .41$, but not stimulus condition, $F(2, 46) = 2.09$, $MSE = 0.01$, $p = .135$, $\eta_p^2 = .08$, or the task by condition interaction, $F(2, 46) = 0.80$, $MSE = 0.01$. Thus, backward counting caused a similar shift to a more negative response bias across all conditions.

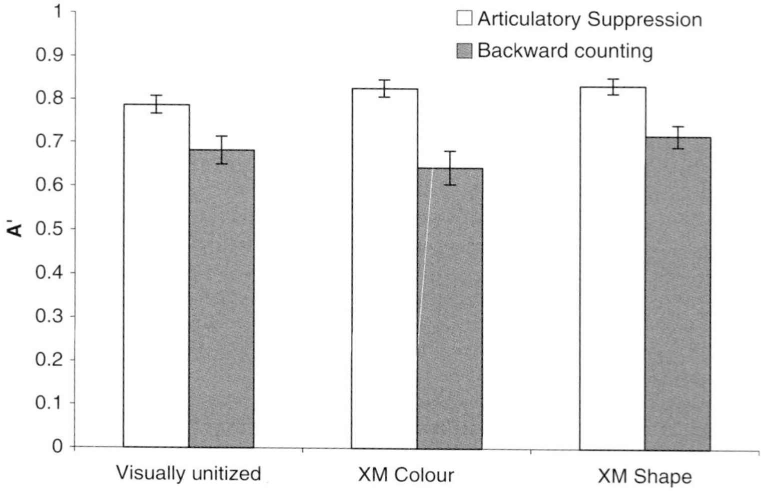

Figure 4. Mean accuracy (A') in each condition in Experiment 3 (with standard error).

Articulatory suppression and backward counting. Responses in the simple articulatory suppression task and in backward counting were scored in the same way. Thus, each production of three digits received a score of 1, with the production of each further digit adding 0.3 to the counting score. For example, following the start number 652, the backward counting response sequence "six five two, six four nine, six four six, six four, . . ." would receive a score of 3.6. Counting scores in the simple suppression and backward counting tasks, and also error rates in the latter task, are displayed in Table 2.

A 4 × 2 ANOVA on simple suppression and counting backwards scores revealed significant effects of binding condition, $F(3, 69) = 40.28$, $MSE = 0.09$, $p < .001$, $\eta_p^2 = .64$, task, $F(1, 23) = 83.87$, $MSE = 1.56$, $p < .001$, $\eta_p^2 = .79$, and the interaction, $F(3, 69) = 5.17$, $MSE = 0.07$, $p < .01$, $\eta_p^2 = .18$. Participants were faster and so scored more highly in the articulatory suppression task than in backward counting. The Task × Condition interaction was explored via separate ANOVAs for each task.

An ANOVA on simple suppression scores (in baseline and concurrent task conditions) revealed a significant effect of condition, $F(3, 69) = 20.69$, $MSE = 0.11$, $p < .001$, $\eta_p^2 = .47$. Further analyses, with Bonferroni corrections applied, revealed significant differences between baseline articulatory suppression and performance during the visually unitized condition, $t(23) = 3.44$, $p < .005$, effect size $d = 0.24$, the cross-modal auditory colour condition, $t(23) = 5.03$, $p < .001$, $d = 0.36$, and the cross-modal auditory shape condition, $t(23) = 7.91$, $p < .001$, $d = 0.62$. Thus, fewer responses were made when simple suppression was performed as a concurrent task, relative to the baseline measure. Comparing the different concurrent task conditions, there were also significant differences in simple suppression scores between visually unitized and the cross-modal auditory colour condition, $t(23) = 3.10$, $p < .008$, $d = 0.13$, and between the visually unitized and cross-modal auditory shape condition, $t(23) = 3.76$, $p < .005$, effect size $d = 0.33$. The two cross-modal conditions did not differ significantly after correcting for multiple comparisons, $t(23) = 2.18$, $p > .008$. To summarize, articulatory suppression was slower during the cross-modal conditions than during the visually unitized condition, though the effect sizes in each case were small.

TABLE 2

Performance scores for simple suppression and backward counting and backward counting error rates in each condition (standard errors in parentheses)

	Baseline	*Visual*	*XM colour*	*XM shape*
Simple suppression score	5.81 (0.24)	5.51 (0.26)	5.34 (0.27)	5.10 (0.22)
Backward counting score	4.22 (0.11)	3.69 (0.12)	3.60 (0.13)	3.66 (0.13)
Backward counting error rate	0.03 (0.01)	0.07 (0.01)	0.07 (0.01)	0.08 (0.01)

Turning to the backward counting scores obtained during the baseline condition and each of the concurrent task conditions, an ANOVA revealed a significant effect of condition, $F(3, 69) = 34.32$, $MSE = 0.03$, $p < .001$, $\eta_p^2 = .60$. Further comparisons of baseline and concurrent task performance (Bonferroni corrected) revealed that significantly more counting responses were made in baseline trials than during the visually unitized condition, $t(23) = 6.83$, $p < .001$, $d = 0.93$, the cross-modal auditory colour condition, $t(23) = 6.88$, $p < .001$, $d = 1.05$, and the cross-modal auditory shape condition, $t(23) = 6.97$, $p < .001$, $d = 0.96$. Thus, backward counting was slower when performed as a concurrent task. However, there were no significant differences between counting during visually unitized presentation and either cross-modal auditory colour, $t(23) = 1.74$, $p = .095$, $d = 0.15$, or cross-modal auditory shape, $t(23) = 0.485$, $d = 0.05$. The two cross-modal conditions did not significantly differ, $t(23) = 1.46$, $p = .158$, $d = 0.11$.

Finally, an ANOVA on error rates during backward counting revealed a significant effect of condition, $F(3, 69) = 13.23$, $MSE = 0.01$, $p < .001$, $\eta_p^2 = .37$. Further comparisons of baseline and concurrent task conditions (Bonferroni corrected) revealed that significantly fewer counting errors were made in baseline trials than during either the visually unitized condition, $t(23) = 7.64$, $p < .001$, $d = 0.95$, the cross-modal auditory colour condition, $t(23) = 5.67$, $p < .001$, $d = 0.85$, or the cross-modal auditory shape condition, $t(23) = 4.94$, $p < .001$, $d = 0.68$. Thus, backward counting was more prone to error when performed as a concurrent task. However, there were no significant differences in error rates between any of the concurrent task conditions ($p > .3$ in all cases).

Discussion

Once again there was no evidence that cross-modal presentation of stimuli led to poorer memory than unitized presentation. Indeed, the present data showed a slight difference in the opposite direction.

Turning to dual-task effects, we consider first the effect of backwards counting on performance of the memory task. As expected, backward counting generated substantial dual-task interference, relative to articulatory suppression, indicating the role that executive resources have in processing incoming information. However, the dual-task decrement was not greater for cross-modal than unitized stimuli.

The effects of the memory task on concurrent articulatory suppression and backwards counting were somewhat unexpected. Unsurprisingly, both tasks were performed less well relative to the single task baseline. However, the effect on backward counting was the same in the unitized and cross-modal conditions, whereas the effect on articulatory suppression was greater in the cross-modal conditions.

GENERAL DISCUSSION

Three experiments all demonstrated that participants are able to bind the features of shape and colour across the visual and auditory modalities. Experiment 2 showed that performance was not disrupted by a spatial tapping task. Experiment 3 showed clear overall memory impairment when the attentionally demanding task of counting back in threes was required concurrently. However, the degree of disruption was no greater for the cross-modal than for the unitized presentation conditions. Both articulatory suppression and backward counting were slower when combined with the memory task. The slowing of counting was greater for articulatory suppression when combined with cross-modal binding, but no such difference occurred in backward counting speed.

Our original hypothesis was based on the Baddeley (2000) model of working memory, which assumed a close link between the episodic buffer and the central executive, with both relying on a limited pool of attentional capacity. Binding was assumed to depend on this capacity. Hence, an attentionally demanding task was expected to disrupt the binding process, particularly when this required cross-modal manipulation. As in our previous within-modality studies (Allen et al., 2006; Karlsen et al., 2008), this prediction was not supported. The failure to find an interaction between binding and concurrent load suggests a modification of the Baddeley (2000) model. Allen et al. (2006) suggested the possibility that binding might be automatic, and hence independent of attentional demand. However, the fact that binding can occur across locations, across time (Karlsen et al., 2008) and across modalities makes this unlikely. Any system that automatically bound features as widely and promiscuously as this would surely lead to perceptual chaos.

A second approach is to assume that binding and storage within the buffer operate independently. One way of conceptualizing this is through the classic distinction made by William James (1890/1981) between two types of attention. One of these, ambient attention, is implicit and automatic, the other, focused attention, is dependent on executive control. Ambient attention allows us to continue to be aware of our surroundings, without explicitly focusing on them, whereas focused attention allows us to emphasize one aspect over others if necessary. Binding features within ambient attention does not appear to depend on explicit attentional focus, hence objects do not break up into separate features when we switch our attention from a scene to our internal thoughts. The distribution of focused attention almost certainly changes, through a shift in the balance between externally and internally focused attention.

Let us suppose that the episodic buffer serves as a basis for ambient attention, providing a passive store that may be fed from a range of features and modalities. Focused attention may be used to bias the contribution made by different features, either within modality as in picking out a meaningful shape from a noisy background, or between, as in responding to a verbal cue that disambiguates a visual object. Executive focus is not, however, essential for bound shapes to be represented as objects.

How might such a system operate? Stein (1992) has proposed a mechanism that serves a broadly similar interactive function, that of coordinating the range of sensory inputs that combine to represent egocentric space. These involve visual, auditory, and somaesthetic sensory inputs, which must be coordinated with oculomotor, limb, head, and body motor signals, with both being modulated by motivational factors. The situation is further complicated by the fact that the mapping of the environment onto the cortex is highly nonlinear, with the tongue and fingers for example occupying considerably more cortical space than the toes and the nose for example, hence requiring a degree of rescaling to reproduce an accurate egocentric spatial representation. Stein rejects the idea of a simple map, preparing instead "a distributed system of rules for information processing that can be used to transform signals from one co-ordinate system to another", proposing that this is subsumed by a network within the posterior parietal cortex. Although we would not wish to speculate at this point regarding anatomical location, we suggest that this proposal of a distributed representational network could be applied to the concept of an episodic buffer.

We have so far discussed our results as if there was no evidence of any cost of cross-modal binding. We did, however, find a greater degree of slowing in rate of articulatory suppression when cross-modal binding was required. The fact that this did not occur with the more attentionally demanding backward counting condition suggests that response frequency rather than processing load is likely to be the crucial factor. One possibility is that participants attempt to interleave verbal rehearsal between articulations. Backward counting was slower and hence left larger gaps between verbal responses, during which the subtractions were made; this may have allowed brief rehearsals to occur without slowing down overall counting rate, in contrast to the more rapid suppression condition. Rehearsal mechanisms other than the verbal type may well be possible, despite the relatively small inter-articulatory gaps (Barrouillet, Benardin, & Camos, 2004), with rate of interruption being a critical factor, possibly because of a response bottle-neck, with rehearsal being given priority over concurrent articulation. More articulatory responses would increase the probability of such response clashes, resulting in a greater sensitivity to competition.

However, despite this rather modest evidence to the contrary, the striking feature of our data is how effectively participants were able to bind features across modalities. Does this imply that unitized and cross-modal representations are identical? Not necessarily, although they do suggest that the two forms of representation are equally effective. Both could be stored in a passive episodic buffer, but could be supported by different off-buffer processes. In the case of the cross-modal conditions this could include both a phonological and a semantic component. Although articulatory suppression will hinder verbal rehearsal, it does not prevent auditory spoken material being registered in the phonological store, which is likely to be somewhat more durable than its visual equivalent (Baddeley, 2007). Furthermore, the cross-modal task requires the semantic translation of a spoken colour name into its meaning, hence providing another source of support for multi-dimensional representation in the episodic buffer. Regarding how features are bound together in each case, it may be plausible to suggest that mechanisms based around temporal synchrony play a role both within and across modalities, though it is likely that the nature of these representations varies considerably between conditions. In short, our results suggest that visual object binding may contain rather more than meets the eye.

REFERENCES

Allen, R. J., & Baddeley, A. D. (2008). Memory for prose: Mechanisms of binding in verbal working memory. In A. Thorn & M. Page (Eds.), *Interactions between short-term and long-term memory in the verbal domain*. Hove, UK: Psychology Press.

Allen, R. J., Baddeley, A. D., & Hitch, G. J. (2006). Is the binding of visual features in working memory resource-demanding? *Journal of Experimental Psychology: General*, *135*, 298–313.

Andrade, J., Werniers, Y., May, J., & Szmalec, A. (2002). Insensitivity of visual short-term memory to irrelevant visual information. *Quarterly Journal of Experimental Psychology*, *55A*, 753–774.

Baddeley, A. D. (1986). *Working memory*. Oxford, UK: Oxford University Press.

Baddeley, A. D. (1996). Exploring the central executive. *Quarterly Journal of Experimental Psychology*, *49A*(1), 5–28.

Baddeley, A. D. (2000). The episodic buffer: A new component of working memory? *Trends in Cognitive Sciences*, *4*(11), 417–423.

Baddeley, A. D. (2007). *Working memory, thought and action*. Oxford: Oxford University Press.

Baddeley, A. D., & Hitch, G. J. (1974). Working memory. In G. A. Bower (Ed.), *Recent advances in learning and motivation* (Vol. 8, pp. 47–89). New York: Academic Press.

Baddeley, A. D., Hitch, G. J., & Allen, R. J. (2008). Working memory and binding in sentence recall. *Manuscript submitted for publication*.

Baddeley, A. D., & Logie, R. H. (1999). Working memory: The multiple component model. In A. Miyake & P. Shah (Eds.), *Models of working memory: Mechanisms of active maintenance and executive control* (pp. 28–61). Cambridge, UK: Cambridge University Press.

Barrouillet, P., Benardin, S., & Camos, V. (2004). Time constraints and resource sharing in adults' working memory spans. *Journal of Experimental Psychology: General*, *133*, 83–100.

Bower, G. H. (1970). Analysis of a mnemonic device. *The American Scientist*, *58*, 496–510.

Dell'Acqua, R., & Jolicoeur, P. (2000). Visual encoding of patterns is subject to dual-task interference. *Memory and Cognition*, *28*(2), 184–191.

Duncan, J. (1984). Selective attention and the organization of visual information. *Journal of Experimental Psychology: General*, *113*, 501–517.

Egly, R., Driver, J., & Rafal, R. D. (1994). Shifting visual attention between objects and locations: Evidence from normal and parietal lesion subjects. *Journal of Experimental Psychology: General*, *12*, 161–177.

Gajewski, D. A., & Brockmole, J. R. (2006). Feature bindings endure without attention: Evidence from an explicit recall task. *Psychonomic Bulletin and Review*, *13*(4), 581–587.

Grier, J. B. (1971). Nonparametric indexes for senstitivity and bias: Computing formulas. *Psychological Bulletin*, *75*, 424–429.

James, W. (1981). *The principles of psychology* (E. Burkhardt & F. Bowers, Eds.). Cambridge, MA: Harvard University Press. (Original work published 1890)

Karlsen, P. J., Allen, R. J., Baddeley, A. D., & Hitch, G. J. (2008). Binding across space and time in visual working memory. *Manuscript submitted for publication*.

Logie, R. H. (1995). *Visuo-spatial working memory*. Hove, UK: Lawrence Erlbaum Associates Ltd.

Luck, S. J., & Vogel, E. K. (1997). The capacity of visual working memory for features and conjunctions. *Nature*, *390*, 279–281.

Miller, G. A. (1956). The magical number seven, plus or minus two: Some limits on our capacity for processing information. *Psychological Review*, *63*, 81–97.

Morey, C. C., & Cowan, N. (2004). When visual and verbal memories compete: Evidence of cross-domain limits in working memory. *Psychonomic Bulletin and Review*, *11*(2), 296–301.

Norman, D. A., & Shallice, T. (1986). Attention to action: Willed and automatic control of behaviour. In R. J. Davidson, G. E. Schwarts, & D. Shapiro (Eds.), *Advances in research and theory: Vol. 4. Consciousness and self-regulation* (pp. 1–18). New York: Plenum Press.

O'Reilly, R. C., Busby, R. S., & Soto, R. (2003). Three forms of binding and their neural substrates: Alternatives to temporal asynchrony. In A. Cleeremans (Ed.), *The unity of consciousness: Binding, interaction, and dissociation* (pp. 28–61). Oxford, UK: Oxford University Press.

Pollack, I., & Norman, D. A. (1964). A non-parametric analysis of recognition experiments. *Psychonomic Science*, *1*, 125–136.

Quinn, G., & McConnell, J. (1996). Exploring the passive visual store. *Psychologische Beitrage*, *38*, 355–367.

Raffone, A., & Wolters, G. (2001). A cortical mechanism for binding in visual working memory. *Journal of Cognitive Neuroscience*, *13*, 766–785.

Rossi-Arnaud, C., Pieroni, L., & Baddeley, A. D. (2006). Symmetry and binding in visuo-spatial working memory. *Neuroscience*, *139*, 393–400.

Stein, J. F. (1992). The representation of egocentric space in the posterior parietal cortex. *Behavioral and Brain Sciences*, *15*, 691–700.

Treisman, A. M., & Gelade, G. (1980). Feature-integration theory of attention. *Cognitive Psychology*, *12*, 97–136.

Vogel, E. K., Woodman, G. F., & Luck, S. J. (2001). Storage of features, conjunctions, and objects in visual working memory. *Journal of Experimental Psychology: Human Perception and Performance*, *27*(1), 92–114.

Wheeler, M. E., & Treisman, A. M. (2002). Binding in short-term visual memory. *Journal of Experimental Psychology: General*, *131*, 48–64.

VISUAL COGNITION, 2009, 17 (1/2), 103–119

Psychology Press
Taylor & Francis Group

Binding hardwired versus on-demand feature conjunctions

Rufin VanRullen

Université de Toulouse, CerCo, UPS, and CNRS, UMR5549, Faculté de Médecine de Rangueil, Toulouse, France

Binding denotes the process by which features represented in early stages of the visual system are brought together within a meaningful representation that can support recognition, action, or consciousness. It is often considered that binding requires attentional resources. However, recent results have demonstrated that recognition of natural and familiar objects or scenes—as opposed to more arbitrary, meaningless conjunctions of features—can be done while attention is distracted. Surprisingly, the same discriminations do not lead to efficient "pop-out" visual search. These seemingly opposite conclusions can be reconciled by postulating the existence of two modes of binding in the brain: "Hardwired" binding of frequently encountered, natural objects through a hierarchy of increasingly complex feature detectors, as in classic computational models inspired by neurophysiological results; and "on-demand" binding mediated by attention for more arbitrary or meaningless feature conjunctions, as advocated in classic psychological theories. The former system can function without attention, but is challenged by spatial competition within neuronal receptive fields when multiple objects are presented. Thus, while on-demand binding always requires attention, hardwired binding only does when receptive field competition occurs. New experimental data using multiple stimuli and variable interstimulus distance supports this theoretical dissociation.

Keywords: Attention; Natural scenes; Feed-forward model; Competition; Pre-attentive recognition

When contemporary scientists describe "the binding problem" to less knowledgeable peers, they generally (1) evoke the well-known fact that early stages of visual processing decompose the visual scene into a number of elementary features represented in separate maps (colour, orientation, motion direction, and so on), and then (2) conjure up an example in which, say two cars driving past one another might be easily confounded (does the red paint belong to the eastbound or the westbound car?). Separated features must be "bound" back together at some point.

Please address all correspondence to Rufin Vanrullen, CNRS, UMR5549, Faculté de Médecine de Rangueil, 31062 Toulouse, France. E-mail: rufin.vanrullen@cerco.ups-tlse.fr

© 2008 Psychology Press, an imprint of the Taylor & Francis Group, an Informa business
http://www.psypress.com/viscog DOI: 10.1080/13506280802196451

Accounts might diverge, however, regarding the nature of the feature binding process. For computational neuroscientists, higher level neurons can "simply" bind elementary features into hardwired[1] combinations, within the limited spatial extent of their receptive fields. Many state-of-the-art models of object recognition are based on such feedforward feature combinations—and the approach works remarkably well (Delorme & Thorpe, 2001; Fukushima & Miyake, 1982; Riesenhuber & Poggio, 1999b; Serre et al., 2005; Serre, Oliva, & Poggio, 2007; VanRullen, Gautrais, Delorme, & Thorpe, 1998; VanRullen & Thorpe, 2002). Many cognitive scientists, on the other hand, tend to consider that the sum of all arbitrary conjunctions of two or more elementary features must be a large number (the "combinatorial explosion"), too large for each conjunction to merit its own "map". They are thus led to the unavoidable conclusion that higher level perception must rely not on any "hardwired" binding of features into objects, but on a flexible, "on-demand" strategy. Attention is generally offered as the key to solving the binding problem (Treisman, 1996). This would imply that no object recognition, no scene comprehension or categorization can occur outside of the focus of attention, a classic view that has been supported by much experimental evidence (Chun & Marois, 2002; Nakayama & Joseph, 1998; Treisman & Sato, 1990; Treisman & Souther, 1985; Wolfe, 1998; Wolfe & Bennett, 1997). But upon more careful scrutiny, there are also findings that are difficult to reconcile with this framework. Attentional deployment should take time and effort, yet natural scene or object categorization can be remarkably fast (Kirchner & Thorpe, 2006; Potter & Faulconer, 1975; Potter & Levy, 1969; Thorpe, Fize, & Marlot, 1996; VanRullen & Thorpe, 2001); more recent work even suggests that it could occur with little attentional effort (Fei-Fei, VanRullen, Koch, & Perona, 2005; Li, VanRullen, Koch, & Perona, 2002; Reddy, Reddy, & Koch, 2006; Reddy, Wilken, & Koch, 2004; Rousselet, Fabre-Thorpe, & Thorpe, 2002; VanRullen, Reddy, & Koch, 2004). Is the dogma floundering? Yes, but only partly. I will present evidence that some forms of object recognition, but not all, can happen without attention. The picture will be further complicated by the finding that different attentional paradigms lead to conflicting results. But in the end, I will show that most of the available data can be reconciled simply by abandoning one of the premises of the previous reasoning: By accepting that hardwired binding, as it is implemented in current computational models, can be a viable strategy for at least some types of object recognition (Riesenhuber & Poggio, 1999a). After all, the complex object selectivities found in inferotemporal neurons (e.g., face-selective cells) (Logothetis & Sheinberg, 1996; Perrett, Rolls, & Caan, 1982) are often preserved in

[1] The term "hardwired" does not imply an innate origin. Here, it indicates a pattern of neuronal connectivity that is, in most cases, the result of experience, and which does not alter significantly from one stimulus presentation to the next.

anesthetized animals, when attention and other top-down factors can only play a minor role (Desimone, Albright, Gross, & Bruce, 1984; Gross, Rocha-Miranda, & Bender, 1972; Kobatake & Tanaka, 1994; Tanaka, 1996).

RECOGNITION WITHOUT ATTENTION

For decades now, attention has been considered as a necessary condition for visual object recognition. In the debate between early (Bergen & Julesz, 1983; Broadbent, 1958; Hillyard, Vogel, & Luck, 1998; Mangun, 1995; Treisman, 1960; Treisman & Gelade, 1980) and late (Allport, Tipper, & Chmiel, 1985; Deutsch & Deutsch, 1963; Duncan, 1980, 1984; Tipper, 1985) selection theories of attention, early selection has more or less taken the prize. This is in no small part the result of the pioneering research programmes of Anne Treisman and Bela Julesz, using visual search arrays (Bergen & Julesz, 1983; Julesz, 1975; Treisman & Gelade, 1980; Treisman & Gormican, 1988; Treisman & Paterson, 1984; Treisman & Souther, 1985; Wolfe, 1994, 1998; Wolfe, Cave, & Franzel, 1989). They clearly and repeatedly demonstrated that the visual system can simultaneously register and compare simple features (oriented bars, coloured patches, moving dots) across multiple spatial locations, as if it was an effortless, cost-free problem; but when more complex objects (i.e., combinations of two or more features such as bicoloured items, Ls vs. Ts, colour-orientation conjunctions, etc.) had to be processed, a performance cost was observed for each additional item in the array, as if some limited resource was becoming more and more in demand: Attention. The interpretation was almost evident: The elementary features being represented in separate, retinotopically organized maps (in early cortical areas) could support the simultaneous representation of multiple items; but no such map existed for the more complex objects and feature conjunctions (due to the "combinatorial explosion" problem), and the required representation had to be constructed on demand—a process mediated by attention, which could only occur for one or a few items at a time. In other words, attention served to select what features of the early, parallel representation stages would be bound into higher level representations (the so-called "object files" of Treisman's theory). But this idea derived from visual search experiments might not have made such an impact if it wasn't also supported by other experimental techniques. For example in dual tasks (another classic and elegant attentional manipulation in which attentional resources are taken away from a target stimulus by a secondary, challenging task), it was observed that a single elementary feature (horizontal vs. vertical bar; red vs. green patch) could be distinguished as target, but a more complex conjunction (L vs. T, bisected red-green vs. green-red disks) could not (Braun & Julesz, 1998; Braun & Sagi, 1990; Lee, Koch, & Braun, 1999). With such a consistent pattern of results, most vision scientists agreed that attention must indeed matter for binding features, and thus for object recognition.

What a surprise then when, more recently, a number of studies started to suggest that this outcome could change if natural[2] scenes and objects were used as stimuli, instead of arbitrary patterns. For example, with a combination of psychophysical and ERP measurements, Rousselet et al. (2002) observed no measurable cost for processing two natural scenes (does each scene contain an animal or not?) compared to a single scene. The same categorization task could be performed easily under dual-task conditions (Li et al., 2002)—those same experimental conditions that prevent observers from discriminating, say a red-green disk from a green-red disk (Braun & Julesz, 1998). This was true even if the natural scene target was a vehicle (Fei-Fei et al., 2005; Li et al., 2002), or if the task involved face gender discrimination (Reddy et al., 2004) or face recognition (Reddy et al., 2006). Thus, when stimuli are taken from natural and familiar object or scene categories, attention matters much less for recognition (Braun, 2003). This could imply that for such categories of objects, a form of automatic binding might exist in the brain.

Whether this form of preattentive binding really supports "true", high-level object recognition is open to debate. For example, Evans and Treisman have suggested that it might only reflect the parallel detection of feature sets (e.g., yellow + stripes + fur + claws ... = tiger) without a precise spatial binding (Evans & Treisman, 2005; Treisman & Kanwisher, 1998). As I will argue later, however, it can be demonstrated that this form of binding is spatially limited in extent, i.e., features are not collected over the entire visual field, but within a well-defined region of more than three degrees and less than eight degrees of visual angle (for a stimulus at five degrees of eccentricity). We cannot conclude yet whether even more spatially precise binding might occur beyond this resolution—but this need not be so problematic: In the real world (as opposed to laboratory situations), when all the relevant features are present within a spatially limited region (yellow, stripes, fur, claws ...), one can bet with almost certainty that the object (tiger) is present. If one is reluctant to equate these object representations that are formed in the absence of attention with "true, high-level objects", then it might be a good compromise to think of them as "proto-objects", as proposed by Rensink (2002).[3]

[2] The term "natural" is used here to refer to ecologically valid stimuli for which the visual system has been optimized throughout its development, as opposed to more arbitrary stimuli that an observer is only likely to encounter in laboratory situations. According to this definition, city scenes, photographs of vehicles, and manmade objects, are all "natural" stimuli.

[3] According to Rensink, proto-objects are "rapidly generated, volatile structures that contain local estimates of scene structure". They can be "quite sophisticated", but have "limited spatial coherence".

The efficient, effortless processing of natural scenes and objects observed under dual-task conditions is a very robust phenomenon: Many recognition and categorization tasks, at different levels of discrimination, can be performed with seemingly little attention. For example, Reddy et al. (2004) observed that face gender discrimination, using faces where obvious external features (e.g., hair, make-up) had been removed, could still be done in dual task. In order to test an even more stringent level of discrimination, they asked observers to recognize a particular male (or female) individual, with distractors being other male (or female) individuals: Still no significant performance decrement occurred when attention was distracted (Reddy et al., 2006)!

THE LIMITS OF EFFORTLESS PROCESSING

On the other hand, a limit to this effortless recognition ability can be observed easily, by placing multiple simultaneous stimuli on the screen. We have already described the experiment by Rousselet et al. (2002) in which two natural scenes could be processed in parallel (for an animal vs. nonanimal discrimination). But in another study where four scenes had to be processed simultaneously, performance started to decrease quite strongly (Rousselet, Thorpe, & Fabre-Thorpe, 2004). In fact, when a whole visual search array of natural scenes (up to 16 distinct elements) was presented to an observer, performance (both in terms of reaction time and proportion correct) greatly decreased with increasing set size, i.e., the number of elements on the screen (VanRullen et al., 2004). This indicates an inefficient "serial" search process, and would generally be interpreted as reflecting the involvement of attention in scene recognition—although other interpretations of serial search have been advanced (Carrasco & Yeshurun, 1998; Eckstein, 1998; Eckstein, Thomas, Palmer, & Shimozaki, 2000; Palmer, 1995; Palmer, Verghese, & Pavel, 2000). These results are very much in line with classic visual search experiments, which to a large extent have failed to show efficient "parallel" search for line drawings of objects—even natural and familiar ones like animals, vehicles, faces (Wolfe, 1998; Wolfe & Bennett, 1997). Some authors have suggested that faces constitute a special class of stimuli, so important ecologically that they could escape the need for serial search (Hansen & Hansen, 1988; Hershler & Hochstein, 2005). But it has later been shown that these "pop-out" effects were mere reflections of spurious low-level differences between the stimuli used[4] (Brown, Huey, & Findlay, 1997; Nothdurft, 1993; Purcell, Stewart, & Skov, 1996; VanRullen, 2006). Whatever the type of object involved (even extremely

[4] This inability of faces to "pop out" does not mean, however, that face stimuli might not be special in other regards.

natural and familiar ones like faces), object recognition in visual search thus appears to be a serial process. Therefore, the visual search paradigm yields the opposite conclusion as before: Attention might be necessary for natural scene and object recognition after all—and so presumably for feature binding.

COMPETITION TO THE RESCUE

How can the same discrimination task (e.g., animal vs. nonanimal scene, male vs. female face, . . .) be "preattentive" in dual-task, but not "parallel" in visual search? Is attention necessary for binding features into natural and familiar object representations, or not? To answer this, let us consider what should happen within the classic computational approach, based on feedforward and "hardwired" feature combinations (see Figure 1, left side). The common architecture in these models mirrors that of the visual system (Felleman & van Essen, 1991) and involves a succession of processing layers in which neurons combine their inputs within a small region (the "receptive field") to represent new features of increased complexity: Small luminance patches are combined to represent oriented bars; bars are combined to represent contours; and so on until "recognition" units at the last level respond selectively to particular object categories (Fukushima & Miyake, 1982; Riesenhuber & Poggio, 1999b; Selfridge, 1959; Serre et al., 2007). Increases of representation complexity are generally accompanied by an increase of receptive field size (as observed in the visual system) (Boussaoud, Desimone, & Ungerleider, 1991; Gattass, Gross, & Sandell, 1981; Gattass, Sousa, & Gross, 1988) in order to provide the network with some spatial invariance.

How would such a model perform in the various experimental paradigms described earlier? Because these feedforward models generally don't include an attention mechanism, dual-task conditions would not change anything to the network behaviour: Recognition would occur as usual, whether or not attention is "distracted". But when a whole visual search array is presented, features corresponding to several distinct objects can fall within each receptive field, preventing the "recognition" neurons from working properly: Parallel search fails, and attentional requirements emerge (Mozer & Sitton, 1998). This is also a form of the binding problem, i.e., a difficulty in assigning the correct features to the correct objects, as proposed in classic theories; but the main difference is that here binding is only a *local* problem: It occurs—or fails to occur—within the receptive fields of the recognition units, because of interference and competition between the inputs. Similar recognition failures are commonly observed in single-unit physiology, when both an effective and an ineffective stimulus are simultaneously presented within a V2, V4, or IT neuron's receptive field: The resulting neuronal response is unselective and intermediate (Luck, Chelazzi, Hillyard, & Desimone, 1997; Moran & Desimone, 1985; Reynolds, Chelazzi, & Desimone, 1999). Drawing attention to one of the stimuli is required to restore the neuronal response, and alleviate the conflict between the inconsistent inputs. Comparable observations have been made in humans using fMRI (Kastner, de Weerd, Desimone, & Ungerleider, 1998) and ERPs, leading Luck and his colleagues to propose an "Ambiguity Resolution" theory of attention (Luck, Girelli, McDermott, & Ford, 1997). In this view, attention would not be necessary for the binding of features per se (and indeed, would not be needed when a single object is to be recognized), but it would only be critical for resolving the competition that ensues (e.g., in visual search situations) from having multiple items in one receptive field (Desimone & Duncan, 1995; Luck & Ford, 1998; Reynolds & Desimone, 1999).

If receptive field competition is truly the main limitation of parallel processing for natural objects and scenes, then the ability to process simultaneous objects should depend on the distance between them: When they fall in a single receptive field, binding should fail; when they fall in separate receptive fields, (parallel) binding should succeed. This is what we proceeded to verify experimentally.

Dual task with two simultaneous stimuli

First, we adapted the dual-task paradigm in order to evaluate the effects of a simultaneously presented, irrelevant item on object recognition without attention (VanRullen, Reddy, & Fei-Fei, 2005). The attention-demanding task that we used for manipulating the availability of attention was a letter search task (singleton present/absent among five randomly rotated Ls or Ts at the centre of the screen), as used in most of the dual-task literature (Braun, 1998; Braun & Julesz, 1998; Lee et al., 1999; Li et al., 2002; Reddy et al., 2004; Reddy et al., 2006). The task of interest was an animal vs. nonanimal natural scene categorization task, or in other sessions an upright vs. inverted face discrimination task. The stimulus of interest was presented at a random peripheral location (5.5 degrees eccentricity), and in some of the trials a second, irrelevant stimulus of the same type (i.e., a natural scene containing an animal, or an upright face, depending on the session) was shown simultaneously (2.5 degrees eccentricity). The subjects were instructed to ignore this irrelevant stimulus, and in order to make this easier we maintained its identity constant throughout the entire experiment (i.e., for several hundred trials). When this distracting stimulus was present, it was either (with 50% probability) shown close to the target stimulus (3 degrees away), or far from it (8 degrees away, with the same 2.5 degrees eccentricity but on the other side of fixation). We obtained identical results for the natural scene categorization and the face discrimination task. When the target stimulus was presented alone, it was recognized easily (at around 90% of the baseline single-task performance), even when attention was distracted by the central letter task; this merely confirms previous reports (Fei-Fei et al., 2005; Li et al., 2002; Reddy et al., 2004; Reddy et al., 2006; VanRullen et al., 2004). The presence of the distracting stimulus had a strong impairing effect on dual-task performance (down to ~ 65%, with chance level at 50%), but *only when it was shown in close proximity to the target*—the remote distracting stimulus had virtually no effect on dual-task performance! This indicates that a binding problem (defined here as interference between two simultaneous items, compared to a situation with a single item) had occurred between the target and the distracting stimulus, but only within a local neighbourhood of the target; a remote distracting stimulus did not trigger this binding problem, and did not impair recognition. Note, finally, that this conclusion is only valid for our natural object or scene recognition tasks: For other, more arbitrary stimuli (e.g., conjunctions of two colours or two orientations), recognition simply cannot occur when attention is distracted, even for a single isolated stimulus (Fei-Fei et al., 2005; Li et al., 2002; VanRullen et al., 2004); it would make little sense in this case to test recognition with two simultaneous stimuli.

Comparison task

In order to confirm and extend these results, we designed another paradigm that would allow us to test attentional requirements and interstimulus distance effects for both natural/familiar and arbitrary/artificial object categories in a comparable way (VanRullen et al., 2005). This paradigm involved the comparison of two simultaneously presented items from a given category: Two natural scenes (animal vs. non-animal), two faces (upright vs. inverted), two colour/colour conjunctions (red-green vs. green-red), or two orientation/orientation conjunctions (rotated L vs. T). The subjects responded by indicating whether the items were of the "same" or of a "different" type (e.g., two Ls, or one L and one T, respectively). Critically, the stimuli were masked and the presentation times (stimulus onset asynchrony, SOA) were determined based on pilot data so that identification performance of a single, isolated stimulus was comparable for all stimulus categories (~ 85% correct). We found that observers could not compare the two arbitrary conjunction stimuli (i.e., rotated Ls and Ts, or red-green vs. green-red disks), for which the comparison performance was near chance (~ 55%), irrespective of the distance between the two simultaneous stimuli. This confirms the idea that attention is an unconditional requirement for binding and recognition of this type of object. On the other hand, the comparison task was easy (i.e., close to 70%, as expected if both stimuli were identified with ~ 85% probability) for the natural object and scene discriminations (animal vs. non-animal; upright vs. inverted face) when the distance between the two stimuli to be compared was 8 degrees of visual angle. This confirms that successful binding can sometimes occur "in parallel" for natural stimuli. But when the interstimulus distance was decreased to 3 degrees, a strong decrement was observed in the comparison performance: This reflected a local binding problem, which we attributed to receptive field competition within the relevant neuronal populations.

Visual search with varying interstimulus distance

To finish, we applied our conclusions to the conundrum raised by visual search for natural objects and scenes. If recognition of these stimuli can (in theory) be done preattentively, but is prevented during visual search by unwanted receptive field competition, then visual search performance should be increased by separating elements within the visual search array—as demonstrated in one previous study (Cohen & Ivry, 1991). Furthermore, this should only be true for natural/familiar object categories (because for them the serial nature of the search is merely due to competition), and not for arbitrary/artificial objects (because for them the serial nature of the search reflects a true attentional need). We tested these predictions by evaluating visual search performance for an upright versus inverted face discrimination and a red-green versus green-red disk discrimination tasks, with varying interstimulus distances (Reddy & VanRullen, 2007). The two tasks are similar, in the sense that distractors are simply obtained by rotating the targets by 180 degrees. To avoid eccentricity confounds, all stimuli were presented on a virtual ring at 1.5 degrees eccentricity. At the smallest interstimulus distance tested (0.75 degrees), both tasks showed a clear and similar serial search behaviour (i.e., performance decreased and RT increased significantly with increasing set size). But when interstimulus distance was increased progressively (up to 3 degrees), search performance increased only for the face discrimination task, while no effect was observed for the two-colour disk discrimination—exactly as we predicted. We also verified, under the same experimental conditions, that classic pop-out search tasks (red vs. green patches, + L vs. T symbols) were not affected by interstimulus distance.

Distinguishing preattentive competition from local attentional interference

At first sight, the results described earlier using the dual task, the comparison task, or the visual search paradigm might seem to merely corroborate the numerous previous reports of a spatial pattern of local suppression around the (facilitatory) attentional spotlight (Bahcall & Kowler, 1999; Cutzu & Tsotsos, 2003; Hopf et al., 2006; McCarley, Mounts, & Kramer, 2004, 2007; Mounts, 2000a, 2000b; Mounts & Gavett, 2004; Muller & Kleinschmidt, 2004). This suppressive pattern has been dubbed "localized attentional interference" (Mounts, 2000a, 2000b). In fact, the phenomenon that we demonstrated is quite different: First, in our case the local interference occurs preattentively (as revealed in the dual-task experiment earlier); second, it occurs only for certain familiar and natural object categories, but is absent in other cases (as shown earlier in the comparison task and the visual search experiment). These two properties would not be expected if the interference reflected the suppressive surround of the attentional spotlight; rather, this interference is more likely to reflect competition within the receptive fields of neuronal populations that are *preattentively* activated. Whether attention, when it finally comes into play, is also accompanied by local suppression, is an interesting question, but one that is orthogonal to our present concern.

TWO TYPES OF BINDING IN THE BRAIN

Putting all these observations together, we suggest that two types of binding might coexist in the brain: Hardwired binding for familiar, natural object categories, and on-demand binding for more arbitrary, artificial, or meaningless conjunctions of features (Figure 1). The former can occur without involving attention, while the latter is directly mediated by attention.

Hardwired binding corresponds to the operation of a system based on a feedforward hierarchy of neurons, which construct their increasingly complex selectivities by pooling the features represented at previous levels. This idea is directly inspired by the organization of the visual system revealed by primate electrophysiology (Barlow, 1972; Felleman & van Essen, 1991; Hubel & Wiesel, 1968). The system is flexible in the sense that it can learn to represent new objects and features over the course of repeated presentations; but for a given stimulus presentation the behaviour of the system is fixed, and fully determined by the existing connectivity between neurons (i.e., it is "hardwired"). Such a system suffers from two main limitations: It can only represent familiar, frequently encountered stimulus categories (and this is probably best if one is to avoid combinatorial explosion problems); and it will fail when the features corresponding to multiple different objects are too close

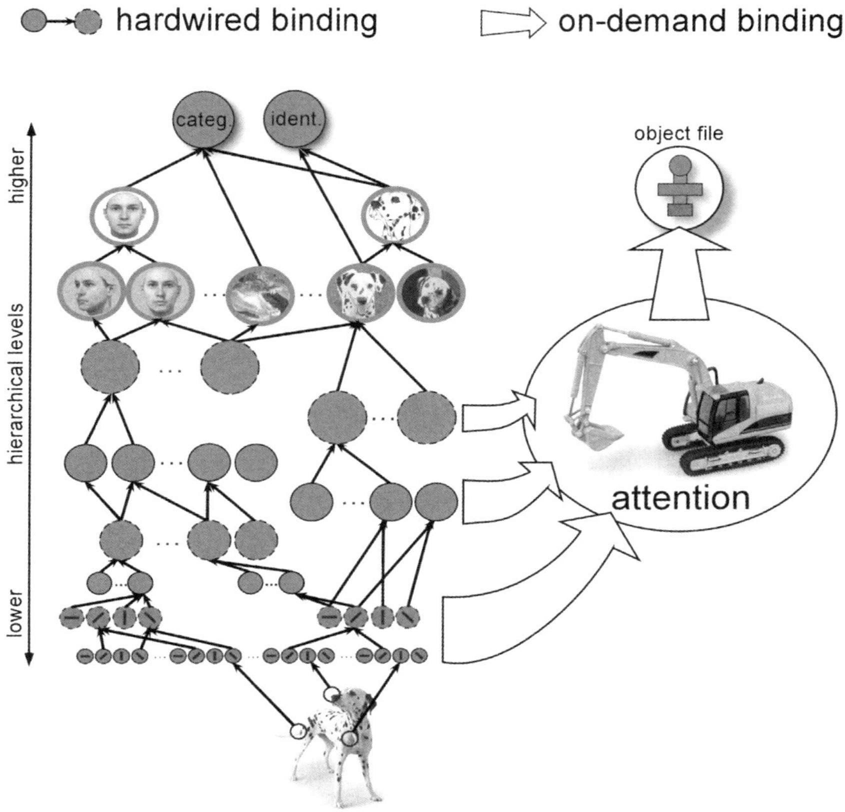

Figure 1. Two types of binding can coexist in the brain. One is automatic and preattentive, based on a hierarchy of hardwired conjunctions of features of increasing complexity, as observed in the primate visual system, and described in classic feedforward models of object recognition. It is limited to the processing of familiar, natural object and scene categories. In this example, adapted with permission from Serre et al. (2005), orientation is the only low-level feature depicted, but other features such as colour, motion, binocular disparity, and so on, can also participate in the early, low-level representation. The other type of binding allows the visual system to deal with previously unknown, unfamiliar or arbitrary conjunctions of features by a costly, on-demand binding process mediated by visual attention. As in the classic Feature Integration Theory of attention, this process results in the formation of a temporary high-level representation or "object file". To view this figure in colour, please see the online issue of the Journal.

in space (as in a visual search experiment), since they will clutter the relevant receptive fields. However, notwithstanding these two caveats, such systems can be very powerful since they have the potential to represent multiple objects simultaneously, as long as they are well separated (as shown for example in the "comparison" task), and can function without involving costly attentional resources (as revealed by the "dual-task" paradigm). Indeed, most state-of-the-art object recognition models are based on this simple idea (Fukushima & Miyake, 1982; Riesenhuber & Poggio, 1999b; Serre et al., 2005; Serre et al., 2007; VanRullen & Thorpe, 2002).

On-demand binding is the form most commonly advocated by psychologists, based on the famous Feature Integration Theory (Treisman & Gelade, 1980). It is the process by which attention combines the various features of a stimulus to construct, one at a time, temporary high-level representations (or "object files" in Treisman's terminology) that will serve as the basis for recognition, categorization, or behavioural responses (and, potentially, conscious perception). The main amendment that we would like to propose is that this costly process is not required for familiar objects.

A corollary of this distinction is that visual attention serves at least two distinct purposes in the brain (VanRullen et al., 2004). Within the context of a hardwired binding system, attention can be called upon to resolve competition within neuronal receptive fields, a role compatible with the "biased competition" (Desimone & Duncan, 1995; Reynolds & Desimone, 1999) and the "ambiguity resolution" theories of attention. Within an on-demand system, attention serves as the medium that binds features into higher level objects. Whether a unique attentional system accounts for both these duties is an open question, but parsimony would suggest that two distinct structures constitute an unnecessary expense. In any case, while the postulated "hardwired" recognition system easily maps onto the known hierarchy of cortical areas and feedforward neuronal selectivities, the biological source(s) and mode(s) of operation of attention is (are) still largely unknown. There is general agreement, however, from both theoretical and experimental perspectives, that attention heavily involves feedback and reentrant processes to resolve competition and/or allow binding to take place (Bullier, 2001; Di Lollo, Enns, & Rensink, 2000; Hamker, 2003; Hochstein & Ahissar, 2002; Lamme & Roelfsema, 2000; Tsotsos et al., 1995). Such a distinction between feedforward hardwired binding and reentrant on-demand binding would then be reminiscent of the separation between "base grouping" and "incremental grouping" postulated by Roelfsema (2006; see also Ullman, 1984).

CONCLUSION

It is important to acknowledge that none of the individual ideas expressed here is fully novel or revolutionary. In particular, the present proposal draws on recognized concepts such as Biased Competition and the Ambiguity Resolution Theory, the Feature Integration Theory, and hierarchical feedforward models of object recognition. No alternative is favoured over another, but I have focused instead on revealing the experimental conditions that tend to promote one or the other mechanisms, and have proposed what seems to be an optimal compromise between two classic, often opposed views of binding. It is thus possible to reconcile computational approaches supporting hardwired binding of natural, frequently encountered object categories, and psychological theories advocating attention-based on-demand binding of arbitrary or meaningless feature conjunctions.

REFERENCES

Allport, D. A., Tipper, S. P., & Chmiel, N. R. J. (1985). Perceptual integration and postcategorical filtering. In M. I. Posner & O. S. M. Marin (Eds.), *Attention and performance XI* (pp. 107–132). Hillsdale, NJ: Lawrence Erlbaum Associates, Inc.

Bahcall, D. O., & Kowler, E. (1999). Attentional interference at small spatial separations. *Vision Research*, *39*(1), 71–86.

Barlow, H. B. (1972). Single units and sensation: A neuron doctrine for perceptual psychology? *Perception*, *1*(4), 371–394.

Bergen, J. R., & Julesz, B. (1983). Parallel versus serial processing in rapid pattern discrimination. *Nature*, *303*(5919), 696–698.

Boussaoud, D., Desimone, R., & Ungerleider, L. G. (1991). Visual topography of area TEO in the macaque. *Journal of Comparative Neurology*, *306*(4), 554–575.

Braun, J. (1998). Divided attention: Narrowing the gap between brain and behavior. In R. Parasuraman (Ed.), *The attentive brain* (pp. 327–351). Cambridge, MA: MIT Press.

Braun, J. (2003). Natural scenes upset the visual applecart. *Trends in Cognitive Science*, *7*(1), 7–9.

Braun, J., & Julesz, B. (1998). Withdrawing attention at little or no cost: Detection and discrimination tasks. *Perception and Psychophysics*, *60*(1), 1–23.

Braun, J., & Sagi, D. (1990). Vision outside the focus of attention. *Perception and Psychophysics*, *48*(1), 45–58.

Broadbent, D. E. (1958). *Perception and communication*. London: Pergamon Press.

Brown, V., Huey, D., & Findlay, J. M. (1997). Face detection in peripheral vision: Do faces pop out? *Perception*, *26*(12), 1555–1570.

Bullier, J. (2001). Integrated model of visual processing. *Brain Research and Brain Research Review*, *36*(2–3), 96–107.

Carrasco, M., & Yeshurun, Y. (1998). The contribution of covert attention to the set-size and eccentricity effects in visual search. *Journal of Experimental Psychology: Human Perception and Performance*, *24*(2), 673–692.

Chun, M. M., & Marois, R. (2002). The dark side of visual attention. *Current Opinion in Neurobiology*, *12*(2), 184–189.

Cohen, A., & Ivry, R. B. (1991). Density effects in conjunction search: Evidence for a coarse location mechanism of feature integration. *Journal of Experimental Psychology: Human Perception and Performance*, *17*(4), 891–901.

Cutzu, F., & Tsotsos, J. K. (2003). The selective tuning model of attention: Psychophysical evidence for a suppressive annulus around an attended item. *Vision Research*, *43*(2), 205–219.

Delorme, A., & Thorpe, S. J. (2001). Face identification using one spike per neuron: Resistance to image degradations. *Neural Networks*, *14*(6–7), 795–803.

Desimone, R., Albright, T. D., Gross, C. G., & Bruce, C. (1984). Stimulus-selective properties of inferior temporal neurons in the macaque. *Journal of Neuroscience*, *4*(8), 2051–2062.

Desimone, R., & Duncan, J. (1995). Neural mechanisms of selective visual attention. *Annual Review of Neuroscience*, *18*, 193–222.

Deutsch, J. A., & Deutsch, D. (1963). Attention: Some theoretical considerations. *Psychological Review*, *70*, 80–90.

Di Lollo, V., Enns, J. T., & Rensink, R. A. (2000). Competition for consciousness among visual events: The psychophysics of reentrant visual processes. *Journal of Experimental Psychology: General*, *129*(4), 481–507.

Duncan, J. (1980). The locus of interference in the perception of simultaneous stimuli. *Psychological Review*, *87*(3), 272–300.

Duncan, J. (1984). Selective attention and the organization of visual information. *Journal of Experimental Psychology: General*, *113*, 501–517.

Eckstein, M. (1998). The lower visual search efficiency for conjunctions is due to noise and not serial attentional processing. *Psychological Science*, *9*(2), 111–118.

Eckstein, M., Thomas, J. P., Palmer, J., & Shimozaki, S. S. (2000). A signal detection model predicts the effects of set size on visual search accuracy for feature, conjunction, triple conjunction, and disjunction displays. *Perception and Psychophysics*, *62*(3), 425–451.

Evans, K. K., & Treisman, A. (2005). Perception of objects in natural scenes: Is it really attention free? *Journal of Experimental Psychology: Human Perception and Performance*, *31*(6), 1476–1492.

Fei-Fei, L., VanRullen, R., Koch, C., & Perona, P. (2005). Why does natural scene categorization require little attention? Exploring attentional requirements for natural and synthetic stimuli. *Visual Cognition*, *12*(6), 893–924.

Felleman, D. J., & van Essen, D. C. (1991). Distributed hierarchical processing in the primate cerebral cortex. *Cerebral Cortex*, *1*(1), 1–47.

Fukushima, K., & Miyake, S. (1982). Neocognition: A new algorithm for pattern recognition tolerant of deformations and shifts in position. *Pattern Recognition*, *15*, 455–469.

Gattass, R., Gross, C. G., & Sandell, J. H. (1981). Visual topography of V2 in the macaque. *Journal of Comparative Neurology*, *201*(4), 519–539.

Gattass, R., Sousa, A. P., & Gross, C. G. (1988). Visuotopic organization and extent of V3 and V4 of the macaque. *Journal of Neuroscience*, *8*(6), 1831–1845.

Gross, C. G., Rocha-Miranda, C. E., & Bender, D. B. (1972). Visual properties of neurons in inferotemporal cortex of the Macaque. *Journal of Neurophysiology*, *35*(1), 96–111.

Hamker, F. H. (2003). The reentry hypothesis: Linking eye movements to visual perception. *Journal of Vision*, *3*(11), 808–816.

Hansen, C. H., & Hansen, R. D. (1988). Finding the face in the crowd: An anger superiority effect. *Journal of Personal and Social Psychology*, *54*(6), 917–924.

Hershler, O., & Hochstein, S. (2005). At first sight: A high-level pop out effect for faces. *Vision Research*, *45*(13), 1707–1724.

Hillyard, S. A., Vogel, E. K., & Luck, S. J. (1998). Sensory gain control (amplification) as a mechanism of selective attention: Electrophysiological and neuroimaging evidence. *Philosophical Transactions of the Royal Society of London, Series B: Biological Sciences*, *353*(1373), 1257–1270.

Hochstein, S., & Ahissar, M. (2002). View from the top: Hierarchies and reverse hierarchies in the visual system. *Neuron*, *36*(5), 791–804.

Hopf, J. M., Boehler, C. N., Luck, S. J., Tsotsos, J. K., Heinze, H. J., & Schoenfeld, M. A. (2006). Direct neurophysiological evidence for spatial suppression surrounding the focus of attention in vision. *Proceedings of the National Academy of Sciences, USA*, *103*(4), 1053–1058.

Hubel, D. H., & Wiesel, T. N. (1968). Receptive fields and functional architecture of the monkey striate cortex. *Journal of Physiology (London)*, *195*, 574–591.

Julesz, B. (1975). Experiments in the visual perception of texture. *Scientific American*, *232*(4), 34–43.

Kastner, S., de Weerd, P., Desimone, R., & Ungerleider, L. G. (1998). Mechanisms of directed attention in the human extrastriate cortex as revealed by functional MRI [see comments]. *Science*, *282*(5386), 108–111.

Kirchner, H., & Thorpe, S. J. (2006). Ultra-rapid object detection with saccadic eye movements: Visual processing speed revisited. *Vision Research, 46*(11), 1762–1776.

Kobatake, E., & Tanaka, K. (1994). Neuronal selectivities to complex object features in the ventral visual pathway of the macaque cerebral cortex. *Journal of Neurophysiology, 71*(3), 856–867.

Lamme, V. A., & Roelfsema, P. R. (2000). The distinct modes of vision offered by feedforward and recurrent processing. *Trends in Neuroscience, 23*(11), 571–579.

Lee, D. K., Koch, C., & Braun, J. (1999). Attentional capacity is undifferentiated: Concurrent discrimination of form, color, and motion. *Perception and Psychophysics, 61*(7), 1241–1255.

Li, F. F., VanRullen, R., Koch, C., & Perona, P. (2002). Rapid natural scene categorization in the near absence of attention. *Proceedings of the National Academy of Sciences, USA, 99*(14), 9596–9601.

Logothetis, N. K., & Sheinberg, D. L. (1996). Visual object recognition. *Annual Review of Neuroscience, 19*, 577–621.

Luck, S. J., Chelazzi, L., Hillyard, S. A., & Desimone, R. (1997). Neural mechanisms of spatial selective attention in areas V1, V2, and V4 of macaque visual cortex. *Journal of Neurophysiology, 77*(1), 24–42.

Luck, S. J., & Ford, M. A. (1998). On the role of selective attention in visual perception. *Proceedings of the National Academy of Sciences, USA, 95*(3), 825–830.

Luck, S. J., Girelli, M., McDermott, M. T., & Ford, M. A. (1997). Bridging the gap between monkey neurophysiology and human perception: An ambiguity resolution theory of visual selective attention. *Cognitive Psychology, 33*(1), 64–87.

Mangun, G. R. (1995). Neural mechanisms of visual selective attention. *Psychophysiology, 32*(1), 4–18.

McCarley, J. S., Mounts, J. R., & Kramer, A. F. (2004). Age-related differences in localized attentional interference. *Psychology and Aging, 19*(1), 203–210.

McCarley, J. S., Mounts, J. R., & Kramer, A. F. (2007). Spatially mediated capacity limits in attentive visual perception. *Acta Psychologica, 126*(2), 98–119.

Moran, J., & Desimone, R. (1985). Selective attention gates visual processing in the extrastriate cortex. *Science, 229*, 782–784.

Mounts, J. R. (2000a). Attentional capture by abrupt onsets and feature singletons produces inhibitory surrounds. *Perception and Psychophysics, 62*(7), 1485–1493.

Mounts, J. R. (2000b). Evidence for suppressive mechanisms in attentional selection: feature singletons produce inhibitory surrounds. *Perception and Psychophysics, 62*(5), 969–983.

Mounts, J. R., & Gavett, B. E. (2004). The role of salience in localized attentional interference. *Vision Research, 44*(13), 1575–1588.

Mozer, M. C., & Sitton, M. (1998). Computational modeling of spatial attention. In H. Pashler (Ed.), *Attention* (pp. 341–393). New York: Psychology Press.

Muller, N. G., & Kleinschmidt, A. (2004). The attentional "spotlight's" penumbra: Center–surround modulation in striate cortex. *Neuroreport, 15*(6), 977–980.

Nakayama, K., & Joseph, J. S. (1998). Attention, pattern recognition and pop-out in visual search. In R. Parasuraman (Ed.), *The attentive brain* (pp. 279–298). Cambridge, MA: MIT Press.

Nothdurft, H. C. (1993). Faces and facial expressions do not pop out. *Perception, 22*(11), 1287–1298.

Palmer, J. (1995). Attention in visual search: Distinguishing four causes of a set-size effect. *Current Directions in Psychological Science, 4*, 118–123.

Palmer, J., Verghese, P., & Pavel, M. (2000). The psychophysics of visual search. *Vision Research, 40*(10–12), 1227–1268.

Perrett, D. I., Rolls, E. T., & Caan, W. (1982). Visual neurones responsive to faces in the monkey temporal cortex. *Experimental Brain Research, 47*(3), 329–342.

Potter, M. C., & Faulconer, B. A. (1975). Time to understand pictures and words. *Nature, 253*(5491), 437–438.

Potter, M. C., & Levy, E. I. (1969). Recognition memory for a rapid sequence of pictures. *Journal of Experimental Psychology, 81*(1), 10–15.

Purcell, D. G., Stewart, A. L., & Skov, R. B. (1996). It takes a confounded face to pop out of a crowd. *Perception, 25*(9), 1091–1108.

Reddy, L., Reddy, L., & Koch, C. (2006). Face identification in the near-absence of focal attention. *Vision Research, 46*(15), 2336–2343.

Reddy, L., & VanRullen, R. (2007). Spacing affects some but not all visual searches: Implications for theories of attention and crowding. *Journal of Vision, 7*(2–3), 1–17.

Reddy, L., Wilken, P., & Koch, C. (2004). Face-gender discrimination is possible in the near-absence of attention. *Journal of Vision, 4*(2), 106–117.

Rensink, R. A. (2002). Change detection. *Annual Review of Psychology, 53*, 245–277.

Reynolds, J. H., Chelazzi, L., & Desimone, R. (1999). Competitive mechanisms subserve attention in macaque areas V2 and V4. *Journal of Neuroscience, 19*(5), 1736–1753.

Reynolds, J. H., & Desimone, R. (1999). The role of neural mechanisms of attention in solving the binding problem. *Neuron*, 24(1), 19–29, 111–125.

Riesenhuber, M., & Poggio, T. (1999a). Are cortical models really bound by the "binding problem"? *Neuron*, 24(1), 87–93, 111–125.

Riesenhuber, M., & Poggio, T. (1999b). Hierarchical models of object recognition in cortex. *Nature Neuroscience, 2*(11), 1019–1025.

Roelfsema, P. R. (2006). Cortical algorithms for perceptual grouping. *Annual Review of Neuroscience, 29*, 203–227.

Rousselet, G. A., Fabre-Thorpe, M., & Thorpe, S. J. (2002). Parallel processing in high-level categorization of natural images. *Nature Neuroscience, 5*(7), 629–630.

Rousselet, G. A., Thorpe, S. J., & Fabre-Thorpe, M. (2004). Processing of one, two or four natural scenes in humans: The limits of parallelism. *Vision Research, 44*(9), 877–894.

Selfridge, O. (1959). Pandemonium: A paradigm for learning. In D. V. Blake & A. M. Uttley (Eds.), *Symposium on the mechanization of thought processes* (pp. 511–529). London: HM Stationery Office.

Serre, T., Kouh, M., Cadieu, C., Knoblich, U., Kreiman, G., & Poggio, T. (2005). *A theory of object recognition: Computations and circuits in the feedforward path of the ventral stream in primate visual cortex* (No. AI Memo 2005-036, CBCL Memo 259). Cambridge, MA: MIT Press.

Serre, T., Oliva, A., & Poggio, T. (2007). A feedforward architecture accounts for rapid categorization. *Proceedings of the National Academy of Sciences, USA, 104*(15), 6424–6429.

Tanaka, K. (1996). Inferotemporal cortex and object vision. *Annual Review of Neuroscience, 19*, 109–139.

Thorpe, S. J., Fize, D., & Marlot, C. (1996). Speed of processing in the human visual system. *Nature, 381*, 520–522.

Tipper, S. P. (1985). The negative priming effect: Inhibitory priming by ignored objects. *Quarterly Journal of Experimental Psychology, 37A*(4), 571–590.

Treisman, A. (1960). Contextual cues in selective listening. *Quarterly Journal of Experimental Psychology, 12*, 242–248.

Treisman, A. (1996). The binding problem. *Current Opinion in Neurobiology, 6*(2), 171–178.

Treisman, A., & Gelade, G. (1980). A feature-integration theory of attention. *Cognitive Psychology, 12*(1), 97–136.

Treisman, A., & Gormican, S. (1988). Feature analysis in early vision: Evidence from search asymmetries. *Psychological Review, 95*, 15–48.

Treisman, A., & Kanwisher, N. (1998). Perceiving visually presented objects: Recognition, awareness, and modularity. *Current Opinion in Neurobiology, 8*(2), 218–226.

Treisman, A., & Paterson, R. (1984). Emergent features, attention, and object perception. *Journal of Experimental Psychology: Human Perception and Performance, 10*(1), 12–31.

Treisman, A., & Sato, S. (1990). Conjunction search revisited. *Journal of Experimental Psychology: Human Perception and Performance, 16*(3), 459–478.

Treisman, A., & Souther, J. (1985). Search asymmetry: A diagnostic for preattentive processing of separable features. *Journal of Experimental Psychology: General, 114*(3), 285–310.

Tsotsos, J. K., Culhane, S. M., Wai, W. Y. K., Lai, Y., Davis, N., & Nuflo, F. (1995). Modeling visual attention via selective tuning. *Artificial Intelligence, 78*, 507–545.

Ullman, S. (1984). Visual routines. *Cognition, 18*, 97–159.

VanRullen, R. (2006). On second glance: Still no high-level pop-out effect for faces. *Vision Research, 46*(18), 3017–3027.

VanRullen, R., Gautrais, J., Delorme, A., & Thorpe, S. J. (1998). Face processing using one spike per neuron. *Biosystems, 48*(1–3), 229–239.

VanRullen, R., Reddy, L., & Fei-Fei, L. (2005). Binding is a local problem for natural objects and scenes. *Vision Research, 45*(25–26), 3133–3144.

VanRullen, R., Reddy, L., & Koch, C. (2004). Visual search and dual-tasks reveal two distinct attentional resources. *Journal of Cognitive Neuroscience, 16*(1), 4–14.

VanRullen, R., & Thorpe, S. J. (2001). The time course of visual processing: From early perception to decision-making. *Journal of Cognitive Neuroscience, 13*(4), 454–461.

VanRullen, R., & Thorpe, S. J. (2002). Surfing a spike wave down the ventral stream. *Vision Research, 42*(23), 2593–2615.

Wolfe, J. M. (1994). Guided Search 2.0: A revised model of visual search. *Psychonomic Bulletin and Review, 1*(2), 202–238.

Wolfe, J. M. (1998). Visual search. In H. Pashler (Ed.), *Attention* (pp. 13–73). London: University College London Press.

Wolfe, J. M., & Bennett, S. C. (1997). Preattentive object files: Shapeless bundles of basic features. *Vision Research, 37*(1), 25–43.

Wolfe, J. M., Cave, K. R., & Franzel, S. L. (1989). Guided Search: An alternative to the feature integration model for visual search. *Journal of Experimental Psychology: Human Perception and Performance, 15*(3), 419–433.

VISUAL COGNITION, 2009, 17 (1/2), 120–140

Psychology Press
Taylor & Francis Group

When an object is more than a binding of its features: Evidence for two mechanisms of visual feature integration

Bernhard Hommel and Lorenza S. Colzato
Leiden University Institute for Psychological Research, and Leiden Institute for Brain and Cognition, Leiden, The Netherlands

People spontaneously integrate the features of visual events into episodic structures that are reactivated if their ingredients match aspects of the current input. Feature integration has been attributed to either the detection of feature conjunctions or the ad hoc binding of feature codes (e.g., by neural synchronization). We report evidence suggesting that both kinds of integration mechanisms coexist. Replicating earlier findings, repeating one visual feature facilitated performance but only if other visual features were also repeated. However, this effect was more pronounced with real objects as compared to arbitrary combinations of shapes and colours. Moreover, the real-object effect was restricted to visual feature integration but did not extend to visuomotor integration, suggesting that the underlying mechanism subserves perception only. We suggest a dual-process feature-integration model that distinguishes between ad hoc binding, which operates on any possible combination of features alike, and conjunction detection, which selectively operates on familiar feature combinations.

Keywords: Object perception; Event file; Feature integration.

Primate brains represent many aspects of the objects and events they perceive and produce in a distributed, feature-based fashion. The human visual cortex, for instance, consists of various neural maps that code for different visual features of perceived objects, such as orientation, shape, or motion (see DeYoe & van Essen, 1988), and the frontal cortex houses maps coding for the direction, distance, and force of intentional actions (see Hommel & Elsner, in press). These observations have been taken to imply various integration or binding problems (e.g., Treisman, 1996), as they raise

Please address all correspondence to Bernhard Hommel, Leiden University, Department of Psychology, Cognitive Psychology Unit, Postbus 9555, 2300 RB Leiden, The Netherlands. E-mail: hommel@fsw.leidenuniv.nl

© 2008 Psychology Press, an imprint of the Taylor & Francis Group, an Informa business
http://www.psypress.com/viscog DOI: 10.1080/13506280802349787

the question how the brain knows which of the feature codes activated at a given time are related to the same event.

Authors differ with respect to how serious they consider these problems to be and how easily they think these problems can be solved. For instance, some authors have claimed that serially operating attentional mechanisms are required to bind related information together (e.g., Treisman & Gelade, 1980), whereas others assume that the retinotopic organization of visual maps provides sufficient information for properly integrating at least visual features (van der Heijden, 1995). Most authors have focused on one of two neural principles that may mediate feature integration and help solving binding problems. One principle is that of *convergence*: Lower level neurons may code for simple features, such as <round> or <green>, and project onto higher level neurons that code for feature conjunctions (e.g., <round> AND <green>). This may lead up to even higher level representations of whole objects (Barlow, 1972). Given the considerable variability of objects in terms of their instances and retinal projections, as well as the numerous ways in which features can be potentially combined, the exclusive reliance on convergence mechanisms would lead to a combinatorial explosion and is therefore not particularly plausible. Accordingly, a second mechanism has been suggested in which integration does not (necessarily) rely on conjunction detectors. The idea is that integration comprises of *synchronizing* the firing patterns of feature-coding neurons, in such a way that the neurons coding for features of the same object act as a unit (Engel & Singer, 2001; Raffone & Wolters, 2001; von der Malsburg, 1999).

Even though these two mechanisms are commonly treated as mutually exclusive alternatives, the benefits and costs they imply suggest that they both play a role in dealing with binding problems (Colzato, Raffone & Hommel, 2006; VanRullen, 2009 this issue). Synchronization-based integration has the advantage of being particularly flexible and parsimonious in terms of long-term memory structures but the disadvantage that even features that are very likely to cooccur would need to be bound anew every time they are encountered. Hence, this integration method would be economical in terms of cognitive structure but wasteful in terms of processing time. In contrast, convergence-based integration has the advantage of allowing for the fast and effortless registration of feature combinations of practically unlimited complexity but the disadvantage that (apart from possible genetically hardwired conjunction detectors) this registration presupposes extensive learning and some degree of separability of conjunctions (as conjunction with too much feature overlap would lead to the activation of too many conjunction detectors). Hence, this integration method would be economical in terms of processing time but wasteful in terms of structure. Given that our environment calls for both the recognition of highly reliable feature combinations (as with natural objects) and the processing of highly arbitrary combinations (as commonly used in psychological experiments), it makes sense to assume that both convergence-based and synchronization-based mechanisms are at work in generating human perception.

The present study was conceived of with this distinction in mind. As we will argue, there is behavioural evidence suggesting that at least two different mechanisms are at work in human visual feature integration, one that operates on any feature conjunction that is encountered (presumably based on synchronization) and another that selectively operates on frequent conjunctions that have been stored (presumably based on convergence). Before addressing the motivation and rationale of our study in more detail we will provide a brief overview of the theoretical background relevant for the study and the experimental paradigm we used.

OBJECT FILES

Most studies addressing feature binding focused on the visual modality. Some studies investigated whether there actually are binding problems in visual feature integration. For instance, Treisman and Schmidt (1982), and many others since then, demonstrated that creating attentionally demanding conditions results in an increasing numbers of incorrect bindings or "illusory conjunctions"—suggesting that feature integration is not a trivial task and raising doubt whether it is solely handled by convergence mechanisms (which have a hard time predicting such observations). Other studies have looked into whether people actually *do* bind features, even under circumstances that do not seem to require any binding. Particularly appropriate for that purpose turned out to be the preview paradigm developed by Kahneman, Treisman, and Gibbs (1992) and used by many others since then.

The simplest, stripped-down form of this paradigm is illustrated in Figure 1 (please ignore the R1 cue and R1 for the moment). The sequence of trial events comprises a nominally task-irrelevant prime or preview display (S1) followed by a probe display (S2). Let's assume in this example that S1 and S2 can either be a circle or triangle, can be red or green, and can be presented in the top or bottom position. The observer's task is simply to identify S2's shape as quickly as possible. Colour and position information are completely irrelevant to the task and can be safely ignored. Because S1 requires no response, it too can be ignored. Critically, S1 may consist of the same or a different shape as S2 and may appear in the same or a different colour and at the same or a different location. Analysing performance on S2 (i.e., R2) as a function of the repetition or alternation of shape, colour, and location (from S1 to S2) may or may not produce main effects, such as better performance if a particular feature repeats. These kinds of effects should

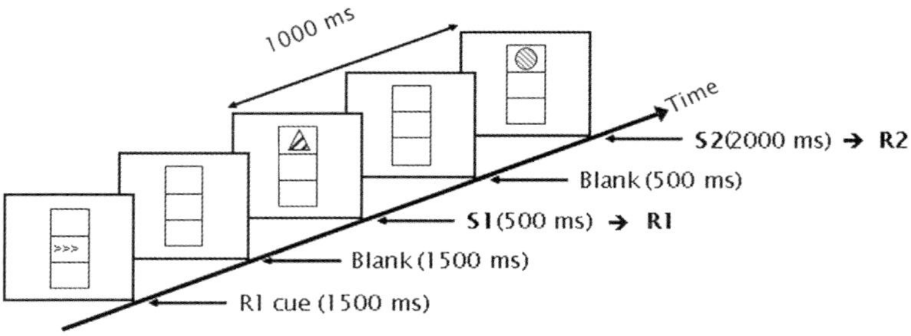

Figure 1. Sequence of events in the present experiment. Participants prepared a left- or right-hand response as indicated by a cue (R1 cue) and carried it out (R1) when the next stimulus (S1) appeared. Then they waited for the next stimulus (S2) and carried out a left- or right-hand response (R2) to its shape. S1 and S2 varied in shape, colour, and location, so that all three features could repeat or alternate. As R1 did not depend on S1 (but on the R1 cue), the response could repeat or alternate irrespective of the stimulus sequence.

reflect the priming of feature codes (e.g., leftover activation in the corresponding codes) and are thus unlikely to reflect binding processes (Kahneman et al., 1992).

Theoretically more interesting are *interactions* between repetition effects, because they indicate that the impact of repeating one feature depends on the identity of the other. Such interactions have been frequently observed: Repeating one feature produces better performance if other features are also repeated (e.g., Kahneman et al., 1992) but worse performance if these other features alternate (e.g., Hommel, 1998). To take our example, responding to a red circle (as S2) is easier following the presentation of another red circle than following a green circle (as S1), but more difficult following a red than a green triangle. Likewise, responding to a top circle is easier following a top than a bottom circle, but more difficult following a top than a bottom triangle. These observations suggest that registering the cooccurrence of two or more given features is sufficient to create some sort of binding between them, so that reencountering one of them tends to reactivate the whole binding in a pattern-completion-like process (Hommel, 2004). As a consequence, partial repetitions induce the retrieval of no longer valid feature codes, which disturbs current coding processes and induces code conflict. There is thus evidence that people do bind features—no matter how plausible one finds the available arguments for or against the logical necessity of feature binding. And they do so even under the most unlikely circumstances, that is, even if neither the bound features nor the object they refer to need to be attended or reported, even in the absence of any attentionally challenging display or task, and even when no more than 250–500 ms are available for creating such bindings (Hommel & Colzato, 2004).

Direct evidence for the retrieval of object files has been obtained in an fMRI study by Keizer et al. (2008). They presented subjects with preview (S1) and probe displays (S2) that both consisted of two blended pictures showing a face and a house. Either the face or the house moved in one of two possible directions, and subjects were to respond to the direction of S2 irrespective of which object moved. Most interesting were the conditions in which S1 showed a moving house and S2 a moving face: If the direction of motion in these two displays was the same more activation of house-related information in the parahippocampal place area was observed than if the motion differed. This suggests that the direction of motion was integrated with the object that moved, so that repeating the motion reactivated the representation of the object that had just accompanied this motion. Hence, binding features creates episodic cognitive structures that tend to be reactivated as a whole as soon as one of their ingredients matches the current input. This is indeed what underlies the original idea underlying Kahneman et al.'s (1992) *object file* concept: Bindings are functional in establishing object constancy by maintaining information about an object even in the absence of current sensory input and by relating this information to later reoccurrences of this object, even though these reoccurrences may only match part of the maintained information. This is why we can track objects over longer periods of occlusion and across changes in a number of visual features.

Interactions between repetition effects indicative of feature binding have been obtained for various features. Shape, colour, and location features have been shown to interact (Hommel, 1998, 2007; Hommel & Colzato, 2004) just as well as face, house, and motion information (Keizer, Colzato & Hommel, 2008)—suggesting that binding can span ventral and dorsal processing streams. An interesting observation in all these studies is that location does not seem to play a particularly dominant role. Some authors have claimed that object files can only be reactivated or reassessed if the current object matches the respective object file in terms of location (Kahneman et al., 1992; Mitroff & Alvarez, 2007). This would suggest that nonspatial matches are insufficient by themselves to retrieve a previous object file, which again implies that nonspatial features can only interact if this interaction is mediated by a location match. Even though it is clear that spatial location and spatial matches are important in multielement displays, simply because location is commonly crucial to track the identity of an object, spatially unmediated interactions between nonspatial features are possible (e.g., Colzato, Raffone, & Hommel, 2006; Hommel, 1998, 2007), which disconfirms approaches that rely on spatial correspondence as a retrieval cue. On the other hand, spatial location clearly plays a central role in the *encoding* of object files. Most studies on feature integration confound the sharing of spatial location with belongingness to the same perceptual object. Van Dam and Hommel (2008) disentangled these factors by testing whether two given features appearing in the same location would be still integrated even if they obviously belonged to two different objects. Indeed, orientation and colour features were bound (i.e., orientation- and colour-repetition effects interacted) irrespective of whether they appeared as part of the same object or of different objects (e.g., one stationary and the other moving continuously, or a banana in a particular orientation overlaying an apple of a particular colour). In contrast, integration was markedly reduced when the two objects were separated in space (cf. Xu, 2006). Thus, spatial location is important for the encoding but not the retrieval or reactivation of object files.

MULTIPLE INTEGRATION MECHANISMS

The available evidence suggests that cooccurring visual features are more or less automatically bound into object files, that is, temporary links between, or pointers to the codes representing, the features of a perceived visual event. To take our example, and following Hommel (2004) and Colzato et al. (2006), this process can be captured by the cartoon model sketched in Figure 2a. Registering a red circle appearing in a top position would lead to the activation of corresponding codes in shape, colour, and location maps, and these codes are cross referenced by creating a temporary object file (symbolized by the folder).

Note that Figure 2 considers a further impact from the current attentional set, which is assumed to prime task-relevant feature dimensions (shape in our example). The reason to include such a top-down mechanism derives from a number of observations. On the one hand, the fact that bindings are created under the most unlikely conditions seems to suggest that feature integration is a highly automatic process. Indeed, systematic manipulations of the amount of attention directed to the to-be-integrated features and available for integration failed to modulate feature integration effects (Hommel, 2005, 2007), suggesting that the encoding of event files is a spontaneous process (cf. Logan, 1988). On the other hand, the retrieval of event files turned out to be rather highly controllable. One indication for that is that features varying on task-relevant feature dimensions are more likely to be involved in interactions with other features. For instance, having participants respond to the shape of S2 yields particularly strong binding-related effects involving shape repetition while having them respond to colour yields particularly strong effects involving colour repetition (e.g., Hommel, 1998). Even trial-to-trial shifts between shape- and colour-relevant versions of the task induce stronger binding-related effects for the currently task-relevant feature dimension, suggesting that attentional set has an immediate impact (Hommel, Memelink, Zmigrod, & Colzato, 2008). As it

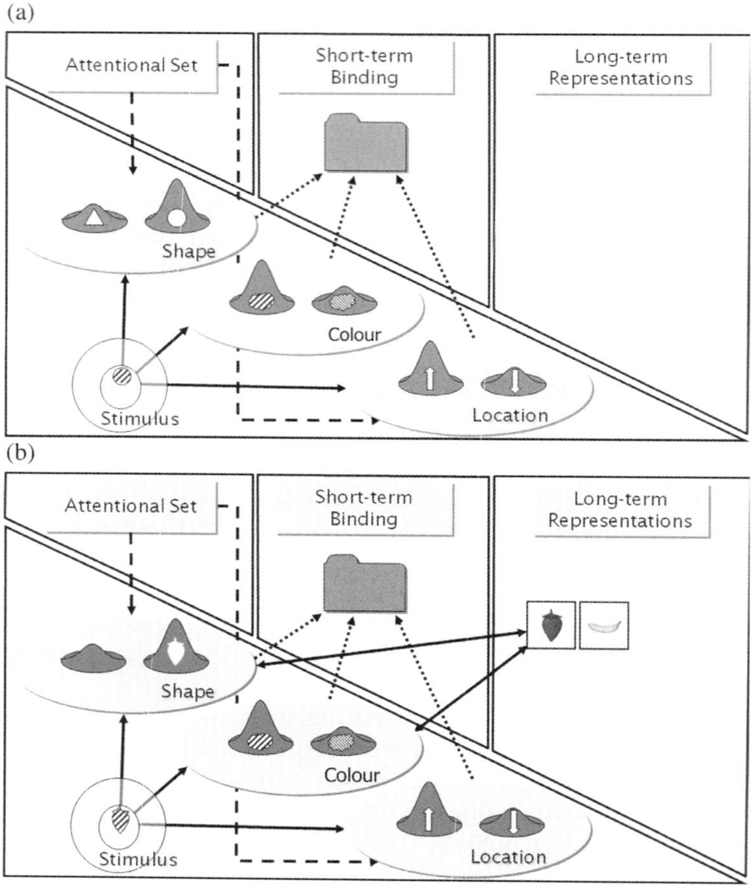

Figure 2. Cartoon model of feature binding and binding retrieval. (a) The coding of arbitrary feature conjunctions (adapted from Colzato et al., 2006). Colours are indicated by fill patterns. Shape is directly task relevant (by having it signalling responses) and location is indirectly task relevant (by defining the responses in terms of spatial locations), so that the shape and location dimensions are primed by the attentional set. Features on primed dimensions are assumed to be more likely integrated with other features and/or retrieved by stimuli that feature-overlap with the respective binding. (b) The coding of highly familiar feature conjunctions or real objects represented in long-term memory. Stimuli that match long-term representations to a sufficient degree activate these representations, which again induce top-down priming of the stimulus features that are coded on object-defining dimensions (shape and colour in the example). Top-down priming may work by increasing the gain of the respective feature dimension, which multiplies the stimulus-induced activation of this dimension's feature codes. Note that short-term bindings and long-term representations relate differently to individual feature codes: Whereas short-term bindings are considered to "point" to, and thus remain linked with the individual codes, long-term representations only respond to the presence of features or feature combinations. Likewise, short-term bindings can reactivate individual feature codes upon retrieval of a code that has been bound with them, whereas the top-down effect of long-term representations is restricted to priming feature dimensions but not individual codes.

does not matter whether the set is established before or after the hypothetical binding process (i.e., before after S1 presentation), it makes sense to assume that the impact of the attentional set selectively targets object file *retrieval* but not encoding (Hommel et al., 2008).

In Figure 2a we have considered two types of impact of the current attentional set. One is rather obvious: Having participants to respond to the shape of stimuli makes the shape dimension task relevant, so that it should receive top-down priming. However, stimuli are not the only events in reaction time tasks; participants also need to prepare and carry out particular actions. Given that actions can be assumed to be cognitively represented in terms of their perceptual effects (reflecting the ideomotor principle; see Hommel, Müsseler, Aschersleben, & Prinz, 2001; James, 1890; Lotze, 1852), preparing and controlling a particular set of actions entails attending the perceptual dimensions on which the actions are defined (Adam, Hommel, & Umiltà, 2003; Fagioli, Hommel, & Schubotz, 2007). If, as in our example, responses are defined by their spatial location (left vs. right keypress), this introduces task relevance of location in general. If we assume that the task relevance of a feature dimension leads to the priming of all feature values defined on it (Fagioli et al., 2007; Found & Müller, 1996; Hommel, 2007), making left and right *response* locations relevant should lead to the priming of any location information (i.e., whether it refers to a stimulus event or a response)—just as indicated in Figure 2a. Accordingly, the impact of (repetitions of) *stimulus* location increases as a consequence of choosing spatial responses. Indeed, Hommel (2007) could provide evidence that repetitions of stimulus location strongly affect binding-related effects with spatially defined response sets but not with nonspatial responses.

The model shown in Figure 2a suffices to account for the basic findings from most studies using the design introduced by Kahneman et al. (1992), and the binding process it implies reflects more characteristics of synchronization-based binding than of convergence-based integration. For one, it is difficult to see how convergence detectors might produce partial-repetition costs. Clearly, activating the same detector twice, as with the complete repetition of a particular shape–colour conjunction, say, should speed up performance and it commonly does. But consider a partial repetition (of either the shape or the colour) and a nonrepetition. Partial repetitions may be thought to also activate the same detector twice, though to a lower degree, or to fail activating the same detector. In the first case one would expect that performance for partial repetitions falls between complete repetitions and nonrepetitions; whereas in the second case one would expect that performance on partial repetitions and nonrepetitions is equally worse than on complete repetitions. As already mentioned, however, the standard finding is that performance on complete repetitions and nonrepetitions is equally good and better than on partial repetitions (e.g., Hommel, 1998). Closer consideration of the possible noise and competition between alternative conjunction detectors helps a bit. For instance, one may assume that encountering one combination of two possible colours and two possible shapes (a red circle, say) leads to the activation of at least three conjunction detectors: A strong activation of the target detector (<red> + <circle>) and some milder activation of feature-sharing detectors (say, <red> + <square> and <green> + <circle>). If the target repeats, all three detectors would be reactivated; this would lead to a particularly strong activation of the target detector, which now dominates the feature-sharing detectors even more. More concretely, if we count three activation units per target-induced activation and one unit per activation through feature overlap, this would mean that the target detector as an activation level of 6 as compared to an activation level of 2 for each of the two main competitors. It is easy to see that this approach correctly predicts worse performance with partial repetitions: If a red circle is followed by a green circle, say, this would first activate the same three detectors (<red> + <circle> = 3, <red> + <square> = 1, and <green> + <circle> = 1) as in the previous example and then the target detector (<green> + <circle> = 3) and the feature-overlapping detectors (<green> + <square> = 1 and <red> + <circle> = 1). Now the activation level of the target detector would be 4, just as much as its main competitor (<red> + <circle>), a situation that should result in impaired performance. The approach can also account for the observation that nonrepetitions produce better performance than partial repetitions. If a red circle is followed by a green square, this would activate (<red> + <circle> = 3, <red> + <square> = 1, and <green> + <circle> = 1) followed by (<green> + <square> = 3) and (<green> + <circle> = 1 and <red> + <square> = 1). The target activation would now add up to 3 and face activation levels of 2 in each of the two main competitors. Even though the target is now exposed to stronger overall competition than with partial repetitions (3:4 as compared to 4:4), the target would be in the position to outcompete each of the two competitors separately. Hence, choosing the right parameters, one may end up with a model that can account for better performance under nonrepetition than partial repetition. But again, it is difficult to see how it can account for *equal* performance under complete repetitions and nonrepetitions.

These difficulties suggest looking for alternative or at least additional mechanisms that are able to integrate features. Particularly promising with regard to the available findings seems the assumption that features are bound by an ad hoc binding mechanism, such as synchronizing the firing patterns of feature codes. If such a mechanism has just bound, say, the feature codes <red> and <circle>, and if this binding has been maintained or stored, repeating one but not the other feature (as with a red square) could retrieve this binding (and thus reactivate the codes <red> and

<circle>), which would result in coding conflict between <circle> and <square> codes (Hommel, 2004). Coding conflict would only occur with partial repetitions but not with complete repetitions (where there is no conflict) or with alternations (where there is no retrieval). Another argument for a role of synchronization derives from the observation that manipulations targeting the muscarinic-cholinergic transmitter system affect both visual binding and synchronization in the visual cortex. Muscarinic-cholinergic agonists and antagonists have been demonstrated to respectively facilitate and impair neural synchrony in the gamma band (~ 30–70 Hz) in the visual cortex of the cat (Rodriguez-Bermudez, Kallenbach, Singer, & Munk, 2004) and muscarinic-cholinergic antagonists were found to interfere with feature binding in the rat (Botly & de Rosa, 2007). Consistent with that, binding-type interactions between repetitions of visual features in humans are boosted by caffeine (a muscarinic-cholinergic agonist) and reduced by alcohol (a muscarinic-cholinergic antagonist), but unaffected by nicotine (a nicotinic-cholinergic agonist that does not affect muscarinic pathways; Colzato, Erasmus, & Hommel, 2004; Colzato, Fagioli, Erasmus, & Hommel, 2005). These parallels are consistent with the assumption that visual feature binding is mediated by neural synchronization processes that are driven by muscarinic-cholinergic neurotransmitters (Colzato et al., 2005).

Recent observations however suggest that the model sketched in Figure 2a is incomplete in important ways. In a series of experiments, Colzato et al. (2006) investigated the relationship between binding and longer term learning. The basic idea was that learning particular feature conjunctions may change the way the features they entail are bound, by either increasing the strength of the binding (because it would find increasing support by long-term associations) or by eliminating binding effects (because online binding would be no longer necessary). Surprisingly, however, even though more frequent feature combinations facilitated performance as such, binding-related effects were not at all affected by learning. This was true for highly frequent arbitrary conjunctions of features, such as orientation and colour, and for real objects, like red strawberries and yellow bananas. Even though performance was better if strawberries appeared in red and bananas in yellow, there was no indication that, say, strawberries are more strongly (or weakly) bound to red than they are to yellow, pink, or purple. These findings suggest that binding and learning are less intimately related then one may think. Interestingly, however, a comparison between the different experiments of Colzato et al. suggested that real objects created larger partial-repetition costs (i.e., binding-related effects) than arbitrary combinations of simple features did, which may point to a contribution from long-term memory.

To account for this pattern of results, Colzato et al. (2006) suggested that feature integration may proceed via two routes, the ad hoc binding of cooccurring features (presumably mediated by synchronization processes) and the registration of previously acquired conjunctions by conjunction detectors stored in long-term memory (presumably using convergence mechanisms). This brings into play long-term memory representations the way we sketched in Figure 2b. Whereas ad hoc integration takes place as described in Figure 2a, overlearning feature conjunctions are thought to establish a conjunction detector in long-term memory. These detectors may be of any complexity and thus function as object representations or cardinal cells in the sense of Barlow (1972). However, establishing a new detector makes sense only, so we suggest at least, under two conditions. First, the conjunction it can detect needs to be *significant* in the sense of reliably indicating a particular stimulus event and, second, the conjunction needs to be *diagnostic* in the sense that it should be functional in discriminating the given stimulus event from other events. The rationale of this reasoning is that devoting (presumably limited) cognitive structure to a task that in principle could also be solved by ad hoc binding presupposes some surplus functionality, which would not be given if a new conjunction detector would be unable to reliably detect the stimulus it stands for or discriminate it from alternative stimuli.

We further assume that, whenever a particular stimulus activates such a conjunction detector, the detector will provide top-down support by facilitating the processing of all the features belonging to the stimulus (Colzato et al., 2006)—which may be achieved by priming the respective stimulus dimensions and thus multiplying any stimulus-induced activation of codes falling on them. This assumption is grounded in evidence coming from several lines of research showing that it is easier to attend multiple features of the same object (e.g., Baylis & Driver, 1993; Duncan, 1984) and more difficult to ignore distractors if they are part of the same object (e.g., Baylis & Driver, 1992; Hommel, 1995; Kahneman & Henik, 1981). This implies that processing one feature of an object automatically opens the attentional gate to other feature dimensions of this object, whether this is useful or not. In the example shown in Figure 2b, this kind of top-down priming would facilitate the processing of shape and colour information, and of any other visual feature belonging to a dimension that defines the stimulus object. Given that stimulus location is not an object-defining feature, location information would not benefit from this top-down priming, however.

Two parallel mechanisms of feature integration could account for the observations of Colzato et al. (2006) in the following way. With arbitrary, not highly overlearned feature combinations that do not signify a unique object (as geometric shapes are commonly not related to or correlated with particular colours), the situation would be as depicted in Figure 2a: Shape coding would be primed, due to the task relevance of shape, but colour coding would not (stimulus location was not varied in that study).

Accordingly, even if shape–colour conjunctions would be automatically integrated, colour-induced retrieval would be weak at best and the corresponding effects would be modest and fragile. Indeed, Colzato et al. found only small effects reflecting shape–colour binding and even these effect tended to disappear with increasing practice (presumably due to increased focusing on the relevant shape information). Real objects with which participants are familiar would be more likely to have led to the creation of reliable and discriminative conjunction detectors or object representations in long-term memory. As depicted in Figure 2b, this would lead to a match between stimuli and the long-term representation and thus induce top-down facilitation of the object features, including both shape and colour. Accordingly, it would matter less that colour is actually not relevant for the task, implying stronger and more stable shape–colour binding effects—exactly what Colzato et al. observed.

AIM OF STUDY

The present experiment was set up to test the post hoc considerations of Colzato et al. (2006) in a more systematic fashion. We used a similar task (as sketched in Figure 1) but compared real objects and arbitrary feature conjunctions that varied on three dimensions (shape, colour, and stimulus location) in a within-subjects design. Shape was directly relevant for the task as participants were to discriminate and respond to the shape of S2. Even though stimulus location varied randomly and could safely be ignored, using spatially defined *responses* (left vs. right keypress) made location indirectly task relevant. Colour was entirely irrelevant. We expected the standard interactions between feature-repetition effects indicative of feature binding but were particularly interested in testing three more specific hypotheses.

First, we expected that interactions between shape and colour repetition (indicating shape–colour binding) would be more pronounced, and perhaps even restricted to, real objects. As explained already, real objects are likely to match representations stored in long-term memory, which should induce top-down priming of all object-related features. As shape is primed by task relevance anyway, it would be colour coding that benefits from this priming process, so that colour codes would interact more strongly with shape codes in the real-object condition.

Second, we expected that the difference between arbitrary feature combinations and real objects would not affect stimulus-location coding and, thus, not mediate location-related interactions. As explained earlier, long-term representations are unlikely to contain information about the location of a given object in space, as location is not an object-defining attribute. Accordingly, location coding would not receive or benefit from top-down priming.

Third, we expected that the hypothetical real-object effect would be restricted to *stimulus-related* feature integration (and/or retrieval). Previous studies have shown that feature binding as such is not restricted to stimulus processing but operates across perception and action. Hommel (1998) has extended the classical preview design to include response repetitions by having participants to respond to the first stimulus (S1) with a previously cued and already prepared response (R1; see Figure 1). As in this design R1 does not correlate with the features of S1, stimulus features and responses can vary independently, so that stimulus–feature repetition and response repetition can be orthogonally manipulated (so to avoid the acquisition of stimulus–response associations). If this is done, the same type of crossover interaction as with stimulus–feature repetitions can be observed: Repeating a stimulus feature facilitates performance if the response also repeats but impairs performance if the response alternates (Hommel, 1998). Again, it seems that the mere single cooccurrence of a stimulus attribute and a response is sufficient to create a binding between their codes, so that repeating either the attribute or the response is sufficient to reactivate both or all members of this binding. Indeed, repeating some of the stimulus attributes induces a tendency to repeat the response as well in a free-choice reaction task (Hommel, 2007). However, visuomotor integration clearly differs from the process responsible for the integration of visual features. Not only do the two integration processes operate at a different point in time (visual binding seems to be stimulus locked, whereas visuomotor binding seems to be response locked; Hommel, 2005) but they are also driven by different neurotransmitter systems: Whereas muscarinic-cholinergic manipulations affect visual but not visuomotor binding (Colzato et al., 2004, 2005), manipulations targeting dopaminergic pathways affect visuomotor but not visual binding (Colzato & Hommel, 2008; Colzato, Kool, & Hommel, 2008; Colzato, van Wouwe & Hommel, 2007a, 2007b). Moreover, if it is true that establishing detectors for highly frequent, unique, and reliable feature conjunctions serves the purpose of facilitating object perception, it makes sense to assume that the impact of such detectors are restricted to perceptual processes—visual integration that is. Accordingly, we expected the standard interactions between visual-feature repetition and action repetition (Hommel, 1998) but no mediation of these effects by the arbitrary-conjunction vs. object manipulation.

METHOD

Thirty students of the Leiden University served as subjects for partial fulfilment of course credit or a financial reward. All reported having normal or corrected-to-normal vision, and were not familiar with the purpose of the experiment.

The experiment was controlled the Experimental Run-Time System (ERTS™) running on a PC attached to a 17-inch monitor. Participants faced three grey square outlines, vertically arranged, as illustrated in Figure 1. From a viewing distance of about 60 cm, each of these frames measured $2.6^\circ \times 3.1^\circ$. A banana ($0.3^\circ \times 0.6^\circ$), a strawberry ($0.5^\circ \times 0.6^\circ$), a triangle ($0.3^\circ \times 0.6^\circ$), and a circle ($0.5^\circ \times 0.6^\circ$) served as S1 and S2 alternatives, which were presented in blue or (close-to-magenta, purplish) pink (to avoid any preexperimental object–colour associations)[1] in the top or bottom frame. The stimuli were taken from Experiment 4 of Colzato et al. (2006; see p. 711 for bitmaps) and presented in the same colours (parameters were red = 0, green = 0, blue = 255, hue = 160, saturation = 240, and luminance = 120, for blue and red = 255, green = 0, blue = 255, hue = 200, saturation = 240, and luminance = 120, for pink). Response cues were also presented in the middle frame (see Figure 1), with rows of three left- or right-pointing arrows indicating a left and right keypress, respectively. Responses to S1 and to S2 were made by pressing the left or right shift-key of the computer keyboard with the corresponding index finger.

The experiment consisted of two sessions of 35 min, one with real objects (banana and strawberry) and one with arbitrary feature conjunctions (triangle and circle). In both sessions participants carried out two responses per trial, a previously cued simple response (R1) and a binary-choice

[1] More specifically, our idea was to get the hypothesized object representations in long-term memory involved—which required the use of stimuli that were likely to have memory representations—without letting them do the integration job on their own (i.e., without the need for ad hoc feature binding)—which required the use of feature combinations that were unlikely to be covered by these representations. Following Colzato et al. (2006), we thus used shapes of real objects (which should suffice to activate the memory representations) but presented them in colours that were unlikely to be part of the memory representation—using two colours that according to the findings of Colzato et al. are not associated with either of the two object shapes. Theoretically speaking, we expected that this manipulation would activate object representations and the corresponding conjunction detectors but still require ad hoc binding of the uncommon shape–colour conjunction. The former was considered to provide top-down priming of the latter with real objects but not with arbitrary feature conjunctions. As an example, facing a banana should activate a banana-related conjunction detector, which would lead to top-down priming of *all* identity-relevant features belonging to the *present* banana (i.e., to both the familiar shape and the in this case unfamiliar colour). This would prime the colour and increase the likelihood that it is being integrated. As the geometric shapes were not considered to have conjunction detectors linking them to particular colours, no top-down priming should occur for these shapes and present their colours.

response (R2) to the shape of the second of two target stimuli (S1 and S2; see Figure 1). They first prepared a left- or right-hand response as indicated by a cue (R1 cue) and carried it out (R1) upon presentation of the next stimulus (S1). S1 thus merely triggered the already prepared response; its features were entirely irrelevant and uncorrelated with the response. Then participants awaited the next stimulus (S2) and carried out a left- or right-hand response (R2) to its shape. Participants were informed that there would be no systematic relationship between S1 and R1, or between S1 and S2, and they were encouraged to respond to the onset of S1 only, disregarding the stimulus' attributes. The mappings of stimuli to response keys (S2 → R2) and the order of sessions were balanced across participants. The sequence of events in each trial is shown in Figure 1. The experiment was composed of 512 trials resulting from a factorial combination of the two possible shapes, colours, and locations of S2, the stimulus-type (real objects vs. arbitrary feature conjunctions) and the repetition vs. alternation of shape, colour, stimulus location, and the response, and three replications per condition.

RESULTS AND DISCUSSION

After excluding trials with missing (> 1500 ms) or anticipatory responses (< 200 ms), mean reaction times (RTs) and proportions of errors for R2 were analysed (see Table 1 for means and Table 2 for ANOVA terms). ANOVAs were run with stimulus type (real objects vs. arbitrary feature conjunctions), the repetition versus alternation of stimulus shape, colour, and location (S1 → S2), and of the response (R1 → R2) as within-participant factors.

In RTs, the main effect of stimulus type indicated that subjects reacted faster to the arbitrary feature conjunctions than to real objects and the stimulus-location repetition costs in RTs and errors reflect "inhibition of return"—the common observation that attending to an irrelevant stimulus impairs later responses to relevant stimuli appearing in the same location (Posner & Cohen, 1984). More interesting for present purposes were the interactions. First, shape repetition interacted with stimulus location (in RTs) and with colour (in RTs and errors)—repeating one object feature but not the other feature impaired performance as compared to complete repetitions and alternations. Importantly, only the shape-by-colour interaction was modified by stimulus type, thus producing a three-way interaction. As suggested by Figure 3, the shape-by-colour interaction was considerably more pronounced with real objects, $F(1, 29) = 28.14$, $p = .0001$, than with arbitrary feature conjunctions, where the interaction was not reliable, $F(1, 29) = 1.39$, $p = .247$. We checked whether the stronger interaction with real objects might be due to the higher RT level in this condition. However, the

TABLE 1
Means of mean reaction times and standard deviations (*SD*) for responses to Stimulus 2 (RT, in ms) and percentages of errors on R2 (PE), as a function of stimulus type (real objects vs. arbitrary feature conjunctions), the match between Response 1 and Response 2, and the feature match between Stimulus 1 and Stimulus 2

	Response							
	Arbitrary feature conjunctions				*Real objects*			
	Repeated		*Alternated*		*Repeated*		*Alternated*	
Match	*RT (SD)*	*PE (SD)*	*RT (SD)*	*PE (SD)*	*RT (SD)*	*PE (SD)*	*RT (SD)*	*PE (SD)*
Neither	482 (19)	10.6 (2.4)	474 (21)	2.3 (1.9)	511 (20)	10.6 (1.9)	482 (22)	2.1 (1.0)
Shape (S)	499 (25)	7.9 (1.7)	492 (21)	10.2 (2.0)	510 (20)	7.7 (1.2)	515 (21)	7.9 (1.7)
Location (L)	522 (27)	9.6 (2.0)	495 (21)	2.7 (0.1)	532 (23)	7.7 (1.9)	509 (17)	5.8 (1.3)
Colour (C)	497 (26)	14.2 (2.9)	463 (21)	2.7 (0.7)	512 (24)	10.8 (2.2)	483 (19)	4.3 (1.2)
S × L	475 (19)	3.9 (1.3)	499 (17)	13.7 (1.9)	497 (20)	4.8 (0.8)	523 (16)	14.6 (2.2)
C × L	512 (24)	10.4 (2.1)	498 (23)	6.9 (1.1)	549 (27)	10.2 (2.5)	528 (22)	7.1 (2.0)
S × C	494 (27)	5.4 (1.4)	478 (22)	8.1 (1.6)	495 (22)	5.2 (0.8)	510 (20)	5.0 (1.1)
S × L × C	462 (20)	3.7 (1.1)	497 (20)	14.6 (3.0)	477 (19)	2.5 (0.9)	499 (20)	12.7 (2.6)

outcome of two analyses speaks against this possibility. First, we median-split participants by their mean RT in the real-object condition and reran the ANOVA with level as additional between-participant variable. Whereas the three-way interaction was still reliable, $F(1, 28) = 4.80$, $p = .04$, there was no hint for any mediation by level, $F(1, 28) < 1$. Second, we computed, for each participant, the increase in shape–colour effect size and the increase in RT from the arbitrary-feature–conjunction condition to the real-object condition.[2] Given that the two measures were uncorrelated, $r = .06$, $p > .7$, it seems safe to conclude that a higher RT level as such does not increase the shape-by-colour interaction. The observation that the interaction is mediated by the type of stimulus fully supports our expectation that real objects provide top-down priming for colour coding that compensates for the lack of task relevance. Accordingly, colour did not interact with any other feature dimensions in the case of arbitrary conjunctions but it did interact with shape, the other object-specific feature dimension, in the case of real objects.

A second cluster of interactions in both RTs and error rates involved response repetition. It interacted with shape repetition and with stimulus-location repetition, and was involved in a three-way interaction with shape

[2] Effect sizes were computed by subtracting the mean RT for complete repetitions and alternations from the mean RT for partial repetitions (i.e., shape repetition and colour alternation or shape alternation and colour repetition). Note that this amounts to the interaction term corrected for possible main effects.

TABLE 2
Results of analysis of variance on mean reaction time of correct responses (RT) and percentage of errors (PE)

	RT_{R2}		PE_{R2}	
Effect	*MSE*	*F*	*MSE*	*F*
Stimulus type (T)	16069.44	5.04*	52.98	0.07
Shape (S)	6254.84	2.39	112.02	0.84
Colour (C)	6909.71	0.58	61.11	0.43
Location (L)	3292.18	8.92**	38.78	6.06*
Response (R)	55221.34	1.32	223.37	0.45
T × S	1362.66	0.50	45.02	0.01
T × C	1991.67	0.10	62.18	0.09
T × L	1902.42	0.05	48.32	0.05
S × C	1277.82	13.62***	47.95	16.16**
T × S × C	916.60	4.97*	31.46	0.25
C × L	1297.17	0.02	81.96	0.87
T × C × L	1523.76	0.13	61.09	1.41
S × L	8461.69	10.01**	65.27	1.56
T × S × L	1800.15	0.36	36.28	0.54
S × C × L	4844.92	0.28	53.57	0.30
T × C × S × L	2747.68	2.06	53.76	1.74
T × R	2574.38	0.08	80.22	0.24
S × R	2005.57	36.98***	169.77	44.73***
T × S × R	1665.66	1.64	54.28	2.74
C × R	1942.08	0.02	47.21	0.22
T × C × R	1374.84	0.37	30.53	0.01
S × C × R	1672.61	0.13	45.61	0.60
T × S × C × R	1450.68	0.05	35.13	0.12
L × R	1281.34	12.20**	132.17	26.25***
T × L × R	1038.80	2.21	49.11	0.48
C × L × R	1715.44	1.36	59.88	1.69
T × C × L × R	3157.48	1.61	48.81	1.76
S × L × R	1086.53	7.92**	44.76	10.21**
T × S × L × R	1759.39	2.56	44.42	0.29
C × S × L × R	2297.17	0.37	55.09	0.29
T × C × S × L × R	862.35	0.01	50.56	1.85

$^*p < .05$, $^*p < .01$, $^{***}p < .001$; $df = 1, 29$ for all effects.

and stimulus location. The latter indicated that location only interacted with the response if shape was repeated, $F(1, 29) = 31.92$, $p < .001$ (RTs), and $F(1, 29) = 24.89$, $p < .001$ (errors), but not if shape alternated, $ps > .4$.The reliable interactions all followed the standard form with better performance for shape repetitions and for stimulus-location repetitions if the response repeated but worse performance for shape repetitions and stimulus-location repetitions if the response alternated. Most interesting for present purposes, stimulus type and response repetition were not involved in any reliable

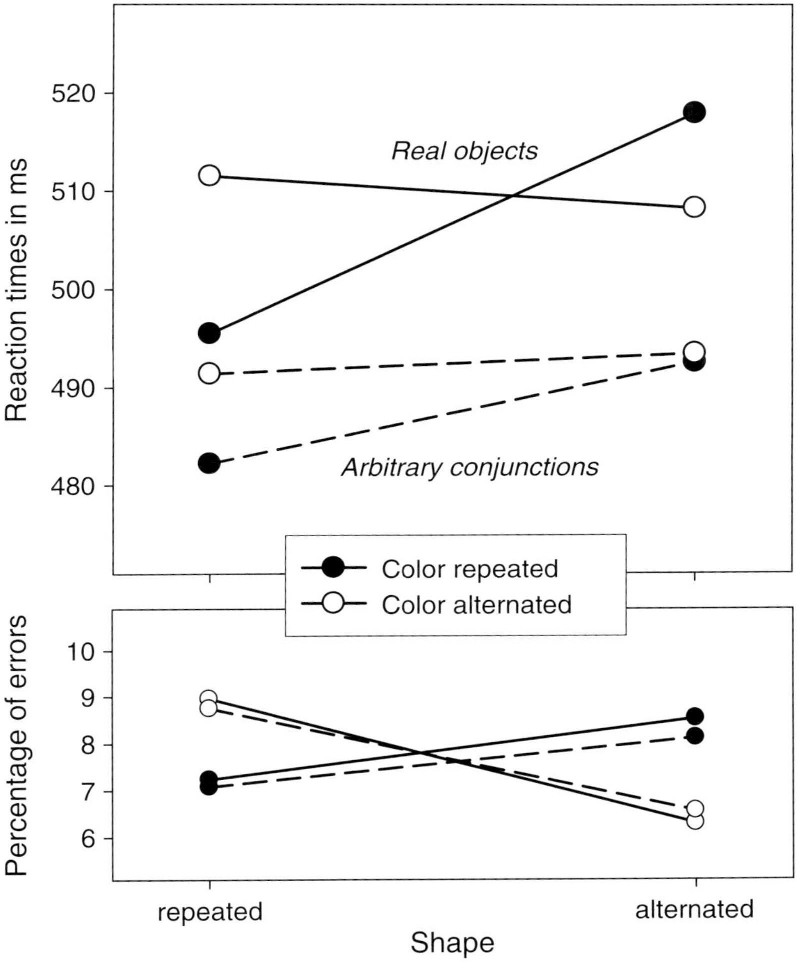

Figure 3. Mean reaction times and error percentages for R2 as a function of stimulus type and of repetition versus alternation of stimulus shape and colour.

interaction. This suggests that visual integration is influenced by stimulus type but visuomotor integration is not.

CONCLUSIONS

Taken altogether, our findings support the assumption of two different feature-integration mechanisms in visual perception (see also VanRullen, 2009 this issue). One mechanism seems to be agnostic about the familiarity or possibility of particular combinations of features and integrates any feature that falls into a given temporal integration window (Akyürek, Toffanin, & Hommel, 2008). We speculate that this mechanism is mediated by, or relies on neural synchronization processes, as is suggested by the observation that both visual integration and synchronization in the visual cortex seem to be driven by the same neurotransmitter system. The other mechanism is sensitive to the familiarity with the stimulus and it seems to provide attentional top-down support for real, familiar objects. Recognizing such objects presupposes a stored detector of the underlying feature combinations, and we speculate that such detectors are created for frequent combinations only—even though we cannot rule out the possibility that the naturalness of the stimulus also plays a role. In any case, there are reasons to assume that feature integration can take place in more than one way and that the principles of integration-through-convergence and integration-through-synchronization do not exclude but complement each other.

More generally speaking, our findings provide support for the assumption that the retrieval of object files is cocontrolled by two types of top-down priming processes. Offline priming, as one may call the impact of the current attentional set, precedes the stimulus and reflects the task relevance of feature dimensions for selecting the stimulus and the response (see Figure 2a and b). This priming is offline in the sense that it can be established any time before a given stimulus or response event occurs. Online priming, as it may be characterized, can be induced by stimuli that have entries in long-term memory, such as familiar real objects. Sensory information coming from these stimuli is likely to access corresponding memory entries in a first fast forward sweep, followed by a recurrent top-down process refining and contextualizing the input (Lamme & Roelfsema, 2000). Whereas the first, bottom-up part of this scenario is likely to be rather nonselective, the recurrent wave will be shaped by the current attentional settings. Given that this wave follows the first contact between the sensory information and the memory content, the outcome of this contact will contribute as well. Accordingly, the eventual representation of the present stimulus and the degree to which this representation is permitted to reactivate available object files will thus be codetermined by the task set and the stimulus-induced memory activation—provided that the stimulus matched some memory content it could activate.

REFERENCES

Adam, J., Hommel, B., & Umiltà, C. (2003). Preparing for perception and action I: The role of grouping in the response-cuing paradigm. *Cognitive Psychology*, *46*, 302–358.

Akyürek, E. G., Toffanin, P., & Hommel, B. (2008). Adaptive control of event integration. *Journal of Experimental Psychology: Human Perception and Performance*, *34*, 569–577.

Barlow, H. B. (1972). Single units and sensation: A neuron doctrine for perceptual psychology. *Perception, 1*, 371–394.

Baylis, G. C., & Driver, J. (1992). Visual parsing and response competition: The effect of grouping factors. *Perception and Psychophysics, 51*, 145–162.

Baylis, G. C., & Driver, J. (1993). Visual attention and objects: Evidence for hierarchical coding of location. *Journal of Experimental Psychology: Human Perception and Performance, 19*, 451–470.

Botly, L. C. P., & de Rosa, E. (2007). Cholinergic influences on feature binding. *Behavioral Neuroscience, 121*, 264–276.

Colzato, L. S., Erasmus, V., & Hommel, B. (2004). Moderate alcohol consumption in humans impairs feature binding in visual perception. *Neuroscience Letters, 360*, 103–105.

Colzato, L. S., Fagioli, S., Erasmus, V., & Hommel, B. (2005). Caffeine, but not nicotine enhances visual feature binding. *European Journal of Neuroscience, 21*, 591–595.

Colzato, L. S., & Hommel, B. (2008). Cannabis, cocaine, and visuomotor integration: Evidence for a role of dopamine D1 receptors in binding perception and action. *Neuropsychologia, 46*, 1570–1575.

Colzato, L. S., Kool, W., & Hommel, B. (2008). Stress modulation of visuomotor binding. *Neuropsychologia, 46*, 1542–1548.

Colzato, L. S., Raffone, A., & Hommel, B. (2006). What do we learn from binding features? Evidence for multilevel feature integration. *Journal of Experimental Psychology: Human Perception and Performance, 32*, 705–716.

Colzato, L. S., van Wouwe, N. C., & Hommel, B. (2007a). Feature binding and affect: Emotional modulation of visuo-motor integration. *Neuropsychologia, 45*, 440–446.

Colzato, L. S., van Wouwe, N. C., & Hommel, B. (2007b). Spontaneous eyeblink rate predicts the strength of visuomotor binding. *Neuropsychologia, 45*, 2387–2392.

DeYoe, E. A., & van Essen, D. C. (1988). Concurrent processing streams in monkey visual cortex. *Trends in Neuroscience, 11*, 219–226.

Duncan, J. (1984). Selective attention and the organization of visual information. *Journal of Experimental Psychology: General, 113*, 501–517.

Engel, A. K., & Singer, W. (2001). Temporal binding and the neural correlates of sensory awareness. *Trends in Cognitive Science, 5*, 16–25.

Fagioli, S., Hommel, B., & Schubotz, R. I. (2007). Intentional control of attention: Action planning primes action-related stimulus dimensions. *Psychological Research, 71*, 22–29.

Found, A., & Müller, H. J. (1996). Searching for unknown feature targets on more than one dimension: Investigating a "dimension weighting" account. *Perception and Psychophysics, 58*, 88–101.

Hommel, B. (1995). Attentional scanning in the selection of central targets from multi-symbol strings. *Visual Cognition, 2*, 119–144.

Hommel, B. (1998). Event files: Evidence for automatic integration of stimulus–response episodes. *Visual Cognition, 5*, 183–216.

Hommel, B. (2004). Event files: Feature binding in and across perception and action. *Trends in Cognitive Sciences, 8*, 494–500.

Hommel, B. (2005). How much attention does an event file need? *Journal of Experimental Psychology: Human Perception and Performance, 31*, 1067–1082.

Hommel, B. (2007). Feature integration across perception and action: Event files affect response choice. *Psychological Research, 71*, 42–63.

Hommel, B., & Colzato, L. S. (2004). Visual attention and the temporal dynamics of feature integration. *Visual Cognition, 11*, 483–521.

Hommel, B., & Elsner, B. (in press). Acquisition, representation, and control of action. In E. Morsella, J. A. Bargh, & P. M. Gollwitzer (Eds.), *The psychology of action, Vol. 2*. Oxford, UK: Oxford University Press.

Hommel, B., Memelink, J., Zmigrod, S., & Colzato, L. S. (2008). How information of relevant dimension control the creation and retrieval of feature–response binding. *Manuscript submitted for publication.*

Hommel, B., Müsseler, J., Aschersleben, G., & Prinz, W. (2001). The theory of event coding (TEC): A framework for perception and action planning. *Behavioral and Brain Sciences, 24*, 849–878.

James, W. (1890). *The principles of psychology*. New York: Dover Publications.

Kahneman, D., & Henik, A. (1981). Perceptual organization and attention. In M. Kubovy & J. R. Pomerantz (Eds.), *Perceptual organization* (pp. 181–211). Hillsdale, NJ: Lawrence Erlbaum Associates, Inc.

Kahneman, D., Treisman, A., & Gibbs, B. J. (1992). The reviewing of object files: Object-specific integration of information. *Cognitive Psychology, 24*, 175–219.

Keizer, A. W., Colzato, L. S., & Hommel, B. (2008). Integrating faces, houses, motion, and action: Spontaneous binding across ventral and dorsal processing streams. *Acta Psychologica, 127*, 177–185.

Keizer, A. W., Colzato, L. S., Theeuwisse, W., Niewenhuis, S., Rombouts, S. A. R. B., & Hommel, B. (2008). When moving faces activate the house area: An fMRI study of object file retrieval. *Manuscript submitted for publication.*

Lamme, V. A., & Roelfsema, P. R. (2000). The distinct modes of vision offered by feedforward and recurrent processing. *Trends in Neuroscience, 23*, 571–579.

Logan, G. D. (1988). Toward an instance theory of automatization. *Psychological Review, 95*, 492–527.

Lotze, R. H. (1852). *Medicinische Psychologie oder die Physiologie der Seele*. Leipzig, Germany: Weidmann'sche Buchhandlung.

Mitroff, S. R., & Alvarez, G. A. (2007). Space and time, not surface features, underlie object persistence. *Psychonomic Bulletin and Review, 14*, 1199–1204.

Posner, M. I., & Cohen, Y. A. (1984). Components of visual orienting. In H. Bouma & D. G. Bouwhuis (Eds.), *Attention and performance X* (pp. 531–554). Hove, UK: Lawrence Erlbaum Associates Ltd.

Raffone, A., & Wolters, G. (2001). A cortical mechanism for binding in visual working memory. *Journal of Cognitive Neuroscience, 13*, 766–785.

Rodriguez-Bermudez, R., Kallenbach, U., Singer, W., & Munk, M. H. (2004). Short- and long-term effects of cholinergic modulation on gamma oscillations and response synchronization in the visual cortex. *Journal of Neuroscience, 24*, 10369–10378.

Treisman, A. (1996). The binding problem. *Current Opinion in Neurobiology, 6*, 171–178.

Treisman, A., & Schmidt, H. (1982). Illusory conjunctions in the perception of objects. *Cognitive Psychology, 14*, 107–141.

Treisman, A. M., & Gelade, G. (1980). A feature-integration theory of attention. *Cognitive Psychology, 12*, 97–136.

Van Dam, W. O., & Hommel, B. (2008). How object-specific are object files? Evidence for integration by location. *Manuscript submitted for publication.*

Van der Heijden, A. H. C. (1995). Modularity and attention. *Visual Cognition, 2*, 269–302.

VanRullen, R. (2009). Binding hardwired vs. on-demand feature conjunctions. *Visual Cognition, 17*, 103–119.

Von der Malsburg, C. (1999). The what and why of binding: The modeler's perspective. *Neuron, 24*, 95–104.

Xu, Y. (2006). Encoding objects in visual short-term memory: The roles of feature proximity and connectedness. *Perception and Psychophysics, 68*, 815–828.

VISUAL COGNITION, 2009, 17 (1/2), 141–159

Psychology Press
Taylor & Francis Group

Overwriting and rebinding: Why feature-switch detection tasks underestimate the binding capacity of visual working memory

George A. Alvarez and Todd W. Thompson

Department of Brain and Cognitive Sciences, Massachusetts Institute of Technology, Cambridge, MA, USA

In these two experiments, we explored the ability to store bound representations of colour and location information in visual working memory using three different tasks. In the location-cue task, we probed how well colour information could be recalled when observers are given a location cue. In the feature-cue task, we probed how well location information could be recalled when observers are given a colour cue. Finally, in the feature-switch detection task, we tested how well observers could detect a recombination of features (e.g., switching the locations of the red and green items). We hypothesized that these tasks might reveal differences in binding capacity limits between switching and nonswitching tests of visual working memory. We also hoped the tasks could provide an explanation for those differences in terms of the component processes of working memory—do failures occur in the encoding, maintenance, or retrieval stages of the task? Experiment 1 showed that performance in the two cued-recall tasks was equally high, and was significantly better than performance in the feature-switch detection task. Thus, the feature-switch detection task underestimates the number of colour–location bindings that can be remembered, but is a useful task for examining the fragile nature of feature binding in working memory. Experiment 2 explored why feature-switch detection underestimates the binding capacity of visual working memory by examining whether the feature switch errors occur at the level of encoding, maintaining, or retrieving binding information from visual working memory. The results suggest that feature switch errors reflect failures to maintain bound objects in working memory, perhaps due to the automatic rewriting and rebinding of information in the face of new perceptual input.

Keywords: Working memory; Binding; Overwriting; Cued recall; Feature switch.

Please address all correspondence to George Alvarez, Department of Brain and Cognitive Sciences, Massachusetts Institute of Technology, 77 Massachusetts Avenue, Cambridge, MA 02139, USA. E-mail: alvarez@mit.edu

GAA was supported by NIH/NEI fellowship no. F32EY016982. TWT was supported by an NDSEG grant from the Office of Naval Research.

© 2008 Psychology Press, an imprint of the Taylor & Francis Group, an Informa business
http://www.psypress.com/viscog DOI: 10.1080/13506280802265496

Perhaps the most basic computation the human visual system carries out is parsing the incoming stream of visual information into meaningful units, such as surfaces, objects, and events. The fact that this seems to be accomplished with little conscious effort belies the challenge the visual system faces of integrating many independent sources of information into these cohesive units. As noted by many previous researchers, the visual system seems to be comprised of specialized, parallel processing streams for different visual feature dimensions (e.g., colour, motion, etc.; for reviews see Cowey, 1985; Zeki, 1993). This gives rise to the perceptual "binding problem": If these features are analysed in separate brain regions, how are they subsequently combined to form meaningful, integrated units? Research on this perceptual binding problem has supported the hypothesis that attention is needed to integrate the features of an object (Treisman, 1996, 1998). Attending to an object binds the features of that object together, whereas withdrawing attention from an object will result in a loss of binding information (Wolfe, Klempen, & Dahlen, 2000) or binding errors such as illusory conjunctions (Treisman & Schmidt, 1982).

In contrast with these previous studies that have investigated the perceptual binding problem, the current study investigates visual working memory for bound objects. However, it is important to consider first whether there exists a binding problem in visual working memory. How can we determine whether errors in a visual working memory experiment reflect true binding errors, or if they simply indicate a failure to retrieve a component feature of a successfully bound object? There would be a stronger case for a specific "binding problem" in visual working memory if it were possible to store the constituent features of an object without remembering how they were bound together. This has in fact been shown in a previous study by Stefurak and Boynton (1986), who showed that it is possible for observers to remember the colours and shapes of objects that were seen, without remembering which colour was bound to which shape. These results suggest that binding operations, and the maintenance of bound object representations, are part of a distinct process or level of representation that can be isolated for further investigation.

One of the central issues addressed in this paper is a methodological question: Do different methods of probing the contents of visual working memory reveal different aspects of binding and feature storage? A variety of methods is employed in the literature for probing visual working memory, including recall, old/new recognition, and change detection. In each of these tasks, a sample display consisting of several multidimensional objects is briefly presented, followed by a retention interval on the order of seconds, which is then followed by a test. A typical recall test would require observers to report the identity of all objects. In cued-recall one feature of the test items is used as a cue to probe recall for other features of that item (e.g., what colour was the square, with shape serving as a cue for colour recall). In old/new recognition tasks, a single test item is presented, and the observer must report whether that item was a member of the memory set. Finally, in change detection, the test display is a second array of objects. On half of the trials all of the items appear identical to the sample display, and on the other half of the trials a single item is different in some way (e.g., in colour, shape, etc.). The task is to report whether the two displays are the same or different.

Change detection is perhaps the most commonly employed task for investigating the capacity of visual working memory (Alvarez & Cavanagh, 2004; Luck & Vogel, 1997). In a seminal study on visual working memory, Luck and Vogel showed that the number of objects that can be remembered is about four, whether observers are required to remember one, two, or even four features per object (Luck & Vogel, 1997). These results were consistent with their claim that visual working memory stores integrated object representations. However, other researchers have noted that in the typical change detection task, features do not have to be bound together to detect a change (Wheeler & Treisman, 2002). In the typical change detection task, only a single feature is probed at test, even when multiple features such as colour and orientation are remembered (Luck & Vogel, 1997). If there were completely independent feature stores for colour and orientation, then a change to either feature dimension could be detected even if there was no binding across dimensions.

To address this limitation of the standard change detection task for investigating feature binding in memory, Wheeler and Treisman (2002) introduced a modified change-detection task, which we will refer to as *feature-switch detection*, in which observers must look for a feature switch. For example, if the task were to remember combinations of colour and shape, then a set of objects with different shapes and colours would be briefly presented (e.g., a red circle, blue square, and green triangle), followed by a brief retention interval, and then by a test display. On half of the trials, the test display would be identical to the sample display. On the other half, two objects would switch features (e.g., the red circle and blue square might change to a blue circle and red square). The task is to determine whether or not any of the features have switched. It is impossible to perform this task simply by remembering which features were presented, because all of the same features appear in both the sample and test displays. Thus, it is necessary to remember how the features were combined to detect a feature switch.

Results using this feature-switch detection task and a dynamic variant in which objects move about the display (Saiki, 2002) have shown that feature switch detection is quite poor (Saiki, 2002, 2003a,2003b; Treisman & Zhang, 2006; Wheeler & Treisman, 2002). The difficulty of feature-switch detection could be due to failures at any stage of working memory, including the encoding, maintenance, or retrieval of information (Atkinson & Shiffrin,

1968). Saiki (2002, 2003b) has interpreted the failure to detect feature switches as evidence for encoding failures, and suggested that working memory storage capacity for feature bindings is more limited than for independent features. Other researchers interpret the difficulty of feature switch detection as evidence for maintenance failures, suggesting that when attention is withdrawn from active maintenance, the stored binding information is lost (Wheeler & Treisman, 2002). Finally, the change detection literature suggests that feature-switch detection errors could also occur due to a failure to retrieve information from visual working memory (Mitroff, Simons, & Levin, 2004; Simons, 2000; Simons, Chabris, Schnur, & Levin, 2002).

Because previous research suggests that feature-switch detection tasks are more difficult than other types of task, such as change detection (Wheeler & Treisman, 2002), we hypothesized that feature-switch detection underestimates the binding capacity of visual working memory. In Experiment 1, we investigated the extent to which the feature-switch detection task underestimates working memory capacity by comparing performance on feature-switch detection to performance on cued-recall within the same group of participants. The results showed that feature-switch detection does indeed underestimate the binding capacity of visual working memory. As already noted, the feature-switch performance alone cannot be used to isolate whether feature-switch errors are due to encoding, maintenance, or retrieval failures. As described by Gajewski and Brockmole (2006), the feature-switch detection task alone enables us to determine when a memory failure occurs, but it does not enable us to determine the nature and extent of the failure (i.e., was the entire object forgotten, or was the binding between two features lost?). In contrast, the cued-recall task enables us to assess exactly what type of memory failure occurs by evaluating which features observers report when they make errors. Thus, Experiment 2 explored whether feature-switch detection errors reflect failures of encoding, maintenance, or retrieval by having observers perform the feature-switch detection task and a cued-recall tasks on the same trial. The results showed that the contents of memory are rapidly overwritten by new perceptual input, suggesting that feature switch detection tasks introduce an additional load at the maintenance stage of visual working memory.

EXPERIMENT 1: FEATURE-SWITCH DETECTION VERSUS CUED RECALL

To test whether the feature-switch task underestimates the binding capacity of visual working memory relative to cued-recall tasks, we had observers remember the binding of colour and location, using a dynamic feature-switch detection task modelled after Saiki's (2002) task. Multiple items of different colours rotated around a fixation point, disappearing and reappearing behind an occluding surface (see Figure 1). This dynamic display places high demands on operations that bind colour to location, as the colour–location combinations are constantly updating, requiring observers to continuously encode

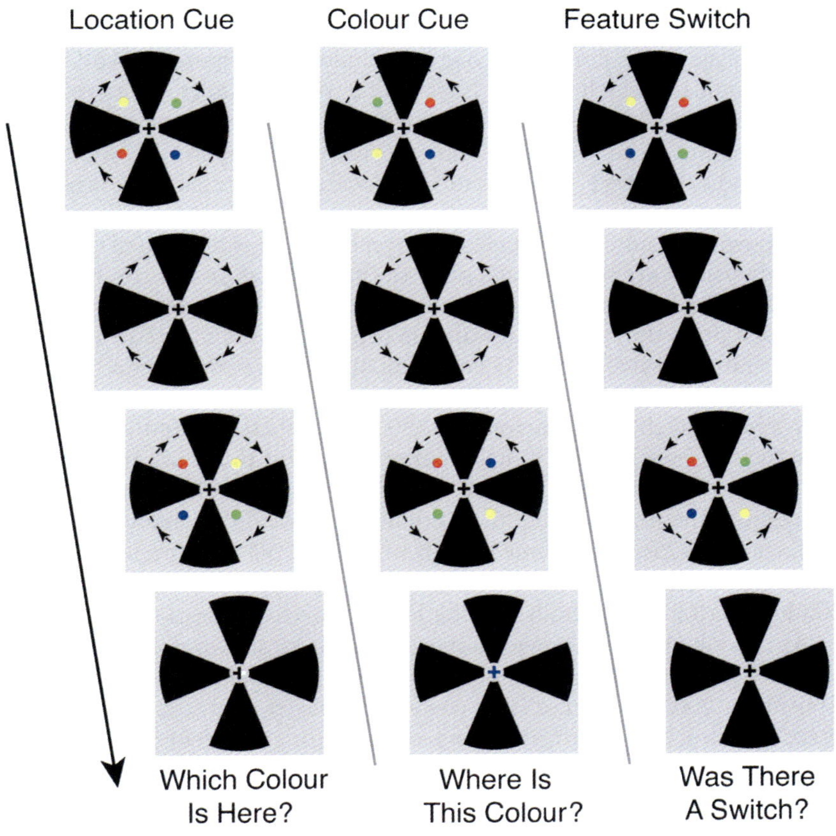

Figure 1. Sample trials for the three different conditions. In each condition, a red, green, blue, and yellow circle rotated either clockwise or counterclockwise (direction chosen randomly for each trial), disappearing and reappearing behind the black occluding surfaces. The task was to keep track of which colour was in which location. In the location-cue condition, all of the items stopped behind the occluders, and one arm of the fixation "+" turned white, prompting the observer to press a key to indicate which colour was in the cued location. In the colour-cue condition, all of the items stopped behind the occluders, and the fixation "+" changed red, green, blue, or yellow, prompting the observer to press an arrow key to indicate where that colour was located. In the feature-switch condition, there was a 50/50 chance that two of the colours would switch places with each other during the trial. In this example, the yellow and blue circles switch places with each other when they reappeared. At the end of the trial, all of the items stopped behind the occluders, and observers indicated whether or not they had detected a switch.

information into visual working memory. Observers monitored these displays and attempted to remember which colour appeared in which location, and simultaneously performed a verbal suppression task to minimize verbal encoding of the stimuli. At the end of each trial, all of the items stopped while hidden behind the occluders. We then probed how well observers were able to remember which colour was in which location using three different tasks (in separate blocks of trials). In the location-cue condition, part of the fixation cross changed white, pointing to one of occluders (see Figure 1a), and the task was to indicate which colour was behind that occluder by pressing the keyboard key corresponding to the colour. In the colour-cue condition, the fixation point turned red, green, blue, or yellow (see Figure 1b), and the task was to indicate where that colour was located by pressing the arrow key corresponding to the correct occluder position (up, down, left, or right). In the feature-switch condition, the task was to report whether any two of the colours had switched locations with each other during the trial. In this condition, 50% of the trials had a feature-switch in which two of the colours switched positions with each other during a disappearance behind the occluders (see Figure 1c). These feature switches only occurred in the feature-switch condition, and occurred only once during a trial. The new feature combination was visible for only a single eighth of a revolution (500 ms). In each condition, observers gave their response to the visual memory task, and then gave their response for the verbal suppression task, typing the letters they had rehearsed throughout the trial. Because these conditions have different levels of chance performance (25% in the cued-recall tasks, and 50% in the feature-switch task), performance was adjusted for chance to enable comparisons across conditions (for more details, see the Data Analysis section).

As described earlier, previous experiments have shown poor performance in this type of feature-switch detection task (e.g., Saiki, 2003a; Wheeler & Treisman, 2002). Because the cued-recall tasks and the feature-switch detection task are identical during the encoding stage of the experiment (see Figure 1), any differences between these tasks must occur during the maintenance or retrieval stages. Thus, to the extent that the feature-switch detection task introduces maintenance or retrieval errors that do not occur in the cued-recall tasks, performance should be worse on the feature-switch detection task (after correcting for differences in chance performance).

Method

Participants

Author GA and 11 naïve observers participated in the experiment. All observers gave informed consent, had 20/20 corrected vision or better, and had normal colour vision.

Apparatus

Experiments were run using the Psychophysics Toolbox extensions (Brainard, 1997; Pelli, 1997), and were conducted on a $35^\circ \times 28^\circ$ CRT monitor running at 60 Hz, viewed from approximately 57 cm. All motion appeared smooth and continuous on this display.

Stimuli

The stimuli were based on a stimulus developed by Saiki (2002) to test binding in visual working memory. As shown in Figure 1, the display consisted of four circles (diameter $= 1^\circ$), each of a different colour (red, green, blue, or yellow), equally spaced on an imaginary ring at an eccentricity of 4°. Four occluding "wedges" were drawn by dividing a black circle (diameter $= 16^\circ$) into eight sectors, erasing a small circular region near the middle (diameter $= 2^\circ$), and erasing every other sector, leaving the north, east, south, and west sectors to occlude the display. A fixation "+" ($1.5^\circ \times 1.5^\circ$) was drawn in black at the centre of the display. On each trial, the small coloured circles rotated at 0.25 revolutions per second, disappearing behind the black wedges, and then reappearing in the gray zones in between. The display rotated for a random total of one to two cycles (in one-eighth of a cycle increments), and always stopped with the circles hidden behind the black occluders. When there was a feature switch, the new feature combination was visible for a single eighth of a revolution (500 ms) and then the circles. The RGB lookup table values of the colours used in these displays were as follows: Red (255,0,0), green (0,245,0), blue (0,0,255), yellow (255,255,0), black (0,0,0), and grey (185,185,185).

Procedure

At the beginning of each trial, two consonants were presented on the screen and the observer began rehearsing the letters, then pressed a key to begin the visual memory trial. This verbal suppression task has been used in previous visual working memory studies to minimize verbal encoding of visual stimuli (e.g., Gajewski & Brockmole, 2006; Vogel, Woodman, & Luck, 2001). During the trial, four circles of different colours (red, green, blue, and yellow) rotated around the fixation point, disappearing and reappearing from behind occluders, eventually stopping while behind the occluders. The observers' task was to keep track of where each colour was located throughout the trial. Memory for colour–location binding was tested in the three different conditions described earlier and shown in Figure 1, in separate blocks of 12 practice trials and 36 test trials, with the order of conditions counterbalanced across observers (switch, location, colour; colour, switch, location; location, colour, switch).

Data analysis

Due to differences in chance performance for the 4AFC tasks (the colour-cue and the location-cue conditions), and the 2AFC task (the feature-switch condition), we computed three different measures which correct for differences in chance performance: (1) Normalized accuracy, (2) sensitivity in d', and (3) a capacity estimate in terms of the number of objects stored, K.

Normalized accuracy. This measure takes the raw percentage correct score and rescales it so that chance performance gives a score of zero, and perfect performance gives a score of 100.

$$\mathrm{NA} = (\mathrm{PC} - \mathrm{chance})/(100 - \mathrm{chance}) \quad (1)$$

Where NA is normalized accuracy, PC is the raw percentage correct score computed directly from the observers' performance, and chance is the chance level of accuracy. An example illustrates how this normalization procedure equates performance for conditions with different chance levels. If Condition A has a chance level of 25% accuracy, then a score of 62.5% would represent a performance level halfway between chance and perfect performance, and would give a normalized score of 50%. If Condition B has a chance level of 50%, then a score of 75% would represent a performance level halfway between chance and perfect performance, and would also give a normalized score of 50%. Thus, according to this procedure, 62.5% correct when chance is 25% is equivalent to 75% correct when chance is 50%.

Sensitivity d'. We used the standard calculation for d' in the feature-switch condition (z(HIT) – z(FA)), where HIT corresponds to the hit rate (probability reporting a feature switch when there was in fact a feature switch), and FA corresponds to the false alarm rate (probability of reporting a feature switch when there was not a feature switch). In the location-cue and colour-cue conditions, d' was calculated based on percentage correct (PC) and the number of response alternatives (M), using the algorithm described by Smith (1982).

Capacity K. We computed capacity in terms of the number of objects stored (K), based on percentage correct on each task (for similar calculations see Cowan, 2001; Pashler, 1988). In the 4AFC location-cue and colour-cue conditions, percentage correct was assumed to be related to K by the following equation:

$$\mathrm{PC} = K/N{*}1 + (N-K)/N{*}1/(N-K) \quad (2)$$

Where PC represents percent correct, K is the number of objects remembered, and N is the total number of items to be remembered. This equation assumes that whenever a remembered item is tested (K/N proportion of the trials), performance will be perfect, but that whenever an item that was not remembered is tested, performance will be at chance guessing. For example, if an observer can remember two out of four items, then percentage correct should be $2/4*1+(4-2)/4 * 1/(4-2)=.75$. This equation assumes that observers perfectly use the information they have remembered, and can be simplified and solved for K as follows:

$$K_{4AFC} = PC * M - 1 \tag{3}$$

For the 2AFC feature-switch condition, the intuition for deriving a K score is that subjects will detect a switch if a remembered item is involved in the switch, so given the probability of detecting a switch, we can solve for the number of objects remembered. Thus, if switch detection is limited only by the number of objects remembered, the HIT rate (reporting a switch when there was one) is related to the number of objects remembered (K) and the guessing rate (or FA, the probability of reporting a switch when there was not a switch) by the following set of equations:

$$T = (N*N-N)/2 \tag{4}$$

$$I = K*N - K*(K+1)/2 \tag{5}$$

$$\text{HIT} = I/T* 1 + \text{FA} \tag{6}$$

Where T is the total number of switches that can occur between pairs of items, and N is the number of items. For four items, there are six possible switches between pairs of items. I is the number of switches that would involve a remembered item if K items were remembered. For example, if only one item out of four items were remembered, $1*4-1*(1+1)/2=3$, indicating that three out of the six possible changes would involve that single remembered item. Thus, 3/6 switches would be detected, and the HIT rate would equal to 3/6 plus the false alarm rate. Given the HIT rate, false alarm rate, and number of items to be remembered, these equations can be simplified to the following:

$$0 = -(K^2) + (2*N+1)*K - 2*T*(\text{HIT}-\text{FA}) \tag{7}$$

In this form (zero $= aK^2 + bK + c$), we can solve for K using the quadratic equation, as follows:

$a = -1$

$b = 2*N + 1$

$c = -2*T*(\text{HIT}-\text{FA})$

$$K_{4AFC} = [-b +/- \text{sqrt}(b^2 - 4*a*c)]/(2*a) \tag{8}$$

There are two solutions to this equation, but one of them will always be outside the range of possible values for K (less than zero, or greater than N), and so the solution that is inside the range of possible K values was taken as the capacity estimate.

Results

Overall, performance on the verbal suppression task was greater than 96% ($SEM = 2.2\%$), and did not differ significantly as a function of the test condition (all $ts < 1.04$, all $ps > .31$). The remaining analyses were conducted on visual memory performance for trials in which both letters of the verbal suppression task were correctly reported.

Raw accuracy. Overall accuracy in the 4AFC colour-cue trials was 83% ($SEM = 4.6\%$), indicating that observers could report the location of a particular colour with fairly high accuracy. Similarly, accuracy in the 4AFC location-cue trials was 84% ($SEM = 4.4\%$), indicating that observers could also report the colour at a cued location with fairly high accuracy. Combined, performance in these two conditions suggests that observers know with high accuracy which colours are bound to which locations. In the 2AFC feature-switch task, observers performed at 79% ($SEM = 3.8\%$). However, due to the difference in chance accuracy (25% for the 4AFC tasks, and 50% in the 2AFC task), these raw accuracy scores cannot be directly compared. To account for this, we computed three performance measures that correct for these differences in baseline accuracy: Normalized accuracy, d', and the number of objects stored (see Method). Comparisons with all three measures indicate that memory performance is worse in the *feature-switch condition than in either the location-cue or colour-cue* conditions.

Normalized accuracy. Normalized accuracy was computed for each condition, as described in the Method section. As shown in Figure 2a, performance was not significantly different in the colour-cue and location-cue conditions, $t(11) < 1$, $p = .463$, $r^2 = .050$, but performance in both of these conditions was better than in the feature-switch condition: Colour-cue vs. feature-switch), $t(11) = 4.19$, $p < .01$, $r^2 = .615$; location-cue vs. feature-switch, $t(11) = 5.14$, $p < .001$, $r^2 = .706$.

d'. Sensitivity in d' units was computed for each condition, as described in the Method section. As shown in Figure 2b, performance was not significantly different in the colour-cue and location-cue condition ($t < 1$), but performance in both of these conditions was better than in the feature-switch condition: Colour-cue vs. feature-switch, $t(11) = 2.33$, $p < .05$, $r^2 = .331$; location-cue vs. feature-switch, $t(11) = 2.86$, $p < .05$, $r^2 = .427$.

Number of objects stored (K). An estimate of the number of objects stored (K) was computed for each condition, as described in the Method section. As shown in Figure 2c, performance was not significantly different in the colour-cue and location-cue condition ($t < 1$), but performance in

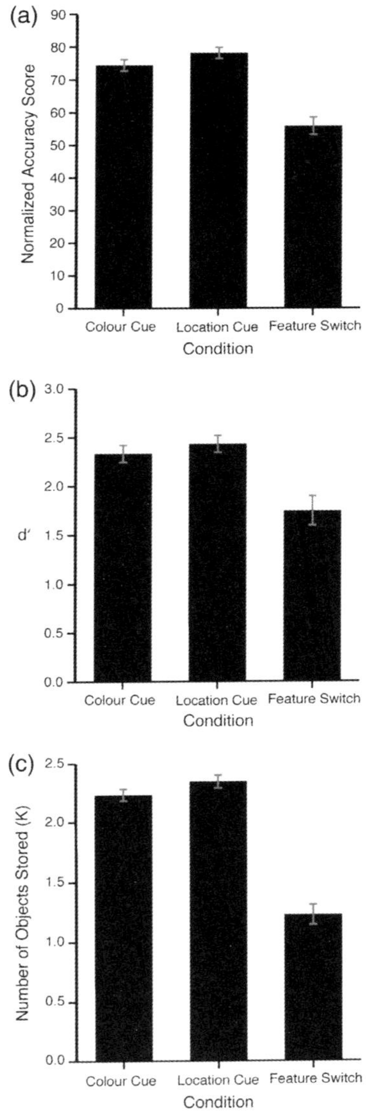

Figure 2. Results of Experiment 1 expressed in three different measures that correct for differences in chance accuracy: (a) Normalized accuracy scores, (b) sensitivity in terms of d', and (c) number of objects stored, K. Each measure shows that performance was not significantly different in the location-cue and colour-cue conditions, but performance in both of these recall conditions was significantly better than in the feature-switch condition. Error bars represent one within-subject standard error of the mean, calculated with Cousineau's (2005) modification of Loftus and Masson's (1994) method.

both of these conditions was better than in the feature-switch condition: Colour-cue vs. feature-switch, $t(11) = 7.47$, $p < .001$, $r^2 = .835$; location-cue vs. feature-switch, $t(11) = 8.45$, $p < .001$, $r^2 = .866$.

Discussion

This experiment tested how well observers could maintain bound representations of colour and location in visual working memory. In the location-cue and feature-cue conditions, which were both cued-recall tasks, observers could report which colour appeared in which location with high accuracy. However, in the feature-switch condition, performance was significantly worse than in either of the cued-recall conditions. In fact, the switch detection task underestimates the number of colour–location pairs that are initially bound and maintained in visual working memory by approximately 90% relative to the cued-recall conditions.

Previous work has interpreted feature-switch errors as evidence that working memory has a relatively limited capacity to store colour–location combinations (Saiki, 2002; Saiki & Miyatsuji, 2007). Although we replicate the difficulty of feature-switch detection, the high level of cued-recall performance indicates that the failure to detect feature switches cannot be attributed entirely to a failure to encode bound features into visual working memory. It appears that the feature switch detection task places additional demands on the maintenance or retrieval of bound objects from visual working memory.

One possible reason observers might miss a feature switch is that the initially bound object representations might not be maintained after a feature-switch occurs. The dynamic displays we employed required observers to constantly update their binding memory, since the colours are constantly changing location. It is possible that when the items are attended, their features are automatically rebound in memory to match the new perceptual input (the *maintenance-failure hypothesis*). Such automatic rebinding could occur if visible stimuli are given priority over the current contents of memory, or if visible stimuli simply have a more robust representation than those maintained in working memory. In fact, previous research suggests that bound representations are fragile and can be interfered with by subsequent encoding of information (Allen, Baddeley, & Hitch, 2006), or by the diffusion of attention during retrieval (Wheeler & Treisman, 2002). We suggest that, due to the fragile nature of these bound representations, the contents of working memory might be particularly susceptible to an automatic rewriting operation. On this view, objects are initially encoded into memory as bound, integrated units, but the contents of visual working memory are automatically rewritten when they are perceived in a new combination.

Another possibility is that the initial binding representation was maintained, but was not retrieved due to time constraints or decision complexity (the *retrieval-failure hypothesis*). Evidence for this type of memory access failure has been observed in change-blindness studies (Mitroff et al., 2004; Simons et al., 2002). In these studies, observers often failed to notice changes to the appearance of objects in a display, and yet were able to answer forced choice questions about what the objects looked like before the changes occurred, as if they had a memory representation which simply had not been retrieved. There are multiple reasons similar memory access failures might occur in the feature-switch detection task. Because all the circles were constantly changing location, observers were required to check each item for a switch each time it reappeared from behind an occluder. Even with perfectly bound representations of each item, this could be difficult if there was not enough time to check each item, or if the decision was simply so complex that observers did not exhaustively check each item. The cued-recall tasks do not share these time constraints, or decision complexity, because only one item must be accessed, via either its location or its colour.

Experiment 2 contrasts the maintenance-failure hypothesis with the retrieval-failure hypothesis directly by requiring observers to perform the feature-switch detection task and a cued-recall task within the same trial.

EXPERIMENT 2: EVIDENCE FOR REWRITING AND REBINDING OF WORKING MEMORY CONTENTS

This experiment explored whether feature switches are missed due to a failure to retrieve information from memory, or due to a failure to maintain the original bindings, perhaps due to an automatic overwriting and rebinding of the contents of memory. To address this question, observers performed both the feature-switch detection task and the cued-recall tasks within the same trial. This enabled us to determine the colour–location binding that observers report when they miss a feature switch. The retrieval-failure hypothesis holds that feature switches are missed because there is not enough time, or it is too difficult, to attempt to retrieve the contents of memory and to detect a feature switch. The maintenance-failure hypothesis assumes that the new combination of features overwrites memory, storing these new colour–location combinations in working memory.

As in Experiment 1, four items of different colours rotated around a fixation point, disappearing and reappearing behind an occluding surface, and observers were required to remember which colour appeared in which location while performing a verbal suppression task. At the end of each trial, all the items stopped while hidden behind the occluders and observers answered the cued-recall question (reporting the location corresponding to the colour cue, or the colour corresponding to the location cue, in separate blocks of trials). Then observers reported whether or not they detected a switch on that trial. When there was a switch, the new colour–location combinations were only seen once for 500 ms (a single eighth of a revolution), so any memory updating must happen within a single interval.

Of principal interest was what colour–location combination observers would report when they missed a feature switch. A tendency to report the old colours in their old locations (the feature combination prior to the switch) would be consistent with the retrieval-failure hypothesis, as successful retrieval of the old features suggests that these features were maintained despite missing the switch. A tendency to report the new colours in their new locations (the feature combination after the switch) would be consistent with the maintenance-failure hypothesis, as the original bindings were not maintained. Finally, an equal probability of reporting the new colours in their new locations, the old colours in their old locations, and the other colour–location combinations that were not involved in the switch would be consistent with an encoding-failure hypothesis (not binding the colours to locations before or after the switch). We found this encoding-failure hypothesis unlikely based on the results of Experiment 1, but included it here for the sake of completeness.

Method

Eight new observers participated in the experiment. The method was the same as Experiment 1 except that observers performed both the feature-switch detection task and a cued-recall task on the same trial, with colour-cue and location-cue trials in separate blocks. Observers completed 24 practice and 144 test trials in each of the cued-recall conditions, with the order of conditions counterbalanced across subjects (colour, location; or location, colour).

Results

On average, observers missed 25% ($SEM = 8\%$) of feature switches. The remaining analyses focused on the distribution of cued-recall responses for these miss trials. Responses were categorized as either new-feature (the postswitch colour in the postswitch location), old-feature (the preswitch colour in the preswitch location), or other-features (averaged over the two colour–location combinations that were not involved in the switch). The results show that in both the colour-cue condition and the location-cue condition, observers reported the new-feature on the vast majority of trials. Figure 3a illustrates that in the colour-cue condition, observers reported the new-feature significantly more than the old-feature, $t(7) = 6.8$, $p < .001$, $r^2 = .87$, or the other-features, $t(7) = 9.4$, $p < .001$, $r^2 = .93$, but there was no significant difference between reports of the old-feature and the other-features ($t < 1$). Similarly, Figure 3b illustrates that in the location-cue condition, observers reported the new-feature significantly more than the old-feature, $t(7) = 6.3$, $p < .001$, $r^2 = .85$, or the other-features, $t(7) = 12.2$, $p < .001$, $r^2 = .96$, but there was no significant difference between reports of the old-feature and the other-feature ($t < 1$).

Discussion

The results indicate that when observers miss feature switches, they report the new colours in their new locations in both cued-recall tasks. Thus, it appears that observers have updated representations of the colour–location combinations, even though they only saw the new feature combinations for 500 ms (one-eighth of a revolution). These results rule out a broad class of explanations for the cause of feature-switch detection errors. Specifically, any

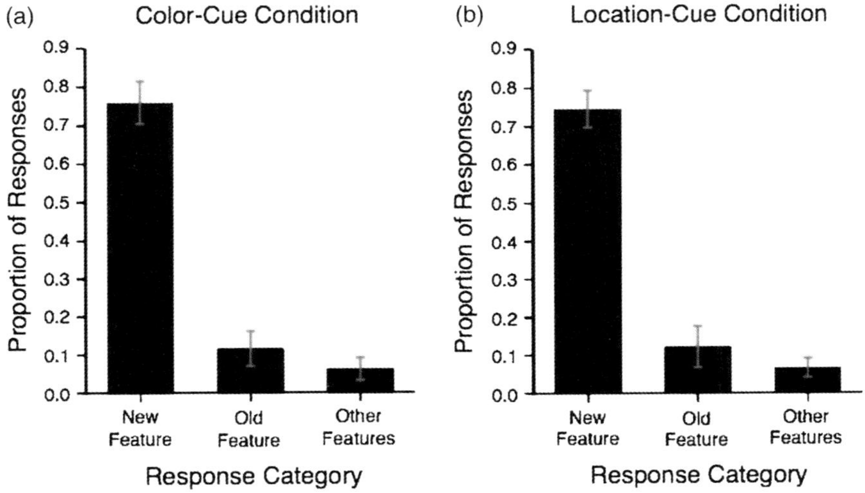

Figure 3. Results of Experiment 2, in terms of the proportion of cued-recall responses in each response category when a feature switch was missed. New-feature corresponds to the new colours in their new locations (the postswitch colours), old-feature corresponds to the old colours in their old locations (the preswitch colours), and other-features corresponds to the other features (those not involved in the feature-switch). (a) The response distribution on colour-cue trials. (b) The response distribution on location-cue trials. Error bars represent one within-subject standard error of the mean, calculated with Cousineau's (2005) modification of Loftus and Masson's (1994) method.

hypothesis that assumes there is not enough time to encode the new feature combinations, or that memory is simply not updated continuously in these dynamic displays, are ruled out by these results. This is consistent with previous research which has shown that colour information can be encoded into visual working memory quite rapidly, on the order of approximately 50 ms per item (Vogel, Woodman, & Luck, 2006). It is possible that stimuli that are encoded this rapidly are particularly susceptible to overwriting and rebinding. The present results are also inconsistent with the hypothesis that feature-switch detection errors are caused by a failure to attempt memory retrieval, as has been shown in previous change-blindness studies (Mitroff et al., 2004; Simons et al., 2002). Although there was a small (nonsignificant) trend for observers to report the old feature combinations more than the other, nonswitch features, the vast majority of cued-recall responses were reports of the new colours in their new locations. Thus, the results are most consistent with the hypothesis that feature-switch detection is difficult because the contents of memory are automatically rewritten and rebound when they are perceived in a new combination. In other words, feature-switch detection errors appear to result from a failure to maintain the initial bindings across the switch.

An alternative possibility is that the initial bindings are maintained, but that there is a bias towards reporting the new feature bindings. On this view, if observers were pressed to report a second guess, the second guess would be more likely to be of the old features (the preswitch colour and location) than the other features (those not involved with the switch). Although it is likely there will be a small trend in this direction, it is unlikely that observers would have maintained the old bindings for a large number of items. Overall accuracy in the cued-recall tasks was nearly the same when there was not a feature switch ($M = 81\%$, $SEM = 4\%$) as when there was a feature switch ($M = 84\%$, $SEM = 4\%$). If the level of accuracy without a feature switch reflects the "full capacity" of memory to store colour–location combinations, then it appears that memory is filled to capacity with the new colour–location combinations after a feature switch (because performance remains at a comparable level). Thus, although there may be some lingering information about the old features, it appears that most of the old information has been displaced by the new feature combinations.

These findings are consistent with previous research, which suggests that bound representations are particularly susceptible to interference from the encoding of new perceptual information (Allen et al., 2006; Wheeler & Treisman, 2002). However, the current results extend these findings by demonstrating that the observed interference is due specifically to an overwriting/rebinding, rather than a more general disruption of stored binding information.

GENERAL DISCUSSION

The current study investigated the ability to encode and maintain colour–location combinations in visual working memory. In Experiment 1, we tested memory for colour–location combinations using two cued-recall tasks (Gajeweki & Brockmole, 2006), and a feature-switch detection task (Saiki, 2002; Wheeler & Treisman, 2002). The results showed that, relative to cued-recall, feature-switch detection underestimates the number of colour–location combinations that can be remembered. These findings indicate that errors in feature switch detection are not due to a failure to encode colour–location bindings into visual working memory (Saiki, 2002, 2003b), but rather indicate a failure at a later stage of working memory processing.

Experiment 2 combined the feature-switch detection task with cued-recall task to determine the nature of feature-switch detection errors by examining which colour–location combinations were remembered when feature-switch detection failed. Observers did not reliably report the preswitch feature combinations (the old colours in their old locations), contradicting the hypothesis that feature-switch errors occur due to a retrieval failure. Instead, observers overwhelmingly reported the postswitch features (the new colours in their new locations), indicating that memory for colour–location combinations had been updated. Thus, it appears that feature-switch detection errors are caused by a failure to maintain the initially bound representations, probably due to the automatic rewriting and rebinding of memory contents in the face of new perceptual input.

Combined, these results clearly indicate that different methods of probing the contents of visual working memory reveal different aspects of feature binding and feature storage. If the goal is to determine the maximum binding capacity of visual working memory (the number of feature combinations that can be remembered), then cued-recall tasks should be preferred over feature-switch detection. Feature-switch detection introduces an additional load at subsequent stages of visual working memory processing, and thus obscures the maximum encoding capacity of visual working memory.

Although feature-switch detection is not ideal for estimating the binding capacity of visual working memory, the difficulty of feature-switch detection is intriguing in its own right, and is worth exploring further. How is it possible to encode the new colour combinations without detecting feature switches? One possibility is that the feature-switch detection task has a higher capacity demand than the cued-recall tasks. For example, one way to detect a feature switch would be to store all of the preswitch features and all of the postswitch features, and then compare them. This would require the storage of eight total colour–location combinations in the current experiments, which clearly exceeds the estimated upper bounds of visual working memory capacity, which appears to be about four items (Alvarez & Cavanagh, 2004; Luck & Vogel, 1997). In contrast, the cued-recall tasks could be performed by only remembering four colour–location combinations at a time. Another possibility is that encoding information into visual working memory is an automatic process (i.e., does not require active cognitive control), but that the detection of recombinations of features is a less natural task that requires active cognitive control. This additional processing demand could increase the likelihood of errors in the feature-switch detection task. Future work will be required to explore these and other possible explanations for the relative difficulty of maintaining bound object representations when a feature switch occurs.

CONCLUSION

The results indicate that feature-switch detection tasks will underestimate the number of bound objects that can be encoded into memory relative to cued-recall tasks, suggesting that cued-recall is the preferred method for determining the maximal binding capacity of visual working memory. However, the feature-switch detection task appears to strain processes involved with maintaining the contents of working memory (due to rewriting and rebinding of memory contents by new perceptual input), making this task valuable for gaining insight into the fragile nature of working memory for bound object representations. These results could have important implications for understanding the nature of storage and access to bound object representations in visual working memory.

REFERENCES

Allen, R. J., Baddeley, A. D., & Hitch, G. J. (2006). Is the binding of visual features in working memory resource-demanding? *Journal of Experimental Psychology: General*, *135*(2), 298–313.

Alvarez, G. A., & Cavanagh, P. (2004). The capacity of visual short-term memory is set both by visual information load and by number of objects. *Psychological Science*, *15*(2), 106–111.

Atkinson, R. C., & Shiffrin, R. M. (1968). Human memory: A proposed system and its control processes. In K. W. Spence & J. T. Spence (Eds.), *The psychology of learning and motivation: Advances in research and theory* Vol. 2 (pp. 89–195). New York: Academic Press.

Brainard, D. H. (1997). The Psychophysics Toolbox. *Spatial Vision*, *10*, 433–436.

Cousineau, D. (2005). Confidence intervals in within-subject designs: A simpler solution to Loftus and Masson's method. *Tutorial in Quantitative Methods for Psychology*, *1*(1), 42–45.

Cowan, N. (2001). The magical number 4 in short-term memory: A reconsideration of mental storage capacity. *Behavioral and Brain Sciences*, *24*(1), 87–114; discussion 114–185.

Cowey, A. (1985). Aspects of cortical organization related to selective attention and selective impairments of visual attention. In M. I. Posner & O. S. M. Marin (Eds.), *Attention and*

performance XI: Attention and neuropsychology (pp. 41–62). Hillsdale, NJ: Lawrence Erlbaum Associates, Inc.
Gajewski, D. A., & Brockmole, J. R. (2006). Feature bindings endure without attention: Evidence from an explicit recall task. *Psychonomic Bulletin and Review*, *13*(4), 581–587.
Loftus, G. R., & Masson, M. E. (1994). Using confidence intervals in within-subject designs. *Psychonomic Bulletin and Review*, *1*, 476–490.
Luck, S. J., & Vogel, E. K. (1997). The capacity of visual working memory for features and conjunctions. *Nature*, *390*(6657), 279–281.
Mitroff, S. R., Simons, D. J., & Levin, D. T. (2004). Nothing compares 2 views: Change blindness can occur despite preserved access to the changed information. *Perception and Psychophysics*, *66*(8), 1268–1281.
Pashler, H. (1988). Familiarity and visual change detection. *Perception and Psychophysics*, *44*(4), 369–378.
Pelli, D. G. (1997). The VideoToolbox software for visual psychophysics: Transforming numbers into movies. *Spatial Vision*, *10*, 437–442.
Saiki, J. (2002). Multiple-object permanence tracking: Limitation in maintenance and transformation of perceptual objects. *Progress in Brain Research*, *140*, 133–148.
Saiki, J. (2003a). Feature binding in object-file representations of multiple moving items. *Journal of Vision*, *3*(1), 6–21.
Saiki, J. (2003b). Spatiotemporal characteristics of dynamic feature binding in visual working memory. *Vision Research*, *43*(20), 2107–2123.
Saiki, J., & Miyatsuji, H. (2007). Feature binding in visual working memory evaluated by type identification paradigm. *Cognition*, *102*(1), 49–83.
Simons, D. J. (2000). Current approaches to change blindness. *Visual Cognition*, *8*(1/2/3), 1–15.
Simons, D. J., Chabris, C. F., Schnur, T., & Levin, D. T. (2002). Evidence for preserved representations in change blindness. *Consciousness and Cognition*, *11*(1), 78–97.
Smith, J. E. K. (1982). Simple algorithms for M-alternative forced choice calculations. *Perception and Psychophysics*, *31*(1), 95–96.
Stefurak, D. L., & Boynton, R. M. (1986). Independence of memory for categorically different colors and shapes. *Perception and Psychophysics*, *39*(3), 164–174.
Treisman, A. (1996). The binding problem. *Current Opinion in Neurobiology*, *6*(2), 171–178.
Treisman, A. (1998). Feature binding, attention and object perception. *Philosophical Transactions of the Royal Society of London*, *353*(1373), 1295–1306.
Treisman, A., & Schmidt, H. (1982). Illusory conjunctions in the perception of objects. *Cognitive Psychology*, *14*(1), 107–141.
Treisman, A., & Zhang, W. (2006). Location and binding in visual working memory. *Memory and Cognition*, *34*(8), 1704–1719.
Vogel, E. K., Woodman, G. F., & Luck, S. J. (2001). Storage of features, conjunctions and objects in visual working memory. *Journal of Experimental Psychology: Human Perception and Performance*, *27*(1), 92–114.
Vogel, E. K., Woodman, G. F., & Luck, S. J. (2006). The time course of consolidation in visual working memory. *Journal of Experimental Psychology: Human Perception and Performance*, *32*(6), 1436–1451.
Wheeler, M. E., & Treisman, A. M. (2002). Binding in short-term visual memory. *Journal of Experimental Psychology: General*, *131*(1), 48–64.
Wolfe, J. M., Klempen, N., & Dahlen, K. (2000). Postattentive vision. *Journal of Experimental Psychology: Human Perception and Performance*, *26*(2), 693–716.
Zeki, S. (1993). *A vision of the brain*. Oxford, UK: Blackwell.

VISUAL COGNITION, 2009, 17 (1/2), 160–179

Psychology Press
Taylor & Francis Group

Bound feature combinations in visual short-term memory are fragile but influence long-term learning

Robert H. Logie and James R. Brockmole
University of Edinburgh, Edinburgh, UK

Annelinde R. E. Vandenbroucke
University of Amsterdam, Amsterdam, The Netherlands

We explored whether individual features and bindings between those features in VSTM tasks are completely lost from trial to trial or whether residual memory traces for these features and bindings are retained in long-term memory. Memory for arrays of coloured shapes was assessed using change detection or cued recall. Across trials, either the same colour-shape (integrated object) combinations were repeated or one feature was repeated while the other varied. Observers became sensitive to the repetition of bindings, but only if it occurred on every trial. Repetition of single features only led to learning in the cued-recall task, and was weak compared to whole-object repetitions. Results suggest that representations in visual short-term memory comprise integrated objects rather than individual features. These representations are readily displaced by new representations formed on subsequent trials. However, when a given representation is not displaced, longer term residual traces can be generated to support long-term learning, and any learning that does occur is based on integrated objects, not individual features.

Keywords: Visual short-term memory; Feature binding; Learning.

Close your eyes and try to recall the colours of the books on your shelves. It is likely that you can only remember a few, even though you have looked at these books many times since they were placed on the shelf. What is it about our immediate visual environment that we actually learn? In this paper, we

Please address all correspondence to Robert H. Logie, Psychology Department, University of Edinburgh, 7 George Square, Edinburgh EH8 9JZ, UK. E-mail: rlogie@staffmail.ed.ac.uk

This research was supported by British Academy grant SG-43564 awarded to JRB and RHL. This study was conducted while AREV was visiting the University of Edinburgh. We thank Graham Hitch and an anonymous reviewer for helpful comments on a previous version of this paper.

© 2008 Psychology Press, an imprint of the Taylor & Francis Group, an Informa business
http://www.psypress.com/viscog DOI: 10.1080/13506280802228411

attempt to answer this question by examining how the properties of object representations in visual short-term memory[1] (VSTM) constrain learning.

Over the last decade, there has been a debate as to whether VSTM representations comprise primarily integrated objects (e.g., Allen, Baddeley, & Hitch, 2006; Brockmole, Parra, Della Sala, & Logie, 2008; Gajewski & Brockmole, 2006; Johnson, Hollingworth, & Luck, 2008; Luck & Vogel, 1997; Vogel, Woodman, & Luck, 2001) or individual features (e.g., Wheeler & Treisman, 2002; Xu, 2002). The fuel for this debate has been in large part the lack of clarity pertaining to the conditions under which the binding of visual features—such as colour, shape, location, or orientation— occurs. For example, Wheeler and Treisman (2002) proposed that individual features are stored in VSTM automatically, but that the process of binding these features or the maintenance thereof requires extra effort and attention. Gajewski and Brockmole (2006) tested this proposal directly by presenting an exogenous cue during the retention interval that directed attention to a subset of to-be-remembered items. Recall of the features for the cued items was superior to that of uncued items, but the uncued items nevertheless continued to be remembered as integrated wholes: Observers tended to recall all the features of the object or none. Therefore, distracting attention between the study display and the recall probe had no effect on memory for bound features. These results suggest that visual attention is not crucial for maintaining integrated objects in VSTM (see also Yeh, Yang, & Chiu, 2005).

A complementary approach to the same question was taken by Allen et al. (2006), who used a change detection paradigm with arrays of shape–colour combinations. Attention was manipulated through the use of secondary tasks, such as generating random sequences of numbers, during the presentation of both the study and the test arrays. The secondary task load affected overall performance but had no greater effect on memory for bound features than it did on memory for individual features (see also Johnson et al., 2008). Again, attention did not seem to be essential for maintaining bindings. In the same series of experiments, however, they found that memory for the binding of features was poorer when objects were presented in a rapid sequence rather than simultaneously. Memory for individual features did not show this same drop in performance with sequential presentation. Allen et al. concluded that although maintaining bindings in working memory does not appear to require attention or

[1] Many vision researchers use the terms *visual working memory* and *visual short-term memory* interchangeably, whereas researchers in working memory view the latter as comprising one of a range of functions of the former (e.g., Logie & van der Meulen, in press). In this paper, we are primarily concerned with representations stored over the short term (within trials) and long term (across trials), and hence we will refer to visual short-term memory without implying a theoretical contrast with visual working memory.

executive functions, the bindings are vulnerable and items early in the sequence may be overwritten by items later in the sequence.

These studies suggest that as long as an object is represented in VSTM, the maintenance of the feature bindings for that object is largely automatic. However, what happens to these bindings once they are no longer immediately relevant to the task of the observer? In most studies of visual feature binding, the combinations of features are randomly varied from trial to trial, but the pool of features on which these combinations are based typically remains the same throughout the experiment. So, for example, on one trial the stimuli might comprise a red triangle, a blue circle, and a green square each in a specific location. On the following trial, one or more of the same locations might be used for a green circle, a red diamond, and a blue triangle. In order to maintain adequate levels of performance throughout the sequence of trials in an experiment, the bindings formed on one trial would have to break apart to allow the formation of a new set of bindings on the next trial. We are aware of only two studies that have systematically investigated whether or not there is any residual trace of the bindings maintained from trial to trial.

One preliminary, but unpublished, study by Dishon-Berkovits and Treisman (described in Treisman, 2006) examined whether particular colour–shape pairings repeated on 80% of trials can be learned and whether participants subsequently benefit from this learning in a VSTM task. The results showed that participants performed better than chance on a surprise postexperiment questionnaire for the combinations that were shown frequently in the VSTM task, but that the performance on the VSTM task itself did not benefit from repeating the same colour–shape configurations. They concluded that bindings were stored in LTM, but that this information from LTM wasn't used in the VSTM task.

In another study about the learning of bound objects, Colzato, Raffone, and Hommel (2006), asked participants to respond to a particular shape with a keypress. The shapes were paired with colours, and to see whether the binding between the colour and the shape could be learned, some colour–shape configurations were repeated more often than others. Colzato et al. predicted that participants would respond faster for repeated colour–shape pairings than for nonrepeated pairings. This effect was found, even though participants only had to respond to a shape regardless of its colour. However, there was no evidence of better memory for the repeated colour–shape pairings in a subsequent memory test. Colzato et al. therefore concluded that binding and learning mechanisms are independent.

From this work, it therefore appears that there is scant evidence for long-term learning of feature bindings within integrated objects. However, each of these studies is limited in important ways. In the Dishon-Berkovits and Treisman (Treisman, 2006) study, each object was repeated in a different location every time it was shown. It could be that location is an important factor when it comes to feature binding (Treisman & Zhang, 2006) and that no benefit was found in the VSTM task as a result (see also Logie, Brockmole, & Jaswal, 2008). In the Colzato et al. (2006) study only one of the visual features was task relevant and binding was not required, perhaps also leading to a limited ability to detect long-term learning of bindings.

The purpose of the experiments reported here, therefore, was to directly address the extent to which bindings created in VSTM leave a longer term memory trace after they are no longer relevant. In each experiment, we adopted a variant of a technique that is referred to as the Hebb (1961) learning paradigm. This technique has been applied primarily to investigate learning of sequences of numbers, words, or letters, and typically involves presenting sequences that exceed short-term verbal memory span (e.g., 16 item lists) for immediate recall. Unknown to the participant, one particular sequence of items is repeated, for example on every third trial. The usual finding is that recall of these repeated lists gradually improves across repetitions compared with recall of the lists that are novel on all other trials (e.g., Caird, 1964; Cunningham, Healy, & Williams, 1984; Hitch, Fastame, & Flude, 2005; Page, Cumming, Norris, Hitch, & McNeil, 2006). A few studies have used a Hebb-type paradigm to investigate learning of sequences of nonverbal items presented visually (e.g., Couture & Tremblay, 2006; Gagnon, Foster, Turcotte, & Jongenelis, 2004; Page et al., 2006; Turcotte, Gagnon, & Poirier, 2005). As with verbal sequences, all of these studies have shown that when the same sequence of pictures or order of appearance of dots is shown repeatedly on some of the trials, participants show improvement in the recall of the repeated sequence compared with the novel sequences on the interpolated trials. This kind of evidence suggests that, although participants expect a series of novel sequences, nevertheless they retain a trace of each sequence after every trial, allowing a strengthening of the trace every time a particular sequence is repeated.

In studies of feature binding, performance is typically based on simultaneous presentation of multiple objects. Our aim here was to use a version of the Hebb repetition paradigm in which these arrays were presented repeatedly. We present three experiments that explore whether individual features and bindings between those features in VSTM tasks are lost from trial to trial or if they show evidence of learning across trials. Across three experiments, observers were to remember an array of multi-feature objects across short retention intervals. Each experiment used a Hebb-type learning procedure where aspects of these to-be-remembered arrays were consistently repeated across trials. In the *repeat-all* condition, the repeated arrays retained the exact same combinations of shapes, colours and locations (i.e., they were identical). In the *repeat-colour* condition, the repeated arrays were composed of the same combination of colours and locations while the shapes in the display were varied across trials. Finally, in the *repeat-shape* condition the repeated array showed the same combination of shapes and locations while the colours in the display varied across trials. If bindings are robust only until the end of a trial, observers should be insensitive to this repetition and show no increase in memory performance over the course of the experiment. This result would be consistent with the findings of Allen et al. (2006) which indicate that bindings in VSTM are fragile and break apart easily, even if they do not require attention for their maintenance. It would also be consistent with the conclusion drawn by Dishon-Berkovits and Treisman (Treisman, 2006; see also Logie, 1995, 2003; Logie & van der Meulen, in press) for a VSTM store that functions rather separately from LTM. On the other hand, any improvement in performance across trials on which the stimulus array is repeated would suggest that some object information is retained across trials. If learning only occurs for bound objects, performance should only improve when the repeated display consists of exactly the same combinations of colour, shape, and location, but performance would not improve when only one of the features is repeated. This pattern of findings would be consistent with the view that integrated objects rather than individual features form the basis for long-term learning.

EXPERIMENT 1

The purpose of Experiment 1 was to examine whether long-term memory traces of repeatedly presented multifeature objects are generated despite the fragility of bound object representations in VSTM. Observers engaged in a change detection task in which they judged whether two sequentially presented arrays were the same or different. When changes were incorporated into the test array, the features of two objects swapped across locations. Repeat-all, repeat-colour, and repeat-shape trials were blocked and the repetitions occurred on every third trial (see Figure 1). The memory arrays on the two intervening trials were completely novel and none were repeated within the experiment.

Method

Participants. Twelve students from the University of Edinburgh participated and were compensated with £6. In this and subsequent experiments, all participants had normal or corrected-to-normal vision.

Stimuli and apparatus. Stimuli consisted of arrays of six objects positioned every 60° around an imaginary circle with a diameter of 8.8 cm. Each object was created by randomly combining six colours and six shapes without replacement from a set of eight colours (black, blue, cyan,

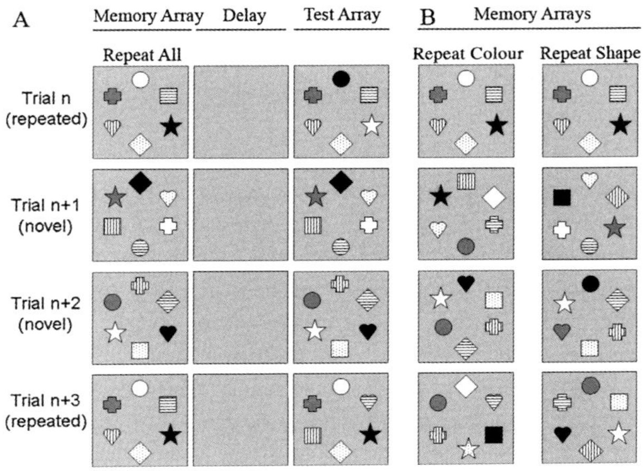

Figure 1. (A) The procedure used in Experiment 1 in the repeat-all condition. On each trial observers judged whether a test array was the same as a memory array. Changes were inserted by swapping either colour (see trial *n*) or shape (see trial *n*+3) features across locations. (B) Example memory arrays used on trials n through *n*+3 of the repeat-colour and repeat-shape conditions. The properties of the delay and test array displays were the same as that illustrated in Panel A. Stimuli were shown in full colour and are not drawn to scale. Experiment 2 used a similar procedure with repetition occurring on every trial.

green, purple, red, white, and yellow) and eight shapes (arrow, circle, diamond, heart, plus, square, star, and triangle). On average, the objects subtended 1.8 cm horizontally and vertically. Stimuli were presented against a grey background on a cathode ray tube (CRT) monitor. Viewing distance was not constrained.

Design and procedure. The experimental procedure is illustrated in Figure 1. To suppress verbal rehearsal, each trial began with the presentation of two digits that the observer vocally repeated throughout the trial. After 1500 ms, a fixation cross appeared for 1000 ms, which was then replaced by the memory display for 200 ms. After a further 2000 ms delay, the test display was presented. On half of the trials, the memory and test displays were identical. On the other half of the trials, changes were made to two of the six objects. On half of these change trials, the colour of two objects were swapped; on the other half of change trials, the shape of two objects were swapped. The test array remained visible until this response was made and the inter trial interval was 2000 ms.

Orthogonal to the no change and change manipulation, two further types of trials were created. A *novel* trial presented a memory array that had not been previously shown in the experiment. A *repeated* trial, however, presented a memory array that contained information that was previously shown to observers. Repeated trials occurred every three trials beginning with the third trial in the experiment (i.e., Trial 3, 6, 9, . . .). The proportion of change and no change trials (see earlier) was the same for both novel and repeated trials.

The experiment was divided into three conditions completed in counter-balanced order across participants. Within each condition the nature of the repeated trials was manipulated. In the *repeat-all block*, repeated memory displays were identical. In the *repeat-colour block*, the same colour-location pairings were used while the shape of each object was randomly selected on each repeated trial. Finally, in the *repeat-shape block*, the shape-location pairings were the same in all repeated memory displays while the colour of each object was randomly selected on each trial. Breaks were provided between each condition, but no information regarding condition structure or the repetition of object information was given to observers. Each condition included 72 trials. The experimental session lasted less than 30 min.

Results and discussion

Change detection performance was analysed with a 2 (repetition) $\times$ 3 (condition) repeated measures ANOVA using both percentage correct and A' as dependent variables. Results are entirely consistent across these measures. No reliable effects were observed (all $F\text{s} < 1$). For novel trials, change detection accuracy averaged 68%, 67%, and 68% ($A' = .76, .77, .75$) in the repeat-all, repeat-colour, and repeat-shape conditions, respectively. For repeated trials, accuracy averaged 68%, 70%, and 67% ($A' = .76, .79, .75$) in the repeat-all, repeat-colour, and repeat-shape conditions, respectively.

The performance levels obtained show that participants could retain visual information within each trial. However, Experiment 1 provided no evidence that the frequent repetition of object information, whether in part or in whole, leads to better change detection performance (cf. Olson & Jiang, 2004; Wolfe, Oliva, Butcher, & Arsenio, 2002). This finding is consistent with the hypothesis that bindings between features are held as temporary representations for the duration of a single trial, but are lost across two intervening trials in a change detection paradigm. That is, each new array displaces any representations of the previous array, and therefore there is no residual trace when the repetition occurs to allow for long-term learning. Therefore, repeating an array on every third trial was insufficient to allow learning even if this frequency of repetition commonly leads to learning in previous studies using the Hebb-type learning paradigm. To explore this possible interpretation of our data, in Experiment 2 we minimized the possible disruption of temporary representations from trial to trial by repeating the same array on every trial. This should maximize the possibilities for learning of feature bindings that lead to improvements in change detection performance.

EXPERIMENT 2

In Experiment 2 we excluded novel trials from the design and repetitions of individual features or of bindings occurred on every trial. This maximized exposure to the repeated arrays (i.e., signal) and minimized any potential distraction from novel arrays (i.e., noise). This provided a scenario in which learning effects within a change-detection task should be optimized. In the absence of novel trials to establish a baseline for comparison, the trial sequence within each condition was divided into three blocks to assess the extent of learning. If observers are sensitive to the across-trial repetition of stimulus information, then change detection accuracy should improve across blocks.

Method

Participants. A new sample of 24 students from the University of Edinburgh participated. They were offered an honorarium of £6. An additional two participants completed the study but were excluded from analysis due to either technical problems or failure to complete the task with above-chance performance.

Stimuli and apparatus. The stimuli and apparatus were the same as in Experiment 1.

Design and procedure. The general procedure replicated that of Experiment 1, except that novel trials were excluded from the design, and the number of trials in each condition (repeat-all, repeat-colour, and repeat-shape) was reduced to 60. The experimental session lasted less than 30 min.

Results and discussion

For analysis, the trial sequence within each condition was divided into three blocks. Change detection performance was analysed with a 3 (condition) × 3 (block) repeated measures ANOVA using both percentage correct and A' as dependent variables (see Figure 2). Results are entirely consistent across these measures and, in the interest of exposition, analyses are only reported for percentage correct.

In contrast to Experiment 1, a main effect of condition was observed, $F(2, 46) = 21.5$, $p < .001$. Planned comparisons demonstrated that performance

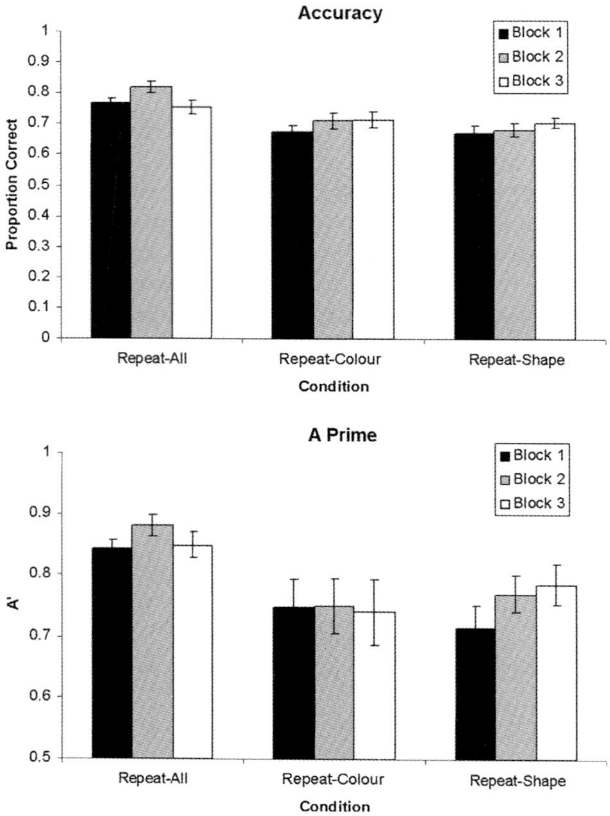

Figure 2. Change detection performance as measured by percentage correct and *A′* across blocks of trials in repeat-all, repeat-shape, and repeat-colour conditions in Experiment 2. Error bars represent standard error.

was better in the repeat-all condition relative to both the repeat-colour, $F(1, 23) = 24.4$, $p < .001$, and repeat-shape blocks, $F(1, 23) = 32.2$, $p < .001$. In addition, within the repeat-all condition, accuracy was reliably superior to that of the novel trials in Experiment 1 ($p < .001$), suggesting that the increased frequency of repetition led to long-term learning when whole objects were repeated from trial to trial. Performance on the repeat-colour and repeat-shape conditions did not differ, $F(1, 23) < 1$, and within both these conditions, performance in Experiment 2 was not reliably different from that on the novel trials in Experiment 1 (colour condition: $p = .42$ shape condition: $p = .94$), suggesting that more frequent repetition did not affect performance in these partial repetition conditions. The main effect of block was not reliable, $F(2, 46) = 1.70$, $p = .20$, nor did the factors interact,

$F(4, 92) = 1.51$, $p = .21$. This lack of an interaction is curious given that performance in the repeat-all condition was superior to that in the repeat-colour and repeat-shape conditions, an effect that one would expect to emerge across trials.

To help resolve this ambiguity and to examine more closely the performance trends in the repeat-all condition over trials, we further decomposed this condition into six blocks of trials ($M = 0.77$, 0.76, 0.79, 0.85, 0.76, and 0.74 in Blocks 1–6, respectively) and analysed change detection performance with a one-way repeated measures ANOVA. The main effect of block was reliable, $F(5, 115) = 2.50$, $p < .05$, and single degree of freedom polynomial tests indicated a reliable quadratic trend in the data, $F(1, 23) = 6.31$, $p < .05$, suggesting that performance improved from Block 1 to Block 4, but declined thereafter. This pattern of performance presents a bit of a puzzle. While the increase in performance across Blocks 1–4 is consistent with learning, what mechanism accounts for the subsequent decline? Although a complete account of this effect is beyond the scope of this paper, we think that it is possible that the diminished repeat-all performance for the later trials may have resulted from a build-up of interference from the varying test arrays on the change trials. However, a post hoc analysis separately comparing change detection accuracy on same and different trials across blocks showed the interaction was not statistically reliable ($F < 1$), so this is a somewhat speculative account, and other explanations may also be possible.

What we can conclude is that Experiment 2 showed some evidence of learning when the study array was repeated on every trial with better overall performance for the repeat-all condition compared to the repeat-colour and repeat-shape conditions in which a set of single features was repeated across trials. This suggests that there is a residual memory trace that carries over from trial to trial, but in contrasting the results of Experiments 1 and 2, it is clear that this learning only occurred when no novel study arrays intervened between repetitions. The fact that learning only occurred for the repeat-all condition also provides evidence consistent with the hypothesis that feature bindings form the VSTM representations used in change detection tasks, and that those bindings can be retained from trial to trial, when no novel arrays intervene. However, the advantage obtained from repeating exactly the same array on every trial was far from dramatic (an increase in accuracy of $< 10\%$), and performance remained well below ceiling even after repeating the same memory array across 60 consecutive trials. Furthermore, the learning effect from repeating the same study array on every trial might not be as robust as suggested from the overall performance levels given that performance started to decline in the repeat-all condition in the last third of the trials. In other words, repeating a stimulus array—even on every trial—yields a very modest impact on change detection performance.

EXPERIMENT 3

The lack of strong evidence from Experiments 1 and 2 that feature bindings are maintained from trial to trial is intriguing, particularly when we consider the evidence from previous studies that feature bindings appear to comprise the representations on which participants base their detection of changes in object arrays. The evidence from Experiments 1 and 2 favours the view that the bindings are maintained for as long as needed and then are discarded in favour of a new set of bindings. However, studies using Hebb-type learning paradigms typically use a measure of recall to test the effect of repetitions, and the limited learning that we observed in Experiment 2, even with repetition on every trial, might stem from our use of change detection to test VSTM (e.g., the test displays which incorporate feature changes on 50% of trials might be a source of interference). Therefore in Experiment 3, we adopted a probed recall procedure (Brockmole et al., 2008; Gajewski & Brockmole, 2006). This also allowed us to look at the impact of repeating stimulus arrays separately on memory for feature bindings and memory for individual features.

Method

Participants. A new sample of 12 University of Edinburgh undergraduate students participated in exchange for course credit.

Stimuli and apparatus. The memory displays were constructed as in Experiments 1 and 2. Memory was probed by placing a white square frame subtending 2 cm at one of the six locations that previously housed an object.

Design and procedure. As in previous experiments, to suppress verbal rehearsal, each trial began with the presentation of two digits that the observer vocally repeated throughout the trial. After 1500 ms, a fixation cross appeared for 1000 ms, which was then replaced by the memory display for 250 ms. After a further 2000 ms delay, a test probe was presented in a location that was previously occupied by one of the objects in the memory display. Observers then ceased repeating digits and verbally reported to the experimenter the colour and shape of the probed item. The test probe remained visible until this response was made and the intertrial interval was 2000 ms. As in Experiments 1 and 2, the experiment was divided into repeat-all, repeat-colour, and repeat-shape conditions, counterbalanced across participants. As in Experiment 2, the experiment employed repeated trials only. Within each condition, each item was probed an equal number of times, and each condition contained 60 trials. The experimental session lasted less than 30 min.

Results and discussion

Separate analyses considered the accuracy (expressed as percentage correct) with which colour and shape combinations were recalled correctly, and the accuracy with which colour or shape were recalled as individual features. In order to assess learning across trials, the 60 trials in each condition were collapsed into three 20-trial blocks.

Feature binding recall. The accuracy of recalling both colour and shape at the probed location was submitted to a 3 (condition) × 3 (epoch) repeated measures ANOVA (see Figure 3a). The main effect of condition was reliable, $F(2, 22) = 20.7$, $p < .001$. Consistent with Experiment 2, feature recall was more accurate in the repeat-all condition than in both the repeat-colour, $F(1, 11) = 43.6$, $p < .001$, and repeat-shape condition, $F(1, 11) = 18.0$, $p < .001$, while performance did not differ between the repeat-colour and repeat-shape conditions, $F(1, 11) = 1.85$, $p = .20$. A main effect of block was also observed, $F(2, 22) = 31.3$, $p < .001$. The factors interacted, $F(4, 44) = 6.65$, $p < .01$. To explore the nature of this interaction we conducted three separate one-way ANOVAs to assess the effect of block within each condition.

In the repeat-all condition, accuracy reliably varied across epochs, $F(2, 22) = 29.4$, $p < .001$. Single degree of freedom polynomial tests revealed both positive-slope linear, $F(1, 11) = 41.7$, $p < .001$. and quadratic trends, $F(1, 11) = 7.48$, $p < .05$. across blocks. Accuracy did not vary reliably across epochs for the repeat-colour, $F < 1$, or the repeat-shape conditions, $F(2, 22) = 1.22$, $p = .32$. These results suggest a strong effect of learning when entire objects are repeated across memory arrays that is absent when only single features are repeated. To obtain a more precise measure of this improvement, we further decomposed the repeat-all condition into six 10-trial blocks ($M = 41\%$, 58%, 72%, 86%, 88%, and 87% in Blocks 1–6, respectively). It is clear from these data that accuracy improved in a linear fashion from Block 1 to Block 4 (on average, accuracy increased 15% per block), after which an asymptotic level of performance (87%) was achieved.

Colour recall. The accuracy of colour recall, regardless of whether or not shape was recalled correctly, was submitted to a 3 (condition) × 3 (epoch) repeated measures ANOVA (see Figure 3b). The main effect of condition was reliable, $F(1, 22) = 20.3$, $p < .001$. Consistent with Experiment 2, feature recall was more accurate in the repeat-all condition than in both the repeat-colour, $F(1, 11) = 20.3$, $p < .001$, and repeat-shape conditions, $F(1, 11) = 44.6$, $p < .001$, while performance did not differ between the repeat-colour and repeat-shape conditions, $F(1, 11) = 2.65$, $p = .13$. A main effect of block was also observed, $F(2, 22) = 23.5$, $p < .001$. Interestingly, however, the

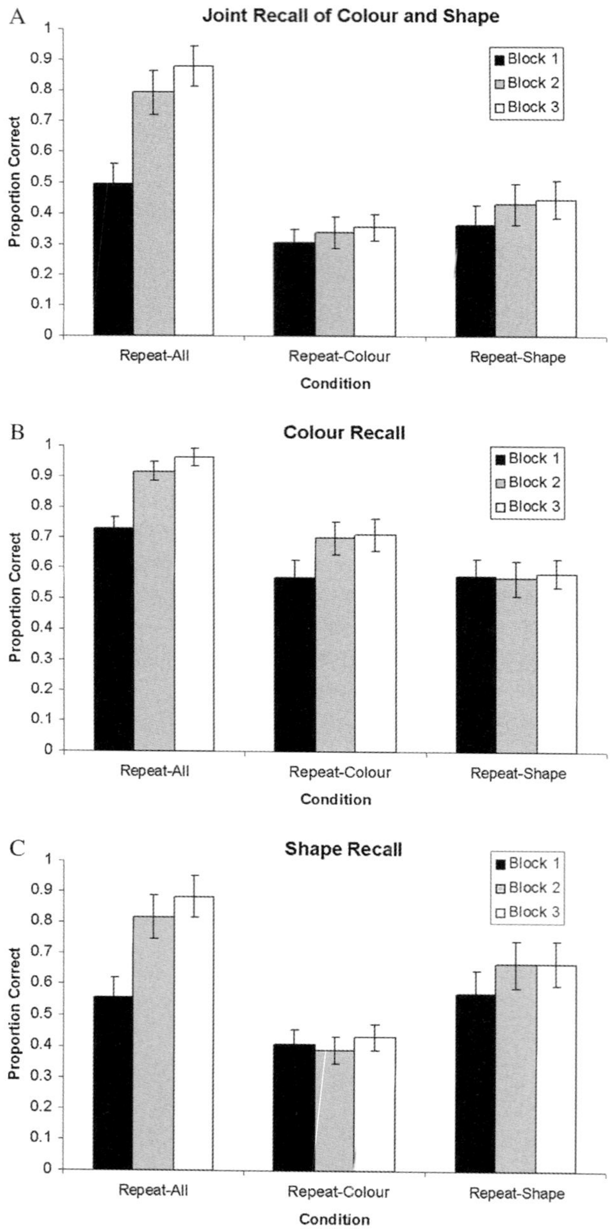

Figure 3. Recall performance across trial blocks in the repeat-all, repeat-colour, and repeat-shape conditions in Experiment 3. (A) Recall of shape and colour combinations. (B) Recall of colour independent of shape. (C) Recall of shape independent of colour. Error bars represent standard error.

factors interacted, $F(4, 44) = 3.41$, $p < .05$. To explore the nature of this interaction we conducted three separate one-way ANOVAs to assess the effect of block within each condition.

In the repeat-all condition, accuracy reliably varied across epochs, $F(2, 22) = 28.4$, $p < .001$. Single degree of freedom polynomial tests revealed both positive-slope linear, $F(1, 11) = 33.1$, $p < .001$, and quadratic trends, $F(1, 11) = 13.3$, $p < .01$, across blocks. In the repeat-colour condition, accuracy also reliably varied across epochs, $F(2, 22) = 28.4$, $p < .001$. This variance was again explained by both positive-slope linear, $F(1, 11) = 8.72$, $p < .05$, and quadratic trends, $F(1, 11) = 6.99$, $p < .05$, across blocks. However, in the repeat-shape condition, no reliable effect of block was observed, $F(2, 22) < 1$. Considering colour recall independent of shape recall, we therefore obtained some evidence that the repetition of a single feature can be learned. However, this rate of learning was smaller (increase in accuracy of 14% over the course of the experiment) compared to cases where both an object's colour and shape repeat across trials (23% increase over the experiment).

Shape recall. The accuracy of shape recall was submitted to a 3 (condition) × 3 (epoch) repeated measures ANOVA (see Figure 3c). The main effect of condition was reliable, $F(1, 22) = 16.6$, $p < .001$. Consistent with Experiment 2, feature recall was more accurate in the repeat-all condition than in both the repeat-colour condition, $F(1, 11) = 37.1$, $p < .001$. The repeat-all condition was not, on average, different from the repeat-shape condition, $F(1, 11) = 2.73$, $p = .13$. Shape recall was reliably better in the repeat-shape condition compared to the repeat-colour condition, $F(1, 11) = 17.8$, $p < .001$. A main effect of block was also observed, $F(2, 22) = 14.6$, $p < .001$. Interestingly the factors interacted, $F(4, 44) = 4.10$, $p < .01$. As with colour recall, to explore the nature of this interaction we conducted three separate one-way ANOVAs to assess the effect of block within each condition.

In the repeat-all condition, accuracy reliably varied across epochs, $F(2, 22) = 21.0$, $p < .001$. Single degree of freedom polynomial tests revealed both positive-slope linear, $F(1, 11) = 27.2$, $p < .001$, and quadratic trends, $F(1, 11) = 7.08$, $p < .05$, across blocks. In the repeat-shape condition, although shape recall improved by 10%, the effect of block was not reliable, $F(2, 22) = 1.24$, $p = .31$. In the repeat-colour condition, no reliable effect of block was observed, $F(2, 22) < 1$. Thus, independent consideration of shape recall provides no evidence that repetition of a single feature leads to robust learning.

Summary

To summarize, when using a probe recall procedure and repeating the complete stimulus array on every trial, improvements in recalling bindings between colour and shape can be obtained across trials. Indeed, performance approaches ceiling, but only after 40 trials. Small effects of learning on recall of colour were found for repeating colours, but there was no equivalent effect on shape. These results are consistent with the hypothesis that bound object representations in VSTM are the primary determinant of long-term learning.

GENERAL DISCUSSION

In the present study, we examined how long-term memory traces for repeatedly presented multifeature objects are generated, and whether these traces are constrained by the representational format of VSTM. Across three experiments, observers were asked to remember an array of coloured shapes across a short retention interval. Previous work has suggested that in such tasks objects are stored in VSTM as integrated, singular, bound units rather than as caches of individual features (Allen et al., 2006; Gajewski & Brockmole, 2006; Johnson et al., 2008; Luck & Vogel, 1997; Vogel et al., 2001). As such, one might expect that bound object representations may serve as the basis for long-term learning. Using a Hebb-type learning procedure, object features were consistently repeated across trials. To the extent that observers are sensitive to this repetition, performance on the short-term memory task should improve over trials. In separate conditions, repetitions involved colour (repeat-colour), shape (repeat-shape), or the combination of colour and shape (repeat-all). If the contents of VSTM constrain learning and learning only occurs for bound objects, performance should only improve when the repeated display consists of exactly the same combinations of colour and shape.

Experiment 1 adopted a change detection paradigm and memory arrays were repeated on every third trial. Change detection performance was well above chance, but was no better on the repeated trials than on the intervening novel trials, suggesting that neither the repetition of individual features nor bindings were learned. By increasing the frequency of repetition to every trial in Experiment 2, change detection performance in the repeat-all condition improved, an effect that was absent in the repeat-colour and repeat-shape conditions. The amount of learning was very modest, however, and was not consistent for the later trials. Much clearer evidence of learning of repeated object information was observed in Experiment 3 in which the study array was presented on every trial and memory was tested using a probed recall method. Learning was most robust when colour–shape bindings were repeated, but developed rather slowly as performance improved linearly over the course of 40 repetitions before reaching asymptote. There was some evidence that repeating a set of colours while varying shape from trial to trial led to modest improvements in colour memory, but there was not an equivalent effect on recalling shape when shape information was held constant across trials.

Collectively, these experiments support the following conclusions. First, our results are broadly consistent with previous demonstrations that bindings in VSTM are fragile as they are susceptible to interference generated by the creation of new multifeature object representations in VSTM (Allen et al., 2006). When novel objects arrays were interleaved between repeated arrays, no learning was obtained. The fact that some learning is possible when repetitions occur on every trial suggests that the fragility arises from overwriting of the contents of VSTM. This result is consistent with the view that VSTM can support temporary representations required for performance on a trial by trial basis, and functions separately from long-term memory.

Second, despite their fragility, feature bindings created in VSTM influence the nature of long-term learning. Due to the complexity of visual objects and the myriad features that define and discriminate them, representations in VSTM combine multiple features into singular object representations. It appears from our experiments that this representational format of VSTM constrains long-term learning about objects and features that we encounter many times. Across experiments, learning effects were generally absent in the repeat-colour and repeat-shape conditions, and when present, they were much smaller than learning effects in the repeat-all conditions. This pattern of data suggests that integrated objects are more likely to be transferred into long-term memory than individual object features.

Third, location might be an important feature of objects. In a study with similarities to our own, Dishon-Berkovits and Treisman (reported by Treisman, 2006) found no evidence that long-term memory for feature bindings improves change detection within trials. However, repeated objects were not always presented in the same spatial location. In contrast, presenting repeated visual features in the same locations on each trial, we did obtain short-term memory benefits from longer term learning, at least for colour-shape conjunctions, in both change detection and cued-recall. Therefore, our data suggest that bound representations that include location along with shape and colour can be the basis for long-term learning, although these results do not suggest that location must be a prerequisite for learning of bindings to occur. Moreover, recent evidence from our own and other laboratories has suggested that if location cannot function as a memory cue, then it does not play any special role in binding once bound object representations are generated in VSTM (Logie et al., 2008; Treisman & Zhang, 2006). The role of location in long-term learning therefore remains an interesting question for future research.

Fourth, although short-term memory and long-term memory may be regarded as separate constructs (e.g., Baddeley, 1986, 2000; Logie, 1995, 2003; Logie & van der Meulen, in press), the present results suggest ways in which they are related. Observers' learning of repeated objects reciprocally benefited short-term memory for those objects. This is consistent with the notion that acquired knowledge can influence short-term visual memory. This is analogous to the well-established finding that verbal short-term memory for letter sequences is better for sequences that resemble real words represented in long-term memory (e.g., Baddeley, 1971). Returning to our own data, the finding that bound objects constrain both VSTM and long-term learning further suggests that VSTM and visual long-term memory share a common representational format. The results of the present study are not, however, consistent with the hypothesis that VSTM is merely a temporarily activated subset of LTM (Anderson, 1983; Cowan, 1995, 1999; Postle, 2007; Ruchkin, Grafman, Cameron, & Berndt, 2003). Performance on the VSTM tasks was well above chance levels even when no evidence for learning was obtained in Experiment 1, and it is extremely unlikely that there were representations in long-term memory of the specific combinations of features used in our experiments that could be used to support performance. Both of these facts suggest that VSTM can operate independently of LTM. Indeed, based on the activated LTM hypothesis, one could reasonably predict that more robust learning should have been present in the single-feature repetition conditions: LTM would hold representations for the individual colours and shapes used in the study, each presentation of a particular colour or shape should lead to repeated activation of those representations, and this in turn should lead to evidence that access to the representations was facilitated across trials. There was some evidence that this might have occurred for colour in Experiment 3, but the evidence for learning was much stronger for representations of feature bindings that would have been encountered for the first time on starting the experiment.

In addition to refining our understanding of the relationship between VSTM and LTM, the current experiments raise new and interesting questions for future research. First, despite identical memory arrays and retention intervals, the strength of long-term learning depended on the manner in which short-term memory was tested with location-cued recall in Experiment 3 resulting in much stronger evidence for long-term learning than did change detection. Why might this have occurred? In general terms, this result suggests that learning is not simply a product of repeated generation of similar VSTM representations, but is also affected by the way in which those representations are subsequently interrogated. With specific reference to the tasks used in this study, one possible explanation for the observed task-discrepancies is that the test displays used in change detection tasks are a source of interference which is not present in the cued recall procedure. Another possibility is that performance in the cued-recall task was driven not only by visual memory for the objects, and the use of location as a cue, but also memory for the verbal responses made during the recall process. Future research will be required to disentangle these (and potentially other) possibilities in an effort to systematically characterize the role of task constraints on the quality of both short- and long-term memory representations.

A second issue for future research concerns the role of explicit memory and awareness in the learning mechanisms tapped in this study. In other visual processing domains such as visual search, researchers have shown that observers become sensitive to target location probabilities as well as repeated covariation between a particular search target and its surrounding context. Several researchers have suggested that these contingencies are represented implicitly in long-term memory (e.g., Chun & Jiang, 1998; Geng & Behrmann, 2005; Walthew & Gilchrist, 2006). The extent to which learning in the change detection and cued recall tasks used in this study depends on explicit memory is therefore an interesting question. Although we did not formally assess the extent to which observers were aware of our manipulations, at the conclusion of each experiment we asked observers whether they noticed anything unusual about the displays. In Experiment 1 (no learning), none of the participants had noticed that certain displays repeated over trials. In Experiment 2 (limited learning), fewer than half of the participants noticed the repetition. In Experiment 3 (robust learning), almost all observers noticed the repetitions. These trends suggest a possible correlation between awareness and learning, and that awareness might arise when there is a residual trace from a previous trial against which the current trial can be compared. If there is no residual trace, then there would be no basis on which to build an awareness of the repetition. However, we were not able to identify any obvious performance differences between observers that were and were not aware of repetitions. A focused and systematic investigation into the role of awareness in the long-term learning of repeated objects is therefore an important avenue for future consideration.

In summary, the results of three experiments suggest that representations in visual short-term memory comprise integrated objects rather than individual features. These representations are readily displaced by new representations formed on subsequent trials. However, when a given representation is not displaced, longer term residual traces can be generated to support long-term learning, and any learning that does occur is based on integrated objects, not individual features.

REFERENCES

Allen, R. J., Baddeley, A. D., & Hitch, G. J. (2006). Is the binding of visual features in working memory resource-demanding? *Journal of Experimental Psychology: General, 135*, 298–313.

Anderson, J. A. (1983). *The architecture of cognition*. Cambridge, MA: Harvard University Press.

Baddeley, A. D. (1971). Language habits, acoustic confusability and immediate memory for redundant letter sequences. *Psychonomic Science, 22*, 120–121.

Baddeley, A. D. (1986). *Working memory*. Oxford, UK: Oxford University Press.

Baddeley, A. D. (2000). The episodic buffer: A new component of working memory? *Trends in Cognitive Sciences, 4*, 417–423.

Brockmole, J. R., Parra, M. A., Della Sala, S., & Logie R. H. (2008). Do binding deficits account for age-related decline in visual working memory? *Psychonomic Bulletin and Review, 15*, 543–547.

Caird, W. K. (1964). Reverberatory activity and memory disorder. *Nature, 201*, 1150.

Chun, M. M., & Jiang, Y. (1998). Contextual cueing: Implicit learning and memory of visual context guides spatial attention. *Cognitive Psychology, 36*, 28–71.

Colzato, L. S., Raffone, A., & Hommel, B. (2006). What do we learn from binding features? Evidence for multilevel feature integration. *Journal of Experimental Psychology: Human Perception and Performance, 32*, 705–716.

Couture, M., & Tremblay, S. (2006). Exploring the characteristics of the visuospatial Hebb repetition effect. *Memory and Cognition, 34*, 1720–1729.

Cowan, N. (1995). *Attention and memory: An integrated framework*. Oxford, UK: Oxford University Press.

Cowan, N. (1999). An embedded-process model of working memory. In A. Miyake & P. Shah (Eds.), *Models of working memory* (pp. 62–101). New York: Cambridge University Press.

Cunningham, T. F., Healy, A. F., & Williams, D. M. (1984). Effects of repetition on short-term retention of order information. *Journal of Experimental Psychology: Learning, Memory, and Cognition, 10*, 575–597.

Gagnon, S., Foster, J. K., Turcotte, J., & Jongenelis, S. (2004). Involvement of the hippocampus in implicit learning of supra-span sequences: The case of SJ. *Cognitive Neuropsychology, 21*, 867–882.

Gajewski, D. A., & Brockmole, J. R. (2006). Feature bindings endure without attention: Evidence from an explicit recall task. *Psychonomic Bulletin and Review, 13*, 581–587.

Geng, J. J., & Behrmann, M. (2005). Spatial probability as an attentional cue in visual search. *Perception and Psychophysics, 67*, 1252–1268.

Hebb, D. O. (1961). Distinctive features of learning in the higher animal. In J. F. Delafresnaye (Ed.), *Brain mechanisms and learning* (pp. 37–51). Oxford, UK: Blackwell Scientific Press.

Hitch, G. J., Fastame, M. C., & Flude, B. (2005). How is the serial order of a verbal sequence encoded? Some comparisons between models. *Memory, 13*, 247–258.

Johnson, J. S., Hollingworth, A., & Luck, S. J. (2008). The role of attention in the maintenance of feature bindings in visual short-term memory. *Journal of Experimental Psychology: Human Perception and Performance, 34*, 41–55.

Logie, R. H. (1995). *Visuo-spatial working memory*. Hove, UK: Lawrence Erlbaum Associates Ltd.

Logie, R. H. (2003). Spatial and visual working memory: A mental workspace. In D. Irwin & B. Ross (Eds.), *Cognitive vision: The psychology of learning and motivation* (Vol. 42, pp. 37–78). San Diego, CA: Elsevier Science.

Logie, R. H., Brockmole, J. R., & Jaswal, S. (2008). Feature binding in visual working memory is unaffected by task-irrelevant changes of location, shape and color. *Manuscript submitted for publication.*

Logie, R. H., & van der Meulen, M. (in press). Fragmenting and integrating visuo-spatial working memory. In J. R. Brockmole (Ed.), *The visual world in memory*. Hove, UK: Psychology Press.

Luck, S. J., & Vogel, E. W. (1997). The capacity of visual working memory for features and conjunctions. *Nature, 390*, 279–281.

Olson, I. R., & Jiang, Y. (2004). Visual short-term memory is not improved by training. *Memory and Cognition, 32*, 1326–1332.

Page, M. P., Cumming, N., Norris, D., Hitch, G. J., & McNeil, A. M. (2006). Repetition learning in the immediate serial recall of visual and auditory materials. *Journal of Experimental Psychology: Learning, Memory, and Cognition, 32*, 716–733.

Postle, B. R. (2007). Activated long-term memory? The basis of representation in working memory. In N. Osaka, R. H. Logie, & M. D'Esposito (Eds.), *The cognitive neuroscience of working memory* (pp. 333–349). Oxford, UK: Oxford University Press.

Ruchkin, D. S., Grafman, J., Cameron, K., & Berndt, R. S. (2003). Working memory retention systems: A state of activated long-term memory. *Behavioral and Brain Science, 26*, 709–728.

Treisman, A. M. (2006). Object tokens, binding, and visual memory. In H. D. Zimmer, A. Mecklinger, & U. Lindenberger (Eds.), *Handbook of binding and memory: Perspectives from cognitive neuroscience* (pp. 315–338). Oxford, UK: Oxford University Press.

Treisman, A. M., & Zhang, W. (2006). Location and binding in visual working memory. *Memory and Cognition, 34*, 1704–1719.

Turcotte, J., Gagnon, S., & Poirier, M. (2005). The effect of old age on the learning of supraspan sequences. *Psychology and Aging, 20*, 251–260.

Vogel, S. J., Woodman, G. F., & Luck, S. J. (2001). Storage of features, conjunctions, and objects in visual working memory. *Journal of Experimental Psychology: Human Perception and Performance, 27*, 92–114.

Walthew, C., & Gilchrist, I. D. (2006). Target location probability effects in visual search: An effect of sequential dependencies. *Journal of Experimental Psychology: Human Perception and Performance, 32*, 1294–1301.

Wheeler, M. E., & Treisman, A. M. (2002). Binding in short-term visual memory. *Journal of Experimental Psychology: General, 131*, 48–64.

Wolfe, J. M., Oliva, A., Butcher, S. J., & Arsenio, H. C. (2002). An unbinding problem? The disintegration of visible, previously attended objects does not attract attention. *Journal of Vision, 2*, 256–271.

Xu, Y. (2002). Limitations in object-based feature encoding in visual short-term memory. *Journal of Experimental Psychology: Human Perception and Performance, 28*, 458–468.

Yeh, Y.-Y., Yang, C.-T., & Chiu, Y.-C. (2005). Binding or prioritization: The role of selective attention in visual short-term memory. *Visual Cognition, 12*, 759–799.

VISUAL COGNITION, 2009, 17 (1/2), 180–194

Psychology Press
Taylor & Francis Group

Feature binding in attentive tracking of distinct objects

Tal Makovski

Department of Psychology, University of Minnesota, Minneapolis, MN, USA

Yuhong V. Jiang

Department of Psychology, and Center for Cognitive Sciences, University of Minnesota, Minneapolis, MN, USA

To what degree can attentive tracking of objects' motion benefit from increased distinctiveness in the objects' surface features? To address this question, we asked observers to track four moving digits among a total of eight moving digits. By varying the distinctiveness of the digits' colour and identity, we found that tracking performance improved when the eight objects were all distinct in colour, digit identity, or both, compared to when the eight objects were identical. However, when the eight objects were distinct in a combination of colour and digit but targets and nontargets shared colour or digit identity, performance enhancement was not observed. Four follow-up experiments extended the range of the feature dimensions generating the effect and ruled out alternative strategic accounts. We conclude that surface features can be used to enhance tracking performance. This enhancement is feature based, revealing a limited degree of feature binding in attentive tracking.

Keywords: Multiple-object tracking; Attentive tracking; Feature and location binding.

The dynamics of the visual environment pose a significant challenge to human vision. How do we maintain a sense of temporal continuity in a constantly changing environment? One solution to this computational problem is to track objects as they move. Motion tracking is easily achieved when a single object must be tracked, or when the tracked objects differ from the other objects in a salient visual feature. Tracking becomes increasingly difficult when multiple objects are to be tracked among visually similar nontargets (Pylyshyn & Storm, 1988). In this study we investigate the degree

---

Please address all correspondence to Tal Makovski, N218 Elliott Hall, 75 East River Road, Minneapolis, MN 55455, USA. E-mail: tal.makovski@gmail.com

This research was supported in part by NSF 0733764 and NIH 071788. We thank Leah Watson, Khena Swallow, Carrick Williams, Todd Horowitz, and James Brockmole for comments and suggestions.

© 2008 Psychology Press, an imprint of the Taylor & Francis Group, an Informa business
http://www.psypress.com/viscog DOI: 10.1080/13506280802211334

to which attentive tracking can benefit from distinctiveness in object features. We asked observers to track a subset of moving chromatic digits and measured their performance as a function of the objects' distinctiveness in colour, digit identity, and the combination of colour and digit identity. The results are informative of feature binding in attentive tracking. In this introduction, we review the current state of knowledge on this topic and identify a critical gap.

Standard multiple-object tracking tasks have deprived participants of the opportunity to use identity information. In Pylyshyn and Storm's (1988) original paradigm, observers are shown a field of identical objects. A subset of these objects is designated as tracking targets during a cue period, after which the targets and nontargets are identical in shape and surface features. Tracking is accomplished by processing where the targets are and by updating each target's location as it moves. Object identity plays no role in this paradigm.

Although it seems that the standard multiple-object tracking task is unrepresentative of everyday visual activity where moving objects are usually distinct, there are several reasons why identity information has rarely been incorporated (with the exception of a few studies reviewed here). First, spatiotemporal properties are used predominantly when visual continuity must be established. Infants rely primarily on spatiotemporal continuity, rather than shape or colour constancy, to track objects after brief occlusions. At the age of 10 months, infants were not surprised when a toy truck moved behind an occluder and reemerged as a toy duck (Xu & Carey, 1996). Infants also did not treat two objects that differ in surface properties as separate objects until the objects started to move independently (Spelke, Gutheil, & van de Walle, 1995). The heavy reliance on spatiotemporal properties was also observed in visually deprived individuals who recovered vision as adults. These individuals also initially relied heavily on motion continuity to segregate a visual scene and only later incorporated surface properties such as colour or shape discontinuity (Sinha, 2007).

Normal human adults also appear to prefer spatiotemporal information to identity information in updating visual objects. For example, in the object reviewing paradigm (Kahneman, Treisman, & Gibbs, 1992), two letters (e.g., A and B) were presented inside two squares positioned at the 3 and 9 o'clock locations. The letters then disappeared while the squares moved clockwise to the 6 and 12 o'clock locations. After the motion, a probe letter was displayed for participants to name as quickly as possible. Participants were faster to name a formerly presented letter if it appeared in its original square rather than in the other square. Kahneman et al. proposed that spatiotemporal continuity served to maintain the integrity of "object files", allowing participants to update object information after motion. Interestingly, object updating appears to rely primarily on spatiotemporal continuity. In a similar paradigm, if the two letters initially appeared against blue and green background and later the background switched colours, performance in reporting the previewed letters was unaffected (Mitroff & Alvarez, 2007).

Another reason why researchers have focused primarily on tracking "where" rather than "what" is because the use of identity information in multiple-object tracking is highly limited. When objects with different shapes were used and tracking was occasionally interrupted by a question about the characteristics of a target, observers accurately reported the target's direction and speed, but had difficulty reporting its shape (Scholl, Pylyshyn, & Franconeri, 1999). Further evidence that "what" is poorly bound to "where" comes from a study by Pylyshyn (2004), who presented different digits, one in each circle in the cue period for participants to remember. The digits were taken away before the circles began to move. At the end of the motion period, participants were asked to select the target circles and to report the digit originally presented in each circle. This paradigm bears some similarity to Kahneman et al.'s (1992) object updating task, except that there were more objects (eight vs. two moving objects), more identities (four vs. two), more complex motion, and an explicit instruction to bind what with where. Although participants in Kahneman et al.'s paradigm were able to update the identity of two objects after a brief rotation of the placeholders, those in Pylyshyn's (2004) more complex task were unable to do so. Even when they successfully tracked the target circles, memory for the associated digit identities was poor. Similar failures of "what-to-where" binding have been observed when participants tracked objects with apparent, rather than continuous, motion (Saiki, 2003).

Although the binding of what to where is difficult in attentive tracking, some degree of binding has been demonstrated when distinct objects are used for tracking, and when participants are explicitly required to bind what to where. The multiple-identity tracking task usually presents observers with a small number of objects and designates either a subset or the entire set for tracking. Unlike Pylyshyn's (2004) task where the distinct identities are presented only during the cue period, in the multiple-identity tracking task objects are always distinct in shape or colour for the entire tracking period. At the end of the motion period, all objects are masked. One of the locations is then probed for observers to retrieve the associated object identity (Oksama & Hyönä, 2004, 2008). Observers' limited ability to bind identities to locations was dependent upon the speed and number of targets.

Horowitz et al. (2007) employed a further modification of the multiple-identity tracking task, investigating whether distinctive identities are addressable during tracking. Participants were asked to track cartoon animals (e.g., a tiger, a leopard) that moved in straight lines. The unique identities of the animals remained on the screen during tracking. At the end of the tracking period the animals hid behind cactuses. Observers were asked to report either the location of all the targets (*standard* question) or the location of a specific animal (*specific* question). Horowitz et al. found that the estimated capacity was higher when answering the standard question than when answering the specific question, with a capacity estimate of about one object in the specific question. From these data Horowitz et al. concluded that "what" information is accessible during tracking, but only to a limited degree. Consistent with this idea, tracking performance was higher when the moving animals were distinct rather than identical to one another (2007, Exp. 5).

The main goal of the present study is to investigate the extent to which attentive tracking can be enhanced by distinctiveness in object identities. Horowitz et al. (2007) showed that tracking performance is higher when distinct, rather than homogeneous, objects must be tracked. However, their use of cartoon animals makes it difficult to dissociate the role of visual distinctiveness from semantic or name distinctiveness. In addition, it is difficult to isolate the visual features that contribute to tracking of distinct objects observed by Horowitz et al. To understand how object features are integrated with their location during tracking, it is necessary to test tracking of visual objects made of identifiable features.

We conducted a series of five experiments using coloured digits (or coloured shape/orientation) to study how distinctiveness in features or conjunction of features affects attentive tracking. In this paper, we report one of the experiments in full and describe briefly the other experiments that provide converging support for the main findings. In the main experiment, we used an array of coloured digits and asked participants to track a subset of those objects. Unlike the multiple-identity tracking task, participants of the present study were not required to remember object identities. Tracking can be achieved entirely by updating the motion trajectories of objects without remembering their identities. Importantly, we manipulated the objects' distinctiveness. The objects could be distinct in one or two features (e.g., all have different colours) or in a combination of features (e.g., the conjunction of colour and shape made all objects unique). We also tested whether all objects or only the target subset needs to be distinct to facilitate tracking.

Consider two conditions shown in Table 1: The homogeneous condition and the colour-distinct condition, where participants tracked four out of eight objects that were either homogeneous or distinct in colour. Motion trajectory tracking is sufficient for both conditions. If spatiotemporal continuity is the only source of information for attentive tracking, then performance should be comparable between the homogeneous and colour-distinct conditions. In contrast, if distinctiveness in colour is also used to separate targets from nontargets, then performance may be superior in the colour-distinct condition. Similar predictions can be made when comparing

TABLE 1
A schematic illustration of tracking objects used in Experiment 1 (to view this table in colour, please see the online issue of the Journal)

Stimuli type	*# of colours*	*# of digits*	*Targets*	*Nontargets*
Homogenous	1	1	**1, 1, 1, 1**	**1, 1, 1, 1**
Colour-distinct	8	1	**3, 3, 3, 3**	**3, 3, 3, 3**
Digit-distinct	1	8	**2, 4, 5, 7**	**1, 3, 6, 8**
Both-distinct	8	8	**1, 5, 7, 8**	**2, 3, 4, 6**
Conjunction-distinct	4	4	**2, 3, 4, 6**	**2, 3, 4, 6**
Colour-paired	4	1	**4, 4, 4, 4**	**4, 4, 4, 4**
Digit-paired	1	4	**1, 2, 4, 7**	**1, 2, 4, 7**
Conjunction-paired	4	4	**2, 3, 4, 6**	**2, 3, 4, 6**

the homogeneous condition with the digit-distinct condition. Furthermore, the distinctiveness in both colour and digit may convey an added advantage in the both-distinct condition. Thus, the comparison of the homogeneous condition with the colour-distinct, digit-distinct, and both-distinct conditions informs us whether featural information is helpful for tracking when the task does not require identity memory. An advantage in the feature distinct conditions may imply that participants can bind a feature with a moving location.

Now consider the conjunction-distinct condition, where the eight objects were made distinctive because they were distinct in the combination of colour and digit shape. For instance, a target object, such as a blue 3, is the only object that is blue in colour and is "3" in shape. In terms of features, it shares with a distractor (e.g., a blue 4) in colour and with another distractor (e.g., a green 3) in digit identity. If the advantage conveyed by tracking distinct objects over tracking homogeneous objects operates upon a colour-digit integrated object, then it should also enhance performance in the conjunction-distinct condition. In contrast, if the advantage for tracking distinct objects emerges primarily from distinguishing features that are not fully integrated together, then the conjunction-distinct condition may not yield superior performance to the homogeneous condition.

Whether distinctiveness in the conjunction of two features helps attentive tracking is an interesting question not addressed previously. When objects are static, binding of separate features to form an integrated object is easily achieved. Indeed, extensive research has shown that visual attention and visual working memory operate on the basis of integrated objects (Duncan, 1984; Scholl, 2001). For example, participants can remember all four colours and all four orientations as well as remembering only four colours or only four orientations, as long as the colours and orientations conjoin to form four coloured oriented lines (Luck & Vogel, 1997). Feature binding may become much more difficult in attentive tracking, however, where objects are moving and where a subset of objects is not actively attended (Pylyshyn, 1989; but see Cavanagh & Alvarez, 2005). In turn, the conjunction-distinct condition may produce performance similar to one of the paired conditions, where targets and distractors share featural information (see Table 1, colour-paired, digit-paired, and conjunction-paired). Sample trials can be viewed online at http://jianglab.psych.umn.edu/MOTdigits/MOTdigits.htm

In short, by comparing performance in the different identity-distinct conditions with the homogeneous condition, this study informs us how feature binding operates in attentive tracking.

METHOD

Participants

All participants were volunteers from the University of Minnesota between 18 and 33 years old. They all had normal colour vision and normal or corrected-to-normal visual acuity. Twenty participants took part in the main experiment.

Equipment

Participants were tested individually in a room with normal interior lighting. They sat approximately 57 cm away from a 19-inch computer monitor. The experiment was programmed with psychophysical toolbox (Brainard, 1997; Pelli, 1997) implemented in MATLAB (www.mathworks.com).

Stimuli

The moving objects were coloured digits (each fit within a $1.5^\circ \times 1.5^\circ$ imaginary square) presented against a black background. There were eight possible colours (red, green, blue, yellow, orange, azure, white, and pink) and eight possible digits (1–8). The colours and digits were randomly sampled according to a trial's condition.

Procedure

Participants were tested in eight conditions with 15 trials each, presented in a randomly intermixed order. All conditions used similar trial sequences. Participants pressed the spacebar to initiate each trial. Eight coloured digits were presented at randomly selected locations within an imaginary presentation window of 21° × 21°. Four of the objects were surrounded by white frames (1.9° × 1.9°), which identified their status as tracking targets. After 1330 ms, the frames disappeared and the objects started moving randomly within the presentation window. The objects moved at a constant speed of 21.9°/s, bounced off the "wall" of the presentation window, and repelled one another when a minimal centre-to-centre distance of 2.1° was reached. Participants were asked to track the cued targets and were encouraged to maintain central fixation during tracking. After the objects moved for 7 s and stopped, they all turned to white disks (1.5° in diameter). Participants were asked to click on the four targets. The correctly selected targets turned green while the missed targets turned red to provide feedback for 1 s.

Design

The eight conditions differed in the distinctness of identity (Table 1). All eight objects were identical in the homogenous condition (e.g., they were all red 2s); the exact colour and digit identity was randomly selected on each trial of that condition.

There were four "distinct" conditions. The eight objects were uniform in digit identity but distinct in colour in the colour-distinct condition (e.g., they were all 4s, but in eight different colours). The objects were the same in colour but distinct in digit identity in the digit-distinct condition (e.g., they were all red, but in eight different digit identities). Or the objects were distinct in both colour and digit identity in the both-distinct condition (e.g., all eight digits and all eight colours were used in random combination). The conjunction-distinct condition involved distinct objects produced by the conjunction of four colours and four digits. In this condition, no two objects were the same in the combination of colour and digit, but a given target (e.g., a blue 3) always shared colour with one of the distractors (e.g., a blue 4) and digit identity with another distractor (e.g., a green 3).

Finally, there were three "paired" conditions in which all four targets were distinct and all four distractors were distinct, but each of the targets was the same as one of the distractors. In the colour-paired condition, for instance, all objects were the same in digit identity, but the four targets were distinct in colour, and the four distractors were distinct in colour, and a target always shared a distractor's colour. Similarly, in the digit-paired condition, the targets and distractors were paired in digit identity but each subset was distinct. In the conjunction-paired condition, the targets and distractors were paired in both digit identity and colour, but each subset was distinct. Note that the conjunction-paired condition included four digits and four colours which were paired to make one target identical to one distractor. The conjunction-distinct condition also included four digits and four colours; however, the features were combined such that all eight objects were distinct in colour-digit combination.

RESULTS

Figure 1 depicts mean tracking accuracy as a function of stimulus condition in the main experiment.

Homogeneous versus distinct identities

Does distinctiveness in feature identities enhance tracking? We addressed this question by comparing performance in the homogeneous, colour-distinct, digit-distinct, and both-distinct conditions using a repeated-measures ANOVA. Distinctiveness in colour enhanced performance, $F(1, 19) = 14.60$, $p < .01$, as did distinctiveness in digit identity, $F(1, 19) = 6.70$, $p < .05$. The interaction between colour distinctiveness and digit distinctiveness was marginally significant, $F(1, 19) = 3.20$, $p = .09$, as the two factors were slightly underadditive. Pairwise *t*-tests showed that each of the three feature-distinct conditions was significantly higher in accuracy than the homogeneous condition, all $ps < .001$. These results clearly showed that attentive tracking was influenced by objects' distinctive identities, even when participants were not required to remember what the objects were (see also Horowitz et al., 2007).

Did the enhancement from distinct identities extend to a condition where the objects were distinct in terms of a combination of colour and digit, but not in colour or digit alone? Our results clearly showed that it did not. To the contrary, the conjunction-distinct condition had significantly lower accuracy than the homogeneous condition, $t(19) = 3.30$, $p < .004$. The accuracy of the

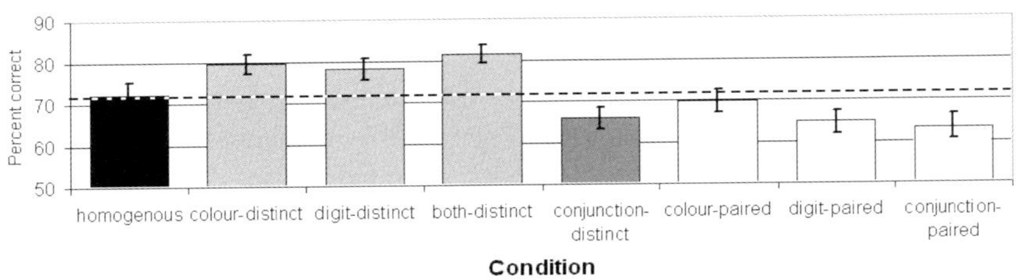

Figure 1. Tracking accuracy as a function of stimulus conditions (error bars show ±1 standard error of the mean). The dashed line represents performance in the homogenous condition.

conjunction-distinct condition was also significantly lower than any of the three feature-distinct conditions, all $ps < .001$.

Homogeneous versus paired identities

The three paired conditions were designed such that objects had distinct features within each subset, but one target was always identical to one distractor. In these cases, tracking on the basis of distinct identity (e.g., a red 7) can only help distinguish between different targets, or between each specific target and three of the distractors. It does not help distinguish a target and its paired distractor. Our results showed that accuracy in the paired condition was lower than the accuracy in the homogeneous condition. The impairment was significant in the digit-paired condition, $t(19) = 4.10$, $p < .001$, and the conjunction-paired condition, $t(19) = 5.40$, $p < .001$, but was insignificant in the colour-paired condition, $t(19) = 1.60$, $p > .10$. These results suggest that the advantage afforded by distinguishing the target from other targets or from three of the distractors was outweighed by the disadvantage of confusing the target with an identical distractor.

Conjunction-distinct versus conjunction-paired

Both the conjunction-distinct and the conjunction-paired conditions were produced by conjoining four colours with four digits to form eight objects. The only difference was that the combination of digits and colours produced eight distinct objects in the former but four pairs of target–distractor in the latter. Does distinctiveness in feature conjunction produce any advantage in the former? No, the conjunction-distinct condition was not significantly better than the conjunction-paired condition, $t(19) = 1.30$, $p > .20$.

FOLLOW-UP EXPERIMENTS

In addition to the main experiment, we conducted four control experiments to verify the generality of the results. The control experiments were similar in procedure to the main experiment, so we included a brief description of the methods and results. Descriptive statistics and p-values for these experiments are provided in Table 2. Our main focus was to show that objects distinct in feature conjunction (but not in single features) are not tracked better than homogeneous objects.

TABLE 2

Mean percentage correct in the four control experiments (standard error in parenthesis). The *p*-values correspond to the *t*-tests comparing each condition with the homogenous condition

Control experiment	*Homogeneous*	*Colour-distinct*	*Shape-distinct*	*Both-distinct*	*Conjunction-distinct*	*Colour-paired*	*Shape-paired*	*Conjunction-paired*
1. Variable trial duration	73 (4)	83 (4)	78 (5)	79 (5)	65 (5)	73 (4)	68 (5)	70 (5)
		$p = .03$	$p = .02$	$p = .09$	$p = .02$	$p = .93$	$p = .17$	$p = .40$
2. Blocked design	70 (4)	78 (4)	79 (4)	77 (4)	68 (4)	N/A	N/A	N/A
		$p = .02$	$p < .01$	$p = .04$	$p = .42$			
3. Novel shapes	80 (3)	86 (3)	82 (3)	87(3)	80 (3)	76 (3)	79 (3)	78 (3)
		$p < .01$	$p = .22$	$p < .01$	$p = .57$	$p = .03$	$p = .50$	$p = .21$
4. Line orientations	70 (5)	77 (4)	69 (5)	77 (5)	71 (5)	71 (6)	73 (5)	69 (6)
		$p < .01$	$p = .62$	$p < .01$	$p = .43$	$p = .41$	$p < .01$	$p = .57$

Control Experiment 1: Variable trial duration

The unpredictable trial duration was used to discourage participants from using a strategy of not tracking until the final moments of a trial.[1] Seven participants were tested in this experiment which was a replication of the main experiment, except that the duration of tracking was unpredictable. Each trial ended after 3.0, 3.8, 4.9, 6.3, or 8.0 s of motion. Similar to the main experiment, each distinctiveness condition contained 15 trials, divided randomly and evenly into the five possible trial durations. The basic pattern of results (Table 2) was the same as the main experiment: Distinctness in features enhanced performance but distinctness in a combination of features did not. Compared with the homogeneous condition, accuracy was enhanced in the colour-distinct and digit-distinct conditions, $ps < .03$, but impaired in the conjunction-distinct condition, $p < .02$.

Control Experiment 2: Blocked design

This experiment was designed to investigate whether effects of feature and conjunction distinctiveness held with a blocked (rather than mixed) design. Eleven participants were tested using coloured digits as in the main experiment. They completed five conditions presented in separate blocks of trials; the order of blocks was randomized. The conditions were homogeneous, colour-distinct, digit-distinct, both-distinct, and conjunction-distinct. There were 15 trials in each condition. Blocking the distinctive conditions did not produce an advantage in the conjunction-distinct condition compared with the homogeneous condition ($p > .40$), which was significantly lower in accuracy than the feature-distinct conditions ($ps < .05$).

Control Experiment 3: Colour and novel shapes

Thirteen participants were tested in this experiment where digits were replaced by novel shapes that were difficult to name. Otherwise the experiment was identical to the main experiment. Again, the results were qualitatively similar to those of the main experiment. Distinctiveness in a combination of features failed to facilitate performance compared with the homogeneous condition, $p > .55$.

---

[1] We thank Todd Horowitz for suggesting this possibility.

Control Experiment 4: Colour and line orientations

Line orientation is a simple visual feature that may be better integrated with colour than digits or novel shapes.[2] Ten participants were tested in this experiment where eight oriented lines (20–160° in units of 20°) replaced the digits. Still, the use of two simple features (colour and line orientation) did not change the results. The conjunction-distinct condition again did not yield higher accuracy than the homogeneous condition, $p > .43$.

DISCUSSION

Everyday visual experience suggests that we track moving objects not only on the basis of their motion trajectories but also on the basis of their surface features. Our study confirms this intuition. Attentive tracking of a subset of moving objects was more accurate when all objects were distinct in colour or digit identity than if they were identical in colour and digit identity. The enhancement by distinctive features was confined to conditions where at least a single feature differentiated all objects, as when all objects had different colours, but not when a combination of features differentiated all objects. In addition, even when the targets were distinct from one another, tracking was not enhanced if the distractors shared the targets' colours or digit identities. Four follow-up experiments demonstrated the robustness of these effects by ruling out strategic biases (Control Experiments 1–2) and by extending the range of the dimensions generating the effect (Control Experiments 3–4). Together these findings have significant implications for feature binding in attentive tracking.

First, the finding that distinctiveness in features enhances tracking apparently contradicts previous results, where participants were found to have poor memory for surface properties in a multiple-object tracking task (Scholl et al., 1999). Indeed, trying to remember object identities may actively interfere with the ability to track (Fougnie & Marois, 2006). The discrepancy can be accounted for by an important difference between our study and the previous studies. Namely, we did not require participants to remember object identities. If we had stopped our participants occasionally to probe their memory of object identities, we might also have observed poor performance. Nonetheless, distinctiveness in features may help segregate targets from nontargets, a critical component of attentive tracking (Yantis, 1992).

We also found that performance was impaired in the paired-identity conditions compared with the homogeneous condition, a finding that was

[2] We thank Todd Horowitz for this suggestion. Digits, rather than orientations, were used in the main experiment because the eight digits were more distinctive than the eight orientations.

observed in one but not another of Horowitz et al.'s (2007) experiments. The effect was not always statistically reliable (Table 2), but it had been observed several times (see also Makovski & Jiang, 2008). The impairment was somewhat surprising because the paired-identity conditions were more distinctive than the homogeneous condition, as each object was distinctive in feature from all but one other object. One might expect that distinctiveness would enhance, rather than impair, performance in the paired-identity condition. In a subsequent study, we found that the impairment for paired conditions was observed only when the paired condition was randomly intermixed in presentation with the distinct and homogeneous conditions (Makovski & Jiang, 2008). Testing these conditions in separate blocks of trials removed impairment in the paired condition. Our current conclusion is that the use of identity information in multiple-object tracking is not obligatory, but is under strategic control. A tendency to rely on identity was also applied to the paired condition when trials were randomly intermixed, because identity information helped performance on distinct trials. This strategy sets up a competition between two types of perceptual grouping: Grouping on the basis of attentional set (tracking targets vs. nontargets), and grouping on the basis of surface features (red objects vs. green objects, and so on). The competition from feature grouping impaired the effectiveness of attentional grouping. Competition for the two kinds of grouping cannot explain the lack of a benefit in the conjunction-distinct condition, however, as blocking conditions did not facilitate its performance compared with the homogeneous condition.

The results of the current study clearly demonstrate that feature rather than conjunction distinctiveness enhances tracking performance. Does this benefit reflect improved tracking abilities, or that distinctiveness provides additional information for recovering lost targets (Horowitz et al., 2007)? On the one hand, tracking ability may be directly improved because observers can tolerate closer distance between a target and a distractor when they have distinct identities. On the other hand, identity information may be held in a separate system, such as visual working memory, which allows participants to recover a lost target. To disassociate these possibilities, in a recent study we asked participants to track distinct objects whose colour changed once every 260 ms (Makovski & Jiang, 2008). The objects were always distinct from one another at any given moment, but the continuity of identity information over time was destroyed. In this setup, participants could no longer track the distinct condition better than the homogeneous condition. These data are more consistent with the second hypothesis, which asserts that identity information is kept in a system (e.g., visual working memory) that operates in parallel to motion tracking.

Even though features held in visual working memory are typically considered to be bound together to form coherent objects (Luck & Vogel,

1997), our results suggest that they are not properly conjoined during attentive tracking. Distinctiveness in feature-conjunction would have produced as much advantage as distinctiveness in features had they have been properly conjoined. Apparently, motion made such feature binding more difficult to retain, probably because the basis for binding—shared location (Treisman, 1988)—is no longer a perceptually stable property.

In summary, we have shown that multiple-object tracking is sensitive to the distinctness in object identities, even in a task where identity memory is never probed. The enhancement is largely feature based, revealing a limited degree of feature binding in attentive tracking.

REFERENCES

Brainard, D. H. (1997). The Psychophysics Toolbox. *Spatial Vision, 10*(4), 433–436.

Cavanagh, P., & Alvarez, G. A. (2005). Tracking multiple targets with multifocal attention. *Trends in Cognitive Sciences, 9*, 349–354.

Duncan, J. (1984). Selective attention and the organization of visual information. *Journal of Experimental Psychology: General, 113*(4), 501–517.

Fougnie, D., & Marois, R. (2006). Distinct capacity limits for attention and working memory: Evidence from attentive tracking and visual working memory paradigms. *Psychological Science, 17*(6), 526–534.

Horowitz, T. S., Klieger, S. B., Fencsik, D. E., Yang, K. K., Alvarez, G. A., & Wolfe, J. M. (2007). Tracking unique objects. *Perception and Psychophysics, 69*(2), 172–184.

Kahneman, D., Treisman, A., & Gibbs, B. J. (1992). The reviewing of object files: Object-specific integration of information. *Cognitive Psychology, 24*(2), 175–219.

Luck, S. J., & Vogel, E. K. (1997). The capacity of visual working memory for features and conjunctions. *Nature, 390*(6657), 279–281.

Makovski, T., & Jiang, Y. V. (2008). The role of visual working memory in attentive tracking of unique objects. *Manuscript submitted for publication.*

Mitroff, S. R., & Alvarez, G. A. (2007). Space and time, not surface features, guide object persistence. *Psychonomic Bulletin and Review, 14*(6), 1199–1204.

Oksama, L., & Hyönä, J. (2004). Is multiple object tracking carried out automatically by an early vision mechanism independent of higher-order cognition? An individual difference approach. *Visual Cognition, 11*, 631–671.

Oksama, L., & Hyönä, J. (2008). Dynamic binding of identity and location information: A serial model of multiple-identity tracking. *Cognitive Psychology, 56*(4), 237–283.

Pelli, D. G. (1997). The VideoToolbox software for visual psychophysics: Transforming numbers into movies. *Spatial Vision, 10*(4), 437–442.

Pylyshyn, Z. W. (1989). The role of location indexes in spatial perception: A sketch of the FINST spatial index model. *Cognition, 32*, 65–97.

Pylyshyn, Z. W. (2004). Some puzzling findings in multiple object tracking: I. Tracking without keeping track of object identities. *Visual Cognition, 11*(7), 801–822.

Pylyshyn, Z. W., & Storm, R. W. (1988). Tracking multiple independent targets: Evidence for a parallel tracking mechanism. *Spatial Vision, 3*, 179–197.

Saiki, J. (2003). Feature binding in object-file representations of multiple moving items. *Journal of Vision, 3*(1), 6–21.

Scholl, B. J. (2001). Objects and attention: The state of the art. *Cognition, 80*(1–2), 1–46.

Scholl, B. J., Pylyshyn, Z. W., & Franconeri, S. L. (1999). When are featural and spatiotemporal properties encoded as a result of attentional allocation? *Investigative Ophthalmology and Visual Science*, *40*(4), S797.

Sinha, P. (2007). *From fragments to objects: Mechanisms of visual integration*. Paper presented at the 2007 Summer Institute on the Visual Perception and Cognition conference, Minneapolis, MN.

Spelke, E., Gutheil, G., & van de Walle, G. (1995). The development of object perception. In D. Osherson (Ed.), *Invitation to cognitive science: Vol. 2. Visual cognition* (2nd ed., pp. 297–330). Cambridge, MA: MIT Press.

Treisman, A. (1988). Features and objects: The 14th Bartlett Memorial Lecture. *Quarterly Journal of Experimental Psychology: Human Experimental Psychology*, *40A*(2), 201–237.

Xu, F., & Carey, S. (1996). Infants' metaphysics: The case of numerical identity. *Cognitive Psychology*, *30*(2), 111–153.

Yantis, S. (1992). Multielement visual tracking: Attention and perceptual organization. *Cognitive Psychology*, *24*, 295–340.

VISUAL COGNITION, 2009, 17 (1/2), 195–211

Psychology Press
Taylor & Francis Group

Staying in bounds: Contextual constraints on object-file coherence

Stephen R. Mitroff
Department of Psychology and Neuroscience, Center for Cognitive Neuroscience, Duke University, Durham, NC, USA

Jason T. Arita
Department of Psychology, Vanderbilt University, Nashville, TN, USA

Mathias S. Fleck
Department of Psychology and Neuroscience, Center for Cognitive Neuroscience, Duke University, Durham, NC, USA

Coherent visual perception necessitates the ability to track distinct objects as the same entities over time and motion. Calculations of such object persistence appear to be fairly automatic and constrained by specific rules. We explore the nature of object persistence here within the object-file framework; object files are mid-level visual representations that track entities over time and motion as the same persisting objects and store and update information about the objects. We present three new findings. First, objects files are constrained by the principle of "boundedness"; persisting entities should maintain a single closed contour. Second, object files are constrained by the principle of "containment"; all the parts and properties of a persisting object should reside within, and be connected to, the object itself. Third, object files are sensitive to the context in which an object appears; the very same physical entity that can instantiate object-file formation in one experimental context cannot in another. This contextual influence demonstrates for the first time that object files are sensitive to more than just the physical properties contained within any given visual display.

Please address all correspondence to Stephen R. Mitroff, Center for Cognitive Neuroscience, Duke University, Box 90999, Durham, NC 27708-0999, USA. E-mail: mitroff@duke.edu

For helpful conversation/comments, we thank Jim Brockmole, Tao Gao, Robert Gordon, John Henderson, Andrew Hollingworth, Brian Scholl, Mowei Shen, anonymous reviewers, and the members of the Duke Visual Cognition Lab. We thank Melissa Bulkin, Ricky Green, Katie Grant, and Tina Liang for help with data collection. This research was supported by NIH grant R03 MH080849 from the National Institute of Mental Health.

© 2008 Psychology Press, an imprint of the Taylor & Francis Group, an Informa business
http://www.psypress.com/viscog DOI: 10.1080/13506280802103457

As we move about the world and as the world moves about us, we readily track objects as being the same entities from one moment to the next. This invaluable skill underlies our ability to interact with our environment without constantly recreating a representation of every entity. In principle, such object tracking could be carried out by continuously comparing a series of individual visual snapshots (Michels, Saxena, & Ng, 2005) or by storing previous exposures to individuals or groups across an entire encounter (Rosencrantz, Gordon, & Thrun, 2003). However, while these are viable computer vision strategies, they would be an overwhelming proposition for the human brain. Rather than using brute force to achieve the perception of persisting objecthood, our visual system uses several heuristics to both optimize and simplify processing. Yet, much remains unknown about what heuristics are used, how they are used, and when they are used.

A powerful framework within which to reason about and test these issues of object persistence is the *object-file theory* (Kahneman, Treisman, & Gibbs, 1992). "Object files" are episodic, visual representations that store and update information about specific objects and track the objects over time and motion via spatiotemporal information. Object files are thought to be a critical mid-level of visual representation that can track an entity's persisting identity without relying upon either low-level surface features (e.g., colour, shape) or higher level information (e.g., type or category). For example, take the classic American movie line "It's a bird, it's a plane ... It's Superman." Despite changes in low-level information (e.g., a size change as Superman moves closer) and in higher level categorization (e.g., switching from bird to plane), the *it* remains the same—there is never any doubt as to how many objects are present (Kahneman et al., 1992).

The object-file theory has gained empirical support through the *object-reviewing paradigm* wherein specific information presented on a given object is later processed more rapidly when it is presented again on the same object as opposed to on a different object, even if the objects have moved (Kahneman et al., 1992). That is, when the information is initially bound to a specific object, processing of that information at a later time is speeded when the binding is maintained. In a modified version of the object-reviewing paradigm (e.g., Kruschke & Fragassi, 1996; Mitroff & Alvarez, 2007; Mitroff, Scholl, & Noles, 2007; Mitroff, Scholl, & Wynn, 2004, 2005; Noles, Scholl, & Mitroff, 2005; see Figure 1), subjects first view a display containing at least two objects (e.g., two simple frames). Preview information is then briefly presented in each object (e.g., a letter is presented within each frame). After the preview information disappears, the objects move about the display. A final target item (e.g., a letter) is then displayed in one of the objects and subjects are asked to make a speeded response as to whether it is the same as any of the preview items or whether it is novel to that trial. Typically, subjects are quicker to respond when the target item reappears on

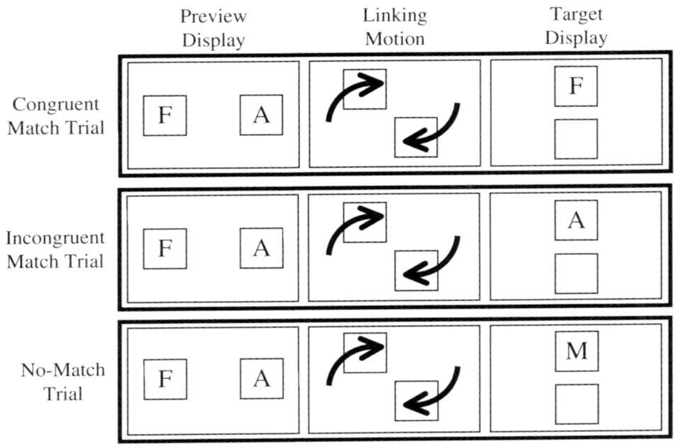

Figure 1. Depiction of the congruent match, incongruent match, and no-match conditions of the object-reviewing paradigm. Faster response times are typically found on congruent than on incongruent match trials and this difference represents the object-specific preview benefit (OSPB). Figures are not drawn to scale and only depict one motion direction and one target letter location.

the same object it was previewed on compared to when it reappears on a different object. This response time benefit has been termed the *object-specific preview benefit* (OSPB). The motion serves to decouple the initial spatial location from object-specific information; thus the OSPB is thought to arise from the preview information being stored in, or bound with, the persisting object-file representation as opposed to a location.

An initial wave of object-file research focused on the nature of an object file's contents (e.g., Kahneman et al., 1992; Gordon & Irwin, 1996, 2000; Henderson, 1994; Henderson & Anes, 1994), establishing that object identity can be maintained in an abstract format. For example, one study found significant OSPBs even if the preview and target items differed in format from words to pictures (Gordon & Irwin, 1996). More recently, object-file research has examined the rules that guide how object files are constructed, maintained, and destroyed (e.g., Mitroff & Alvarez, 2007; Mitroff et al., 2004, 2005; Noles et al., 2005). For example, object files were found to be sensitive to the principle of *cohesion*; to be tracked over time and motion as the same entity, an object should continuously maintain both a single contour and its status as a single unit (Mitroff et al., 2004). When an object split apart into two, the OSPBs for the two resulting objects were significant, but also significantly reduced in magnitude compared to the OSPB from intermixed control trials wherein objects did not undergo a cohesion violation. Thus the cohesion violation of the splitting object played an important role in the object-file maintenance, but perhaps not an "all-or-none" role. An open and important question that remains is to what extent such rules guide object-file processing.

To date, it has been suggested that object-file processing is influenced by the rule of cohesion (Mitroff et al., 2004) and perhaps the rule of *solidity*, that objects can't pass through other objects (Mitroff et al., 2005). Prior infant cognition research directly inspired these suggestions and raises the possibility that other such principles might guide object files. Developmental work has explored whether specific principles constrain how young infants interact with objects in the world around them (e.g., Cheries, Mitroff, Wynn, & Scholl, 2008; Spelke, 1990; Spelke, Kestenbaum, Simons, & Wein, 1995; Wang, Baillargeon, & Paterson, 2005). For example, using looking time procedures, Spelke et al. (1995) found that young infants expect objects to move along continuous paths—objects cannot move from one location to another without traversing the intermediate region. Such principles have also been linked to the adult object-file literature (e.g., Carey & Xu, 2001; Feigenson, Carey, & Hauser, 2002; Richardson & Kirkham, 2004; Scholl & Leslie, 1999). As such, exploring additional developmentally inspired rules in adult mid-level vision provides a natural continuation of this research enterprise.

CURRENT STUDY

In the current paper, we address two previously unexplored rules in the adult object-file literature: *Boundedness*—that an object must have a single continuous boundary, and *containment*—that the properties of the object must be located within the boundaries of the object itself. By exploring these two potential object-based constraints we aim to further establish the rules of how information is bound into object-file representations. As will be addressed in the General Discussion, our investigation into boundedness and containment has also given rise to an intriguing effect—the results suggest that the *context* in which an object is encountered influences the "goodness" of the object for object files; the very same physical entity that can instantiate object-file formation in one experimental context cannot in another context. We explore the contribution of context by assessing boundedness and containment in two different experimental procedures. In the intermixed condition, trials containing bounded objects (see Figure 2) are randomly interleaved with trials containing unbounded objects (likewise for containment in Experiment 2). In the pure condition, only trials with unbounded objects are presented (again, likewise for containment in Experiment 2). If the general context within which a stimulus is presented affects object-file processing, we should see a difference between the intermixed and pure conditions. This is exactly what we found and it

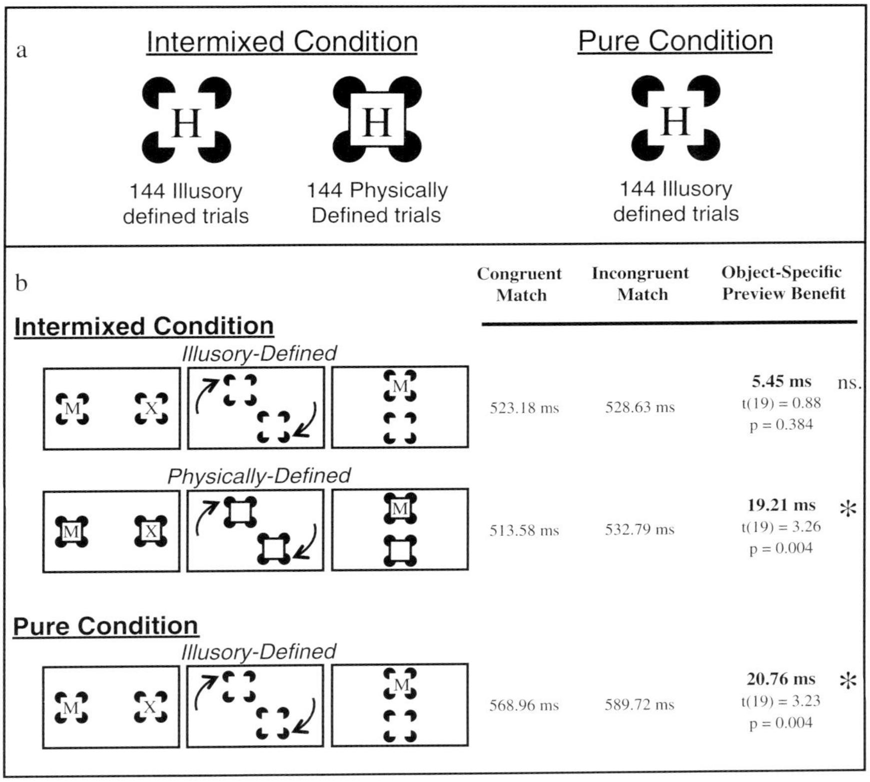

Figure 2. The (a) stimuli and (b) response times of Experiment 1.

represents a sharp deviation from existing lines of research that have focused specifically on the role of visual characteristics for object files.

EXPERIMENT 1: THE ROLE OF BOUNDEDNESS

Previous investigations have found that the principle of cohesion influences what the adult mid-level visual system will consider the same object over time and motion (Mitroff et al., 2004). Yet, why exactly such cohesion violations disrupt object files remains an open question. On one hand, the deleterious effects of a cohesion violation could stem from the breaking of an already established boundary or the instantiation of a new object. On the other hand, the mere presence of an ambiguous boundary at any point during the object tracking process could result in such disruptions. Here we address this open question by exploring the principle of boundedness—that an entity must have and maintain a single continuous boundary. Must an object be "bounded" to be represented as a true object and to be tracked over time and motion as the same? This is an intriguing topic of enquiry since both prior infant (e.g., Xu, 1997) and adult (e.g., Marino & Scholl, 2005) research has suggested that boundedness can influence object perception. However, it remains unclear how this specific constraint influences object-file calculations and object tracking.

To address the role of boundedness for object files, we use an especially apt visual stimulus—objects constructed with illusory contours (e.g., Kanizsa, 1955/1987; see Figure 2). Objects defined by illusory contours behave much like objects defined by physical contours, and evidence suggests they are completed early and automatically in visual processing (e.g., Davis & Driver, 1994; Smith & Over, 1977; von der Heydt, Peterhans, & Baumgartner, 1984). Since illusory-defined objects do not have a single, continuous boundary, they provide an ideal stimulus for exploring the role of boundedness in object persistence, allowing us to compare the viability of object-file processing for "objects" with and without physical boundaries.

Methods

Participants. Forty members of the Duke University community participated for either payment or course credit (20 in each of the intermixed and pure conditions).

Apparatus and stimuli. The experiment was presented on a Macintosh G4 computer with a 19-inch monitor, programmed with customized software utilizing the VisionShell Graphics Library (Comtois, 2006). Subjects sat approximately 55 cm from the monitor without head restraint. The objects in the "illusory-defined" trials consisted of four equally spaced black notched discs (0.86 deg in diameter) that were aligned inwards creating a Kanizsa-like illusory square that subtended 3.44 deg^2 (see Figure 2). The objects in the "physically defined" trials were identical with the addition of a thin black line (0.17 deg) connecting the discs, creating a physically connected square. Letters were drawn in a black monospaced font subtending 1.72 deg and were centrally presented within an object. Unique preview letters were assigned randomly on each trial from the set [F,H,M,Q,U,X] and the target letter was either one of the preview letters or a novel letter from the same set.

Procedures. Each trial began when subjects pressed the spacebar with their left hand. A "preview" display would appear with two objects horizontally aligned, 4.25 deg to the left and right of centre. A single preview letter appeared in each object for 500 ms. The letters were then removed and the objects traversed a circular path (50% clockwise) for 1000 ms such that they stopped 4.25 deg above and below centre. A single target letter was then presented within one of the two objects (50% of the time in the top object) and subjects were to make a speeded response as to whether it was the same as *either* of the two previously displayed letters (pressing "1" for match and "2" for no match). The target display remained until the response. On 50% of the trials the target letter did not match either of the two preview letters (no-match trials). Of the remaining match trials, 50% of the time the target letter reappeared in the same object in which it was initially displayed (congruent match trials) and 50% of the time it reappeared in the object which initially contained the other preview letter (incongruent match trials).

Subjects participated in one of two experimental conditions. The intermixed condition contained 144 illusory-defined trials and 144 physically defined trials, with trials randomly intermixed. A given trial always contained either two illusory-defined objects or two physically defined objects throughout. That is, there was never a mix of object types within a single trial. The pure condition contained 144 illusory-defined trials. Prior to the experiment, subjects completed 20 practice trials that mirrored their experimental condition.

Results

The subjects were highly accurate on the match/no-match task for both the intermixed ($M = 96.46\%$, $SD = 2.54\%$) and pure conditions ($M = 96.44\%$, $SD = 2.26\%$; see Table 1). Trials with a response time greater than 2000 ms were removed from analyses (0.10% and 0.73% trials removed for intermixed and pure, respectively). All further analyses were conducted only on trials with a response time within 2 *SD*s of each individual subject's global mean (removal of 4.11% and 4.32% of the trials for intermixed and pure) and with a correct response.

The primary measure of interest was the difference in response time between the congruent match trials (when the target letter reappeared in the same object in which it was originally previewed in) and incongruent match trials (when the target letter reappeared in the object it was *not* previewed in). This response time difference represents the object-specific preview benefit (OSPB)—a processing advantage beyond general display-wide priming for information that had previously been associated with a specific object file (Kahneman et al., 1992). The OSPB serves as an operational definition of object persistence such that finding a significant OSPB demonstrates that the object was perceived as the same persisting

TABLE 1
Accuracy and response times (with standard errors) for Experiments 1 and 2 by condition and trial type

		Experiment 1: Boundedness			*Experiment 2: Containment*		
		Intermixed		*Pure*	*Intermixed*		*Pure*
		Illusory defined	*Physically defined*	*Illusory defined*	*Outside trials*	*Inside trials*	*Outside trials*
Accuracy	Congruent match	97.08%	95.42%	95.56%	95.14%	95.83%	96.53%
	Incongruent match	95.42%	92.50%	94.58%	94.58%	94.58%	95.69%
	No match	97.57%	98.06%	97.36%	97.78%	97.92%	98.61%
Response time	Congruent match	523.18 ms (18.15 ms)	513.58 ms (18.95 ms)	568.96 ms (21.50 ms)	545.28 ms (17.14 ms)	537.15 ms (14.89 ms)	545.54 ms (23.59 ms)
	Incongruent match	528.63 ms (17.09 ms)	532.79 ms (16.73 ms)	589.72 ms (21.81 ms)	549.13 ms (13.82 ms)	561.09 ms (18.77 ms)	558.35 ms (25.10 ms)
	No match	536.70 ms (19.96 ms)	531.41 ms (18.79 ms)	581.94 ms (24.20 ms)	538.89 ms (15.94 ms)	553.35 ms (16.63 ms)	571.77 ms (26.24 ms)

entity across the trial. As shown in Figure 2, the intermixed condition revealed a significant OSPB of 19.21 ms for the physically defined trials, $t(19) = 3.26$, $p = .004$, yet no significant OSPB (5.45 ms) for the illusory-defined trials, $t(19) = 0.88$, $p = .384$. The pure condition, which consisted solely of illusory-defined trials, did however reveal a significant OSPB of 20.76 ms, $t(19) = 3.23$, $p = .004$; see Yang, 2006, for similar results with "pure" trials). The OSPB for the illusory-defined trials from the pure condition was marginally significantly different from that of the intermixed condition, $t(18) = 1.78$, $p = .091$. The illusory-defined trials produced a significant OSPB when presented in isolation (pure condition) but not when presented in the context of physically defined trials (intermixed condition).

How bounded are unbounded illusory contours?

The differences between the intermixed and pure conditions suggest that illusory-defined objects do not underlie object-file processing as well as physically defined objects. However, an important question is whether illusory-defined, modally completed entities should even be considered "objects". We address this before discussing the implications of this study via an additional experiment. Here we pit illusory-defined objects against entities constructed of the same elements that do not give rise to a subjective object. Twenty new subjects participated in an experiment identical to the intermixed condition described above where half the trials were the illusory-defined trials previously described with pac-men facing each other to create an illusory square and the other half of the trials had the same pac-men rotated 180 deg so each was facing away from the centre. Subjects reported seeing an illusory square when the pac-men faced inwards but not when they faced outwards. The inwards facing, illusory-defined, trials revealed an OSPB of 11.98 ms (congruent and incongruent match mean RTs = 595.19 ms and 607.17 ms, respectively), $t(19) = 2.06$, $p = .053$. However, the outwards facing, nonillusory-defined, trials did not produce a significant OSPB (1.83 ms; congruent and incongruent match mean RTs = 609.44 ms and 611.27 ms, respectively), $t(19) = 0.16$, $p = .867$. Any concern over the relative visibility of the preview and target letters between the inwards and outwards facing trials due to physical differences is alleviated by identical performance in accuracy ($M = 96.91\%$ and 96.28%, respectively) and in no-match trial RT (612.54 ms and 613.89 ms, respectively). The results suggest that the illusory-defined trials in Experiment 1 do represent object-based processing—the mere grouping of inducing elements into a coherent entity is not as sufficient as an "object" in producing object-specific preview effects.

Discussion

Objects constructed of illusory contours do not always underlie the formation and/or maintenance of object files. This is quite surprising given that illusory contours are processed early in visual perception and that the stimuli in this experiment adhered to several strong grouping cues that have previously been shown to underlie object tracking (e.g., vanMarle & Scholl, 2003; Yang, 2006). Since the only difference between the illusory- and physically defined objects was the lack of a physical boundary, these results suggest that the developmentally inspired rule of *boundedness* may in fact influence adult computations of object persistence. Importantly, it is not the case that the illusory-defined objects can never support object files—they did produce a significant OSPB when presented in isolation with no physically defined objects presented in the experiment. Thus boundedness may be an important rule for forming and/or maintaining object persistence, but not always a necessary rule. An intriguing outcome of this study is that the *context* in which illusory-defined objects are presented (in isolation vs. intermixed with physically defined objects) can impact whether or not object-file representations are instantiated. We return to this issue of context in the General Discussion after first exploring the principle of containment in Experiment 2.

EXPERIMENT 2: THE ROLE OF CONTAINMENT

Experiment 1 provided two findings—object files are sensitive to the principle of boundedness and this sensitivity can be modulated by contextual information. Here we look to further explore the role of context by investigating the independently important question of whether or not object files are sensitive to the principle of *containment*—that an object's features must be located within the boundaries of the object itself for it to be tracked over time and motion as a single persisting entity. Containment has been explored in the developmental literature (e.g., Hespos & Baillargeon, 2001; Wang et al., 2005) but has yet to be explored in the adult object persistence literature. As well, we also hope to provide converging evidence for Experiment 1's intriguing implication that the object-file system is sensitive to contextual information.

Methods

Participants. Forty members of the Duke University community participated for either payment or course credit (20 in each of the intermixed and pure conditions).

Apparatus, stimuli, and procedures. The experimental paradigm was identical to Experiment 1 except for the following. The objects in the "inside" trials were outlined squares (2.87 deg^2, 0.17 deg frame thickness) and had the preview and target letters drawn at their centre. The "outside" trials were identical to the inside trials except the letters were drawn 2.87 deg to the left of each object's centre (see Figure 3). Subjects in the intermixed condition completed 144 inside trials randomly intermixed with 144 outside trials. Subjects in the pure condition completed 144 outside trials.

Results and discussion

As for Experiment 1, the subjects were highly accurate on the match/no-match task for both the intermixed ($M = 98.61\%$, $SD = 2.25\%$) and pure

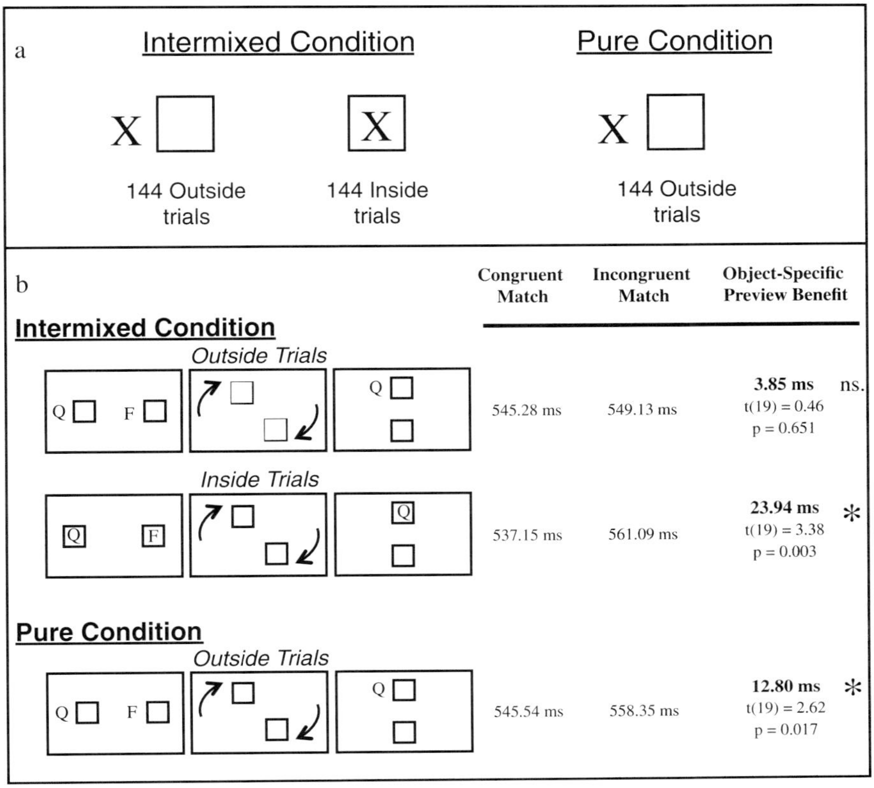

Figure 3. The (a) stimuli and (b) response times of Experiment 2.

conditions ($M = 97.27\%$, $SD = 3.02\%$; see Table 1). Outlying data were removed using the criteria described in Experiment 1: Trials were removed with a response time over 2000 ms (0.38% and 0.43% for intermixed and pure, respectively) and for a response time over 2 *SD*s from the individual subject's mean (4.46% and 4.43% removed for intermixed and pure, respectively). As depicted in Figure 3, the intermixed condition revealed a significant OSPB of 23.94 ms for the inside trials, $t(19) = 3.38$, $p = .003$, yet no significant OSPB (3.85 ms) for the outside trials, $t(19) = 0.46$, $p = .651$. However, in the pure condition, there was a significant OSPB of 12.80 ms for the outside trials, $t(19) = 2.62$, $p = .017$.

The intermixed condition of Experiment 2 provides the first evidence that the principle of *containment* can affect object-file calculations. When the preview and target letters were simply moved outside the objects, the corresponding object files were attenuated such that they failed to produce a significant OSPB. This offers a surprisingly specific adherence to the principle of containment since an OSPB was found when all other aspects of the display were identical except that the letters appeared inside the objects. This finding also highlights the fact that object files are not driven solely by a simple association between the preview information and the objects in the displays; such an association would predict no difference between the inside and outside trials.

However, the object file adherence to containment appears to be contingent upon the nature of the objects present in the experiment since the outside trials did produce a significant OSPB in the pure condition. Beyond the theoretical implications that will be discussed in the General Discussion, the pure condition also serves to alleviate concerns that simple, atheoretical differences between the inside and outside displays may be driving the intermixed trial results. It is not that the outside trials (those violating containment) can never underlie object files, it is that they do not successfully do so in the context of more canonical object relationships.

GENERAL DISCUSSION

Three novel findings are presented here. First, object files, episodic mid-level visual representations that bind identity information to visual objects, are sensitive to the principle of boundedness—objects without complete closure do not support object files as well as objects with complete closure. Second, object files are influenced by the principle of containment—objects without all of their identifying information residing within their physical boundaries do not support object files as well as objects that do contain all their parts. Third, the global context created by the types of objects presented across an experiment can modulate the influence of these two principles. We discuss the broader impact of these issues in turn.

Object file rules

The current findings combine with past work to suggest that distinct principles can guide the formation and maintenance of object files. The influence of these principles on object-file processing mirrors infant cognition research; when entities violate certain principles of persisting objecthood, infants do not treat those entities as "real" objects (e.g., Chiang & Wynn, 2000; Huntley-Fenner, Carey, & Solimando, 2002). For example, young infants have specific expectations about the qualitative and quantitative properties of objects hidden behind occluding surfaces: Wynn (1992) found that when infants are shown two objects placed behind a screen, they expect there to be two items when the screen is removed. However, Huntley-Fenner et al. (2002) found no such expectations with piles of noncohesive sand.

Each principle tested within the object-file framework to date (cohesion, boundedness, containment, and solidity) has been explored with young infants and has been found to directly guide how infants reason about persisting objecthood. As such, it will be highly beneficial for both fields to explore other developmentally inspired principles in adult mid-level vision (e.g., object support; Needham & Baillargeon, 1993) and to re-explore these principles with infants. For example, based upon the findings of Mitroff et al. (2004), Cheries et al. (2008) returned to the principle of cohesion in infants and found that even very simple cohesion violations could disrupt infants' ability to track objects through occlusion.

The contingency of object file rules

An important aspect of both of the current experiments is that they suggest a contingency to how object files obey specific rules—violations of boundedness and containment adversely affect object files, but not in every situation. The illusory-defined and outside trials produced significant OSPBs when presented in isolation but not when intermixed with the physically defined and inside trials. It remains an open question whether this contingency takes a graded form or an all-or-none form; object files might be formed for the illusory-defined and outside objects but formed to a lesser degree, or not at all, for the violation trials in the intermixed conditions. Previous findings suggest adherence to the cohesion rule is graded—when objects split into two, the resulting objects produced significant but attenuated OSPBs (Mitroff et al., 2004). Work outside the object-file literature has also demonstrated a graded aspect to object-based effects. For example, visual attention can spread through a single object more efficiently when the object obeys the boundedness principle; object-based attention effects can be found for entities lacking closure (Avrahami, 1999), but the effects are enhanced for bounded objects (Marino & Scholl, 2005). The current findings cannot distinguish the exact nature of this contingency, but they do raise several important issues about contextual influences on object files.

Context affects object files

The context within which an object is presented influences the degree to which its object-file representation adheres to specific rules. For example, the rule of boundedness had no clear influence when unbounded objects were presented in isolation but a strong effect when those same unbounded objects were seen in the context of bounded objects. Few object files are maintained at any given moment (Kahneman et al., 1992) so perhaps when less-than-ideal entities are seen in the context of canonical objects, resources are withheld so they can be reserved for the more legitimate objects. This would suggest that object files are not restricted to the "here-and-now" of any given situation since they can be affected by prior information. Note also that the contextual effects operated temporally over the experiment—objects that violated the boundedness or containment principles were never presented in the same visual array as objects that did not violate these principles.

Does context affect perception, attention, or memory? The present finding that object files are sensitive to the nature of the objects seen before them mirrors previous object-based attention research (e.g., Chen & Cave, 2006; Zemel, Behrmann, Mozer, & Bavelier, 2002). Zemel et al. (2002) were able to reverse what subjects perceived as an object or nonobject in an ambiguous display by exposing them to specific visual stimuli. That is, how subjects process objecthood for a single trial can be directly affected by what they have seen before. Previous research has thus revealed experience effects on the ability to parse and distribute attention through static displays, and the present work is the first to demonstrate similar experience effects for object-file representations. However, it remains an important goal to establish when along the process these contextual effects administer their influences. On the one hand, as mostly discussed here, the effects can be at the representational stage, wherein noncanonical entities are not represented as persisting objects in the presence of better objects. On the other hand, the influence could also occur at the perceptual stage, such that the presence of better objects leads to the parts of the noncanonical objects not being perceived as bounded together into a single object. Future work can help to distinguish between these two theoretical possibilities.

Limits of the contextual effects. The effects of context do not seem to be universally administered. We have recently found that object-file tracking relies heavily upon spatiotemporal parameters; in the absence of spatiotemporal continuity, surface feature information (e.g., an object's colour or shape) does not support object-file maintenance (Mitroff & Alvarez, 2007). Analogous to the experimental conditions of the current paper, both "intermixed" and "pure" conditions were tested—feature-defined trials were either intermixed with spatiotemporally defined trials or presented alone. In contrast to the clear differences between the intermixed and pure conditions of Experiments 1 and 2, surface features failed to underlie object-file processing in both conditions (Mitroff & Alvarez, 2007). Whereas spatiotemporal continuity is a necessary condition for object files, the principles studied here appear to operate in a more contingent fashion.

CONCLUSIONS

The current experiments began with the primary goal of exploring the effects of violating the boundedness and containment principles on object files. However, not only did these studies demonstrate novel, nuanced effects of boundedness and containment violations, they also revealed an exciting contextual influence on object files. Whereas object files have been examined and discussed as "here-and-now" representations of a given visual environment, the contextual effects suggest a much broader scope. Combined with prior research there now exist three cases in which context can affect object files (with violations of cohesion, boundedness, and containment) and one case in which object files are immune to context (spatiotemporal violations). These contextual effects speak to the nature of feature binding in visual working memory, highlighting perhaps a special role for spatiotemporal factors where tracking an object relies relatively little on an object's features. Conversely, the effective binding of episodic information (e.g., the presentation of a letter) to a specific object can be influenced by the "goodness" of the object itself. Clearly these results just scratch the surface of this important issue and in so doing they raise several questions. For example, what other aspects of object persistence are context-dependent and context-independent? How malleable are these context effects? Are the context effects interactive (e.g., what would happen when intermixing the illusory-defined trials of Experiment 1 with the outside trials of Experiment 2)? With these and other such questions still unanswered, we have much to learn about object files. Nevertheless, the current findings serve an important role by elucidating the complex nature of object-file processing. To facilitate object persistence, object files both adhere to specific rules and incorporate prior knowledge.

REFERENCES

Avrahami, J. (1999). Objects of attention, objects of perception. *Perception and Psychophysics, 61*, 1604–1612.

Carey, S., & Xu, F. (2001). Infant knowledge of objects: Beyond object files and object tracking. *Cognition, 80*, 179–213.

Chen, Z., & Cave, K. R. (2006). Reinstating object-based attention under positional certainty: The importance of subjective parsing. *Perception and Psychophysics, 68*, 992–1003.

Cheries, E., Mitroff, S. R., Wynn, K., & Scholl, B. J. (2008). Cohesion as a principle of object persistence in infancy. *Developmental Science, 11*, 427–432.

Chiang, W. C., & Wynn, K. (2000). Infants' tracking of objects and collections. *Cognition, 77*, 169–195.

Comtois, R. (2006). VisionShell PPC [Software libraries]. Cambridge, MA: Author.

Davis, G., & Driver, J. (1994). Parallel detection of Kanizsa subjective figures in the human visual system. *Nature, 371*, 791–793.

Feigenson, L., Carey, S., & Hauser, M. (2002). The representations underlying infants' choice of more: Object-files versus analog magnitudes. *Psychological Science, 13*, 150–156.

Gordon, R., & Irwin, D. (1996). What's in an object file? Evidence from priming studies. *Perception and Psychophysics, 58*, 1260–1277.

Gordon, R., & Irwin, D. (2000). The role of physical and conceptual properties in preserving object continuity. *Journal of Experimental Psychology: Learning, Memory, and Cognition, 26*, 136–150.

Henderson, J. (1994). Two representational systems in dynamic visual identification. *Journal of Experimental Psychology: General, 123*, 410–426.

Henderson, J. M., & Anes, M. D. (1994). Roles of object file review and type priming in visual identification within and across eye fixations. *Journal of Experimental Psychology: Human Perception and Performance, 20*, 826–839.

Hespos, S. J., & Baillargeon, R. (2001). Infants' knowledge about occlusion and containment events: A surprising discrepancy. *Psychological Science, 12*, 140–147.

Huntley-Fenner, G., Carey, S., & Solimando, A. (2002). Objects are individuals but stuff doesn't count: Perceived rigidity and cohesiveness influence infants' representations of small groups of distinct entities. *Cognition, 85*, 223–250.

Kahneman, D., Treisman, A., & Gibbs, B. J. (1992). The reviewing of object files: Object-specific integration of information. *Cognitive Psychology, 24*, 174–219.

Kanizsa, G. (1987). [Margini quasi-percettivi in campi con stimulazione omogenea]. In S. Petry & G. Meyer (Eds.),*The perception of illusory contours* (pp. 40–49). New York: Springer-Verlag. (Original work published 1955)

Kruschke, J. K., & Fragassi, M. M. (1996). The perception of causality: Feature binding in interacting objects. In *Proceedings of the eighteenth annual conference of the Cognitive Science Society* (pp. 441–446). Hillsdale, NJ: Lawrence Erlbaum Associates, Inc.

Marino, A. C., & Scholl, B. J. (2005). The role of closure in defining the "objects" of object-based attention. *Perception and Psychophysics, 67*, 1140–1149.

Michels, J., Saxena, A., & Ng, A. Y. (2005). *High-speed obstacle avoidance using monocular vision and reinforcement learning*. Paper presented at the 21st international conference on Machine Learning, Bonn, Germany.

Mitroff, S. R., & Alvarez, G. A. (2007). Space and time, not surface features guide object persistence. *Psychonomic Bulletin and Review, 14*, 1199–1204.

Mitroff, S. R., Scholl, B. J., & Noles, N. S. (2007). Object files can be purely episodic. *Perception, 36*, 1730–1735.

Mitroff, S. R., Scholl, B. J., & Wynn, K. (2004). Divide and conquer: How object files adapt when a persisting object splits into two. *Psychological Science, 15*, 420–425.

Mitroff, S. R., Scholl, B. J., & Wynn, K. (2005). The relationship between object files and conscious perception. *Cognition, 96*, 67–92.

Needham, A., & Baillargeon, R. (1993). Intuitions about support in 4.5-month-old infants. *Cognition, 47*, 121–148.

Noles, N. S., Scholl, B. J., & Mitroff, S. R. (2005). The persistence of object-file representations. *Perception and Psychophysics, 67*, 324–334.

Richardson, D. C., & Kirkham, N. Z. (2004). Multi-modal events and moving locations: Eye movements of adults and 6-month-olds reveal dynamic spatial indexing. *Journal of Experimental Psychology: General, 133*, 46–62.

Rosencrantz, M., Gordon, G., & Thrun, S. (2003). *Locating moving entities in dynamic indoor environments with teams of mobile robots.* Paper presented at the Autonomous Agents and Multi-Agent Systems conference, Melbourne, Australia.

Scholl, B. J., & Leslie, A. M. (1999). Explaining the infant's object concept: Beyond the perception/cognition dichotomy. In E. Lepore & Z. Pylyshyn (Eds.), *What is cognitive science?* (pp. 26–73). Oxford, UK: Blackwell.

Smith, A. T., & Over, R. (1977). Orientation masking and the tilt illusion with subjective contours. *Perception, 6*, 441–447.

Spelke, E. S. (1990). Principles of object perception. *Cognitive Science, 14*, 29–56.

Spelke, E. S., Kestenbaum, R., Simons, D. J., & Wein, D. (1995). Spatiotemporal continuity, smoothness of motion and object identity in infancy. *British Journal of Developmental Psychology, 13*, 113–143.

VanMarle, K., & Scholl, B. J. (2003). Attentive tracking of objects vs. substances. *Psychological Science, 14*, 498–504.

Von der Heydt, R., Peterhans, E., & Baumgartner, G. (1984). Illusory contours and cortical neuron responses. *Science, 224*, 1260–1262.

Wang, S., Baillargeon, R., & Paterson, S. (2005). Detecting continuity violations in infancy: A new account and new evidence from covering and tube events. *Cognition, 95*, 129–173.

Wynn, K. (1992). Addition and subtraction by human infants. *Nature, 358*, 749–750.

Xu, F. (1997). From Lot's wife to a pillar of salt: Evidence for physical object as a sortal concept. *Mind and Language, 12*, 365–392.

Yang, Y. (2006). *The role of gestalt principles in the creation of object file.* Masters dissertation, Zhejiang University, Hangzhou, P.R. China.

Zemel, R. S., Behrmann, M., Mozer, M. C., & Bavelier, D. (2002). Experience dependent perceptual grouping and object-based attention. *Journal of Experimental Psychology: Human Perception and Performance, 28*, 202–217.

VISUAL COGNITION, 2009, 17 (1/2), 212–231

Psychology Press
Taylor & Francis Group

Functional roles of memory for feature-location binding in event perception: Investigation with spatiotemporal visual search

Jun Saiki

Graduate School of Human and Environmental Studies, Kyoto University, Kyoto, Japan

In a dynamic environment full of degraded or missing perceptual information, memory might facilitate or even substitute efficiently for perception. We tested this idea with a "spatiotemporal search" task that required participants to search for a target defined by a binding of two features across a single object, across two points in time. Eight coloured bars moved horizontally until they became partially occluded behind squares. Before the tail of the bar becomes occluded, the head of the bar reemerged with a possibly different colour. Observers were precued a subset of the bars, and judged the presence of a colour changing target among the precued set. A series of three experiments revealed that memory can substitute for perception only for one object, and that the preview of colour-location binding does not facilitate perceptual processing. Cueing location and object features do not have additive effects. Binding memory may have highly limited capacity in substitution and facilitation of perception.

Keywords: Binding; Visual working memory; Visual search; Capacity limit; Spatiotemporal.

Visual cognition is an interaction of perception and memory. What we see is not only a product of visual processing of incoming stimuli, but also a product of their interpretation based on our previous experiences stored in memory. However, how visual perception and memory coordinate to accomplish efficient recognition of visual objects and scenes remains largely unknown.

Please address all correspondence to Jun Saiki, Graduate School of Human and Environmental Studies, Yoshida-Nihonmatsucho, Sakyo-ku, Kyoto, Japan 606-8601. E-mail: saiki@cv.jinkan.kyoto-u.ac.jp

I thank Steve Franconeri, and two anonymous reviewers for helpful comments on the earlier draft of the paper. This work was partially supported from Grants-in-Aid (#13610084, #14019053, and #19500226) from JMEXT, the Global COE Program "Revitalizing Education for Dynamic Hearts and Minds", from JMEXT, and PRESTO from JST.

© 2008 Psychology Press, an imprint of the Taylor & Francis Group, an Informa business
http://www.psypress.com/viscog DOI: 10.1080/13506280802280230

In complex visual cognition tasks in everyday life such as driving, efficient interaction of perception and memory is essential. Because of various disruptions of perceptual input, visual memory must compensate for such disruption. On the other hand, visual memory for an object in current state may facilitate perception of the object in the future. This study investigated how visual working memory of objects affects perceptual processing of a subsequent visual scene, by addressing the two issues: (1) Efficient substitution of disrupted perceptual information by object memory, and (2) facilitation of perceptual processing by object memory.

EFFICIENT SUBSTITUTION OF PERCEPTION BY FEATURE-BOUND OBJECT MEMORY

In the literature of visual working memory, the standard paradigm is change detection, in which memory representation of the previous display is compared with the current visual display. The change detection task is used to address various aspects of visual working memory: Memory for locations (Courtney, Petit, Maisog, Ungerleider, & Haxby, 1998), memory for objects (Courtney, Ungerleider, Keil, & Haxby, 1997; Luck & Vogel, 1997), and capacity of memory representations (Todd & Marois, 2004; Xu & Chun, 2006). However, this task is not suitable for investigating efficient substitution of perception by memory, because it cannot evaluate memory-based processing in comparison to perceptual processing. The issue of substitution addresses not only whether, but also how quickly and efficiently one can utilize memory information compared with perceptual processes, which is relevant for various monitoring tasks where the speed of detection of an unusual event is critical. To evaluate speed and efficiency, we need to compare a situation where both memory and perception are available and one where perceptual information is disrupted.

FACILITATION OF PERCEPTUAL PROCESSING BY FEATURE-BOUND OBJECT MEMORY

Visual search is usually considered a task for investigating visual attention, but it also contains visual working memory component. To find the target object, observers need to maintain the target information in their visual working memory (Chelazzi, Duncan, Miller, & Desimone, 1998). Recently, Wolfe, Horowitz, Kenner, Hyle, and Vasan (2004) addressed this issue, and investigated how fast humans can set up target information in visual working memory (also see Vickery, King, & Jiang, 2005). This line of research shares some empirical findings with research on dimensional weighting (Found & Muller, 1996), and feature-based attention (Moore &

Egeth, 1998; Shih & Sperling, 1996), because these studies show that cueing partial information of search target, just one dimension or feature, facilitates visual search performance. However, it is unclear whether setup of target information in visual working memory facilitates perceptual processing per se, or just selection of a target among distractors, because visual search task inherently contains both components. Previous studies on feature-based attention suggest that the latter may be the case (Moore & Egeth, 1998; Shih & Sperling, 1996).

To evaluate perceptual facilitation, we need to dissociate selection process and perceptual processing of the selected item. For this purpose, cueing both location and identity, instead of either location or identity alone, is necessary. If cueing both location and identity improves task performance compared with a cueing location alone, this should reflect facilitation in perceptual processing of an object, not selection. Standard visual search, however, is not suitable for this purpose, because if both identity and location are cued, there is no need to search!

SPATIOTEMPORAL VISUAL SEARCH: THE PARADIGM

The main theoretical questions of this study are (1) whether visual working memory for objects (defined by a conjunction of location and colour) can enable observers to perform a search task as efficiently as they could do it perceptually, and (2) whether visual working memory can facilitate perceptual processing of a target object in visual search. To answer these questions, I devised a paradigm called spatiotemporal visual search. Stimuli were moving coloured bars behind occluders (or moving occluders in front of coloured bars), and the task was to search for a bar that changed its colour before and after occlusion. Occluders are small so that only part of bars can be occluded. Thus, search for a target event can be executed either of the two ways. First, observers can compare two parts of a coloured bar and detect a target by finding difference in colours of the parts. This is called spatial matching, because observers do not need to use visual memory for object's colour. Second, observers can compare the head colour (the part reappearing from the occlusion) with its colour before occlusion stored in memory. This is called temporal matching, because observers rely on visual memory. Note that all previous works on visual memory are investigating exclusively temporal matching process, because spatial matching is impossible.

Spatiotemporal visual search allows us to investigate the relative contribution of spatial and temporal matching and their interaction by introducing control conditions. Figure 1 schematically illustrates the task structure. In the standard condition (called perception-plus-memory condition), both spatial and temporal matching are possible. For comparisons,

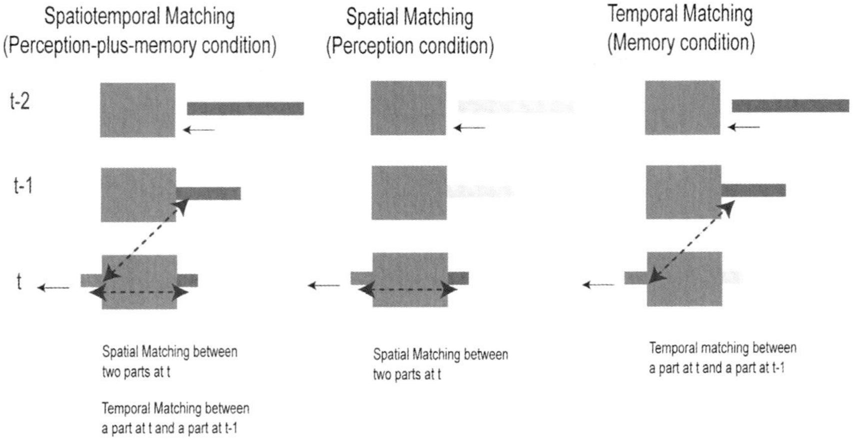

Figure 1. Schematic illustration of spatiotemporal, spatial, and temporal matches and their relations. To view this figure in colour, please see the online issue of the Journal.

conditions where only spatial or temporal matching is possible were introduced. In the perception condition, all bars were achromatic before the occluded part reappears, so that only spatial matching is possible. In contrast, in the memory condition, all colours of unoccluded parts (called tails hereafter) become achromatic at the time of reappearance of occluded parts (called heads hereafter), so that only temporal matching is possible.

Comparison of memory and perception-plus-memory conditions evaluates how visual memory efficiently substitutes for the lack of perceptual information in temporal matching. If visual memory can substitute for perceptual disruption in temporal matching, then performance in the memory condition will be equivalent to that in the perception-plus-memory condition. Comparison of perception and perception-plus-memory conditions evaluates how visual memory for object facilitates perceptual processes in spatial matching. If visual memory facilitates perception, then performance in the perception-plus-memory condition will be more efficient than in the perception condition. Note that the spatiotemporal search primarily measures processing speed in evaluating memory substitution and perceptual facilitation, but, as shown in Experiment 3 with an entire psychometric function, it also shows limits in capacity as reflected by the asymptote level of the psychometric function.

To investigate the effect of object working memory, cue set size was manipulated. Among eight, one to four items were cued as possible targets. Thus, the memory substitution and facilitation is evaluated within capacity limit of visual working memory. Note that the issue of efficient memory substitution is independent of the presence of capacity limit, because the capacity limit merely reflects whether items can be stored or not, whereas memory substitution reflects how efficiency memory can be used. Therefore, within capacity limit, memory may efficiently substitute for perceptual processing with any set sizes, with only small set sizes, or no efficient substitution at all.

EXPERIMENT 1: SPATIOTEMPORAL SEARCH WITH HIGH-CONTRAST STIMULI

Method

Design. There were two experimental factors: Cue set size (one, two, three, or four objects), and search type (perception and memory, perception, or memory).

Materials. Stimulus display was composed of eight pairs of a coloured bar and an occluder, configured on an imaginally circle. Coloured bars were $2.4° \times 0.4°$ horizontal rectangles, and occluders were $0.8° \times 0.8°$ square. Coloured bars were initially placed where their centre was offset 1.8° either rightward or leftward to the corresponding occluder. Thus, there was a 0.2° separation between an object and an occluder at the initial display. Either coloured bars or occluders moved to form occlusion events. Objects and occluders were placed on an imaginally circle centred on the central fixation point with an eccentricity of 4° in visual angle. Their locations were two horizontals, two verticals, and four 45° diagonals.

Four equiluminant colours were used for coloured bars. They were pink (CIE $x = 0.38$, $y = 0.22$), brown ($x = 0.41$, $y = 0.42$), light blue ($x = 0.20$, $y = 0.24$), and purple ($x = 0.22$, $y = 0.11$). The occluders were grey with the luminance of 13.6 cd/m^2. Background was black, so the stimulus contrast was almost 100%.

Stimulus sequence was made up of three periods: Cue period, occlusion period, and reappearance period. In the cue period, initial display was shown for 600 ms, followed by cue display by flashing possible target bars for 600 ms. Possible targets were flashed three times, and the number of cued bars varied across trials. Cues were always valid in the sense that the target bar was always among the cued objects. After the flashing, the display remained stationary for 200 ms before motion onset. Objects or occluders moved at the speed of 1.1°/s, and it took 920 ms from the motion onset until the heads of coloured bars were aligned with the vertical edge of the occluder. Motion continued, so that the heads of coloured bars reappeared from the occluder. After the reappearance period, the stimulus display disappeared with a pattern mask display composed of randomly placed coloured bars and grey squares. Figure 2 illustrates the temporal sequence of each trial.

In the perception-plus-memory condition, colour information for cued bars was available throughout the stimulus sequence. The colour of heads and tails of uncued bars changed to grey in the reappearance period. In the perception condition, all eight bars were grey in the cue and occlusion period, and in the reappearance period, only the cued bars had their colours in both their heads and tails. In the memory condition, cue and occlusion periods were identical to the perception and memory condition, but in the reappearance period, tails of the all bars changed to grey. Figure 3 illustrates occlusion and reappearance periods of three search type conditions. Note that because the perception-plus-memory and memory conditions had the identical cue and occlusion periods, and search type conditions were randomly mixed in the experiment, participants could not use any different strategies between these conditions. In the reappearance period, the head of one of the cued bars changed its colour in half the trials, and there was no colour change in the other half. Experimental programs were written in MATLAB, using Psychophysics Toolbox extensions (Brainard, 1997; Pelli, 1997).

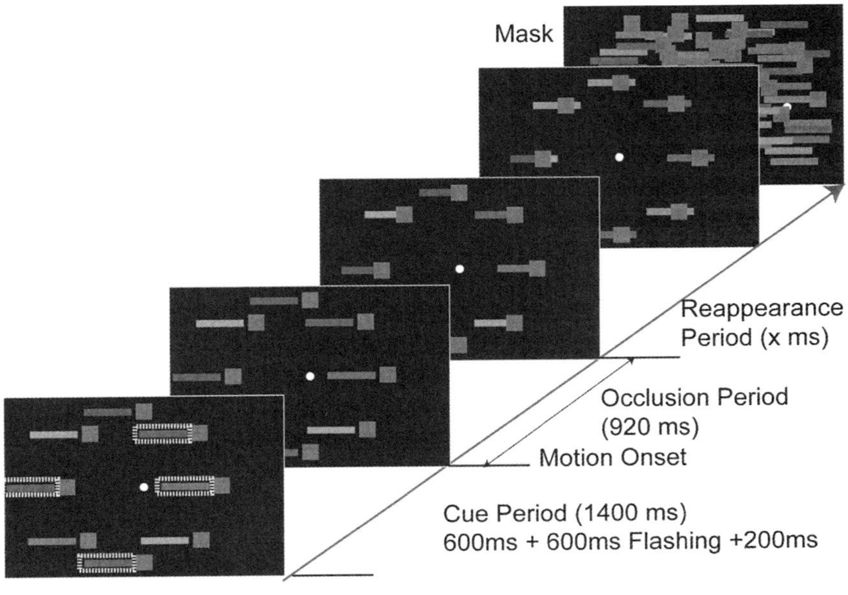

Figure 2. Temporal sequence of each trial in Experiment 1. Yellow markings denote cued objects. To view this figure in colour, please see the online issue of the Journal.

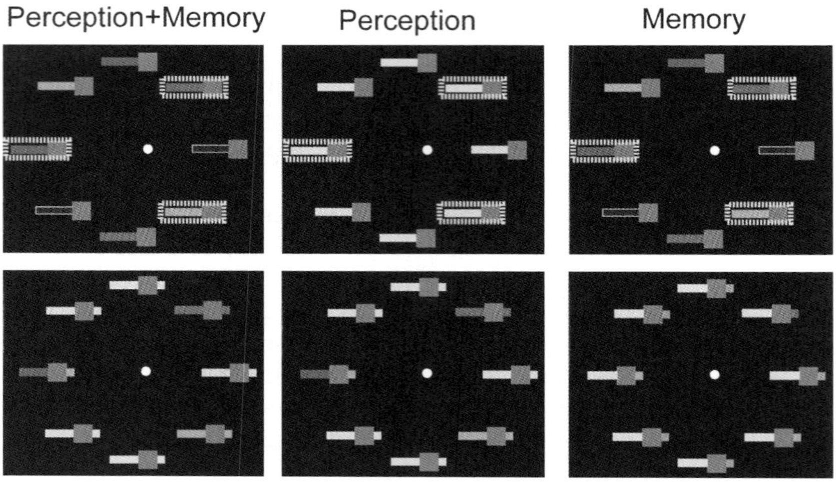

Figure 3. Stimulus configurations for search type conditions. Top and bottom figures illustrate occlusion and reappearance periods, respectively. Yellow markings denote cued objects, but cues were provided in the cueing period in experiments. To view this figure in colour, please see the online issue of the Journal.

Procedure. The task was to judge whether there was any bar whose head and tail had different colours in the reappearance period among cued bars. Each trial began with a keypress by an observer. After 1000 ms, an initial display was presented for 600 ms, followed by a stimulus sequence. Observers made a judgement by a keypress, and they were asked to be as accurate as possible. Response time was not measured. Observers were instructed to keep the central fixation throughout a trial, though eye movement was not monitored. The length of reappearance period was determined by an adaptive procedure called SIAM (a Single-Interval Adjustment-Matrix) procedure (Kärnbach, 1990). This procedure is an unbiased adaptive testing procedure for yes/no task. The experiment composed of eight sessions of 768 trials. Each session contains 12 staircase sequences for each combination of cue set size and search type. Each sequence had 64 trials, and the threshold was estimated by taking the average of durations of the last six reversal points. Initial durations were 235 ms for perception-plus-memory and perception conditions, and 353 ms for the memory condition.

Participants. There were four participants, including the author. The three other participants were naïve to the purpose of the experiment. All four had extensive experience with psychophysical experiments. The three naïve participants received payment for participation.

Results

Table 1 shows mean threshold durations as a function of cue set size for search type conditions. To evaluate memory substitution, performance in the memory condition was compared with that in the perception-plus-memory condition. The cost of memory search monotonically increases as the cue set size. A 2 (search type) $\times$ 4 (cue set size) repeated measures ANOVA for threshold duration showed a significant main effects of search type, $F(1, 3) = 24.21$, $p < .05$, and of cue set size, $F(3, 9) = 49.24$, $p < .01$; and a significant interaction of search type and cue set size, $F(3, 9) = 27.16$, $p < .01$. Planned comparisons revealed a significant main effect of search type under the set size four, $F(1, 3) = 26.19$, $p < .025$, and under the set size three, $F(1, 3) = 24.21$, $p < .025$. For the set sizes one and two, the effect of search type was not significant, $F < 1$.

Next, to evaluate memory facilitation, performance in the perception condition was compared with that in the perception-plus-memory condition. Table 1 shows that the threshold is quite similar between the perception and the perception-plus-memory conditions in all set sizes. Only the main effect of cue set size was significant, $F(3, 9) = 18.34$, $p < .001$, and the main effect of search type was not significant, $F(1, 3) = 1.35$.

Discussion

As shown in Table 1, the estimated threshold increased monotonically as the cue set size, suggesting that the spatiotemporal search task reflects processes similar to visual search. Comparison of memory and perception-plus-memory conditions showed significant difference in search slope, suggesting that object working memory cannot substitute for perceptual processing as the cue set size increases.

As for the effect of facilitation by memory exemplified by comparison between perception and perception-plus-memory conditions, two threshold functions are largely overlapped, suggesting that additional availability of

TABLE 1
Mean thresholds for different search conditions as a function of set size in Experiment 1 (standard errors in parentheses)

	Set size			
Search type	*One*	*Two*	*Three*	*Four*
Perception-plus-memory	127 (11)	144 (6)	174 (12)	227 (22)
Perception	135 (11)	145 (9)	173 (13)	253 (40)
Memory	126 (11)	160 (19)	242 (26)	469 (54)

colour does not facilitate perceptual matching. The lack of facilitation in the set size 1 condition is particularly important, because this result reflects perceptual comparison process alone, unlike larger set sizes.

EXPERIMENT 2: SPATIOTEMPORAL SEARCH WITH LOW-CONTRAST NOISY STIMULI

One possible reason for the lack of memory facilitation effect is a ceiling effect. Because the stimuli used in Experiment 1 were high-contrast, and without noise, the estimated threshold may be at the level of functional ceiling, which may conceal possible advantage of perception-plus-memory condition. To examine this possibility, Experiment 2 used low-contrast stimuli with pixel noise. The visibility of coloured bars was substantially reduced, thus if the results in Experiment 1 reflect a ceiling effect, this experiment will reveal a significant advantage of perception-plus-memory condition over perception condition.

Method

Aspects changed from Experiment 1 are described next.

Design. Cued set size had three levels: One, two, and four. In all, two-factor design was employed: Search type (perception and memory, perception, or memory), and cued set size (one, two, or four).

Materials. Only the object moving sequences were used in this experiment. The stimulus contrast was substantially reduced by using a grey background. The luminance of the background was 16.3cd/m^2, so that contrast was 9%. Furthermore, random noise was added to reduce the discriminability of coloured bars. Coloured noise display was formed in the following way. The display area of 15° square was decomposed to small 2×2 pixel dots. For each dots, the values of linearized R,G,B signals had random variation with the variance of 40%, so that the visibility of coloured bars was lowered. Thus, the coloured noise display had the mean luminance of 16.3 cd/m^2, with various small dots with different colours.

Procedure. The experiment composed of six sessions of 576 trials. Each session contains nine staircase sequences for each combination of cue set size and search type.

Participants. All four participants in this experiment also participated in Experiment 1.

Results

Table 2 shows mean threshold durations as a function of cue set size for search type conditions. For memory substitution effect, comparison between the memory and the perception-plus-memory conditions revealed a significant main effects of cue set size, $F(2, 6) = 13.86$, $p < .01$, and a significant interaction of search type and cue set size, $F(2, 6) = 19.03$, $p < .01$. Planned comparisons revealed a significant main effect of search type under the set size four, $F(1, 3) = 13.68$, $p < .05$. For the set sizes one and two, the effect of search type was not significant, for the size one, $F < 1$, and for the size two, $F(1, 3) = 3.67$, $p = .15$.

To evaluate memory facilitation effect, comparison between the perception and the perception-plus-memory conditions revealed a significant main effect of cue set size, $F(2, 6) = 12.19$, $p < .01$. Again the main effect of search type was not significant, $F < 1$.

Discussion

The pattern of results was similar to those in Experiment 1, suggesting that the lack of memory facilitation was not due to ceiling effects. The reduction of perceptual contrast and addition of noise clearly elevated threshold duration, but the advantage of perception-plus-memory condition over the perception condition was not observed. The memory substitution also showed the results similar to those in Experiment 1. Memory can substitute for perception under set size one and two, but not under set size four. One may argue that differences in results between set size 1 and others reflect observers' eye movement, but it is highly unlikely, because both Experiments 1 and 2 did not show any substantial drop in threshold duration at set size 1, which is expected if observers took advantage of fixating the target when the set size is 1.

As an evaluation of colour-location binding, the task design of Experiments 1 and 2 was not optimal, in that simple detection of a new colour

TABLE 2
Mean thresholds for different search conditions as a function of set size in Experiment 2 (standard errors in parentheses)

	Set size		
Search type	*One*	*Two*	*Four*
Perception-plus-memory	229 (13)	231 (20)	340 (42)
Perception	227 (16)	254 (25)	333 (21)
Memory	219 (21)	331 (54)	790 (161)

could lead to correct judgement, suggesting that Experiments 1 and 2 may overestimate memory for binding colour and its location. The next experiment examined this issue with more carefully controlled stimulus and task design.

EXPERIMENT 3: SPATIOTEMPORAL SEARCH AND COLOUR-LOCATION BINDING

Experiment 3 addressed two issues. First, because previous experiments estimated threshold level reappearance durations, it is unclear whether the lack of facilitation by colour memory holds just at the threshold level performance, or for the entire psychometric function. Experiment 3 utilized the method of constant stimuli, and derived psychometric functions. Second, as discussed earlier, this experiment investigated the effects of memory for colour-location binding in more controlled stimuli and task settings.

To investigate memory for colour-location binding in more detail, this experiment focused on the two-target condition. To achieve the goal of evaluating binding memory, the modified task requires observers to monitor both targets and to maintain colour-location binding simultaneously. The task was to judge whether both target objects changed their colour or not. There were four event types: Colour-switch, double-change, single-change, and no-change, where the correct response for the former two types was "yes". The colour-switch contained a switch in colours of two targets. The double- and single-change contained a change in colour of one or both of the targets to a new colour. Schematic illustration of the task design is shown in Figure 4.

This task design was necessary for the following reasons. As shown by Saiki (2003), Saiki and Miyatsuji (2007), and Wheeler and Treisman (2002), colour-switch manipulation is necessary to evaluate memory for colour-location binding properly. However, if the colour-switch is the only type of change, colour-switch between two-target objects becomes redundant because of the cueing. Observers could judge the presence of colour-switch by monitoring one of the two objects alone. To make sure that observers monitor two target objects simultaneously, two additional change types, single-change and double-change, were introduced. Simultaneous monitoring of two targets is necessary in discrimination of double- and single-changes.

Method

Materials. Cue set size was fixed to be two. The length of the reappearance period was fixed to these six values: 71 ms, 176 ms, 282 ms, 388 ms, 494 ms, and 600 ms. Unlike previous experiments, where a change

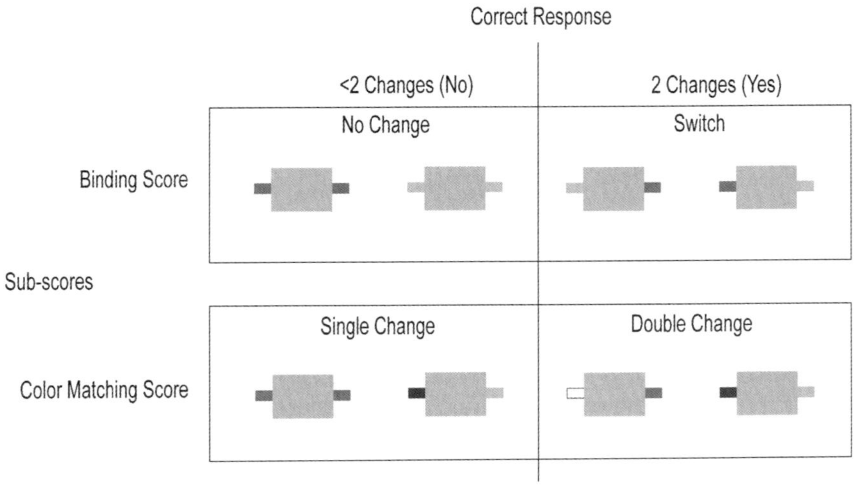

Figure 4. Schematic illustration of binding manipulations used in Experiment 3. To view this figure in colour, please see the online issue of the Journal.

occurred at one object alone, three different patterns of change were used. The first type, called double-change, had both of the two target objects change their colour to new colours. The second type, called colour-switch, switched the colours of the two targets. The third type, called single-change, had one target object change their colour to a new colour. The single-change is similar to the change in previous experiments, except an additional constraint of the changed colour being different from the other target. In addition, there were sequences with no-change.

Procedure. The observers' task was to judge whether both target objects changed their colour or not. Thus, they require to judge yes to double-change, and colour-switch sequences, and no to single-switch, and no-change sequence. The experiment was composed of six sessions of 576 trials. Each session had eight repetitions of experimental conditions (three search types, six durations of reappearance period, and four change types). The order of trials was randomized.

Participants. There were five participants, including the author. Three of them participated in Experiments 1 and 2.

Data analysis. Unlike previous experiments estimating threshold durations, the current experiment evaluated psychometric functions of correct judgement and reappearance duration. To evaluate observers' performance, we used the performance curve relating exposure duration d and performance measure p, based on Busey and Loftus (1994):

$$p = \begin{cases} 0.5 & (d < L) \\ 0.5 + (Y - 0.5)(1.0 - \exp(-(d - L)/C)) & (d \geq L), \end{cases}$$

where Y, L, and C denote asymptotic level (called asymptote hereafter), the maximum duration that gives chance-level performance (called latency hereafter), and exponential growth constant (called slope hereafter), respectively. This descriptive model was used to evaluate the psychometric functions. The parameters Y, L, and C reflect maximum level of performance at long duration (thus related to processing capacity), processing delay, and processing speed, respectively. Thus, difference in threshold between the memory and memory-and-perception conditions in the previous experiments can be further evaluated as to whether it reflects memory capacity, delay in access to memory, or processing speed in memory matching. In addition to proportions correct, two subscores were used: Binding score is defined by combining colour-switch and no-change trials, and colour-matching score is defined by combining single-change and double-change trials. The binding score reflects colour-location binding, and the colour-matching score reflects colour-matching, or counting the number of colours, which does not necessarily requires colour-location binding.

Results

Proportions correct (Figure 5a). Figure 5 shows psychometric curves for three search type conditions based on group means. The fitting of individual data was quite good (range of r^2 is from .930 to .999), and the means of parameter estimates were quite similar to the parameter estimates of the grouped data. To examine memory substitution, performance in the memory condition was compared with that in the perception-plus-memory condition. The asymptote was significantly lower in the memory condition than in the perception-plus-memory condition, $F(1, 4) = 29.49$, $p < .01$, but latency and slope did not show significant difference, $F < 1$. The significantly lower asymptote in the memory condition suggests that even if there are only two targets, memory for objects cannot substitute for perception.

To examine memory facilitation, performance in the perception condition was compared with that in the perception-plus-memory condition. The asymptote parameter was significantly higher in the perception condition than in the perception-plus-memory condition, $F(1, 4) = 17.60$, $p < .05$, but latency and slope parameters did not show significant difference, $F(1, 4) = 0.222$, and $F(1, 4) = 2.55$, respectively. Consistent with the previous results, memory for object did not facilitate perception. Moreover, the whole

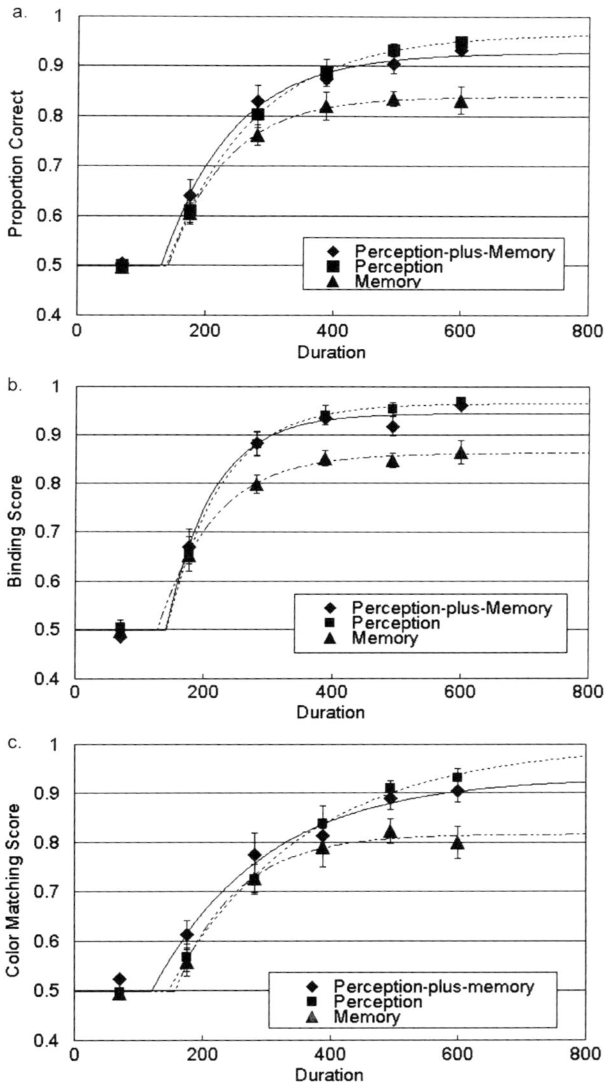

Figure 5. Psychometric functions for different search conditions as a function of reappearance duration. (a) Proportions correct. (b) Binding scores. (c) Colour matching scores.

psychometric functions were quite similar between the perception and perception-plus-memory conditions. If anything, the perception condition showed slight advantage in terms of the asymptote level.

Binding score (Figure 5b). Comparison of memory and perception-plus-memory conditions to examine memory substitution effects revealed significantly lower asymptote in the memory condition, $F(1, 4) = 8.90$, $p < .05$, but no significant differences in latency and slope parameters, $F(1, 4) = 2.08$ and $F < 1$, $p > .1$. The memory cost reflected in the lower estimate of asymptote in the memory condition was observed for the binding score.

Comparison of the perception and perception-plus-memory conditions to examine memory facilitation effects showed a pattern similar to proportion correct data. The perception condition showed significantly higher value of asymptote than the perception-plus-memory condition, $F(1, 4) = 8.21$, $p < .05$. The latency and slope parameters did not show any effect of conditions, $F < 1$.

Colour-matching score (Figure 5c). Comparison of memory and perception-plus-memory conditions to examine memory substitution effects revealed a significantly lower asymptote in the memory condition than in the perception-plus-memory condition, $F(1, 4) = 76.64$, $p < .001$, a significantly larger latency in the memory condition than in the perception-plus-memory condition, $F(1, 4) = 9.56$, $p < .05$, and marginally significant difference in slope parameter, $F(1, 4) = 5.84$, $p = .073$. For the colour-matching score, memory cost was observed in the longer latency, in addition to the lower asymptote.

Comparison of the perception and perception-plus-memory conditions to examine memory facilitation effects showed a pattern similar to proportion correct data. The asymptote difference between the perception and perception-plus-memory condition was marginally significant, $F(1, 4) = 7.35$, $p = .054$. The latency and slope parameters did not show any effects of conditions, $F < 1$.

Finally, I compared the psychometric function of binding and colour-matching scores. The slope parameter was significantly smaller for the binding score than for the colour-matching score, $F(1, 4) = 12.06$, $p < .05$, suggesting that the slope of the psychometric function was steeper for the binding score than for the colour-matching score.

Discussion

Comparison of performance curves between the perception and perception-plus-memory conditions revealed that these two conditions were quite similar to each other, not only in terms of threshold level as measured in previous experiments, but also other parameters such as slope and asymptote. Regarding the asymptote level, the analysis showed that the perception condition tend to have higher asymptote than the perception-plus-memory condition. This small, but significant difference in asymptote may reflect a small interference due to conflict between memory and perceptual representations when memory representation was not veridical. However, this difference may be an artefact in parameter fitting, in that a higher asymptote in the perception condition compensates for small but nonsignificant difference in slope parameter, as shown in Figure 5. Further investigation is necessary to resolve this issue.

Regarding the memory substitution, the present experiment showed a significant cost in asymptote level in the memory condition even when the number of targets was only two, suggesting significant capacity limit on visual working memory maintenance and retrieval. Separate analysis with binding and colour-matching subscores showed that this cost was observed with both subscores. However, the colour-matching score showed memory cost in both asymptote and latency, whereas the memory cost for the binding score was observed only with asymptote, suggesting that additional perceptual representation in the perception-plus-memory condition speed up processes related to colour-matching, not processes related to binding.

GENERAL DISCUSSION

This study investigated the role of working memory for objects in visual search for a spatiotemporal relation of colours. The two issues were addressed: (1) Whether visual memory can efficiently substitute for the lack of perceptual information, and (2) whether visual memory can facilitate perceptual processing. Overall, memory could efficiently substitute for only one object (but not more), when no tail colours were on the screen, but when colours were perceptually available, visual memory showed no facilitation at one object (or any other set size).

For the issue of memory substitution, I compared perception-plus-memory and memory conditions. Overall, memory can substitute for perception when the cue set size is one, but when the set size is two or more, the cost of memory was significant. Although the cost of memory failed to reach statistical significance in the set size two in Experiments 1 and 2, this likely reflects target detection without using memory for feature binding, because memory for colours alone, not colour-location binding was sufficient to detect a target in these experiments.

The significant costs in memory substitution may be specific to the experimental paradigm in this study. First, colour change of the objects' tail into grey in the reappearance period may overwrite memory for target objects. Second, the mixture of memory and perception-plus-memory conditions may discourage observers from memorizing as much information as they could, because of strategic uncertainty. A follow-up experiment showed that neither factors were essential.[1]

Regarding the issue of perceptual facilitation by visual memory, comparison of perception-plus-memory and perception conditions repeatedly showed that there was no facilitation in search performance by preview of colour-location bindings up to four objects. Memory for object colours did not have any benefit additional to the benefit due to memory for object locations. This was the case not only for the threshold level (Experiments 1 and 2), but also for the entire psychometric function (Experiment 3). Although one needs to be cautious about making a strong conclusion from the null results, replications with different settings may allow us to state that the memory facilitation effect, if any, seems to be rather small.

Perceptual facilitation effect investigated by the spatiotemporal search paradigm was dissociated from memory effects on target selection process, because selection is unnecessary. The lack of facilitation in these conditions thus suggests that setup of target colour information in visual working memory does not facilitate perceptual processing of colour comparison, and that previous finding of facilitation in search performance primarily reflects memory effects on target selection. These results are consistent with previous research on feature-based attention (Moore & Egeth, 1998; Shiu & Sperling, 1996), showing that feature-based attention effects reflect prioritization of the allocation of spatial attention.

Relation to other studies

I discuss the implications of the present study in relation to various literature, visual short-term memory, visual search and feature-based attention, and object files.

Visual short-term memory. Compared with a standard change detection task, the unique aspect of the spatiotemporal search task is the evaluation of efficiency of memory matching in comparison with perceptual matching. With the change detection, we could not tell any difference among small set sizes, because the task performance is at the ceiling. The results suggest that

[1] A follow-up experiment ($N = 7$) replicated Experiment 3 with two reappearance durations (200 ms and 680 ms), and without the perception-plus-memory condition to eliminate strategic uncertainty. To evaluate overwriting effect, a long-occluder condition, where objects' tail was occluded at the time of head reappearance, was added. Using accuracy increment from 200 ms to 680 ms conditions as an index, both memory ($M = 0.185$) and long-occluder ($M = 0.208$) conditions showed significantly smaller increment relative to the perception condition ($M = 0.357$) with Tukey's HSD test (both $p < .005$), suggesting that neither overwriting nor strategic uncertainty was primary cause of the memory cost.

object memory is fully functional only for one object, and memory for two or more objects suffer from substantial costs in substituting perceptual processes. These costs can be explained at least in two ways. First, memory representations during maintenance are already degraded due to set size increase. Second, memory representations are intact during maintenance, but temporal match processing during search impairs performance. Another unresolved issue is whether memory substitution in set size one holds regardless of the complexity of object. Further research is necessary to resolve these issues.

Visual search and feature-based attention. Previous studies about the effects of identity cues on search performance could not distinguish facilitation based on target localization and on perceptual processing of localized item. The spatiotemporal search task, by eliminating target localization, showed the lack of facilitation with feature-location cues, suggesting that cueing target location is sufficient for target processing. Feature-based attention may facilitate the guidance of attention to a target object, only when the location information is unavailable (Moore & Egeth, 1998; Shiu & Sperling, 1996). Taken together, space-based attention and feature-based attention may not function additively (McMains, Fehd, Emmanouil, & Kastner, 2007). However, the spatiotemporal search with different colour cues differs from typical feature-based attention experiments with cues with a single feature (one colour, one motion direction, etc.), and it remains unknown whether multiple feature values can produce feature-based attention effects. If the feature-based attention benefit occurs only when a single feature is cued, colour cue will facilitate attentional guidance when all cued objects have the same colour, which needs to be examined in future research.

Object files. The lack of perceptual facilitation in the current study appears inconsistent with object-specific preview benefit by Kahneman, Treisman, and Gibbs (1992). This may be due to a task difference: Whereas Kahneman et al. used a kind of priming as dependent measure, this study required explicit colour comparison to detect a target.

Broader implications

From a broader theoretical perspective, the conclusions drawn from the results seem to support Rensink's proposal on general architecture of visual cognition system (Rensink, 2000). The finding that conditions in which all relevant information is visible yield superior performance to conditions in which memory must be used seems consistent with Rensink's notion that the visual system relies primarily on visible information and only uses memory when absolutely necessary.

Such a consideration also has various applicational implications in various aspects of our daily life including human interface design. If the visual system uses memory information only when absolutely necessary, interface devices counting on our voluntary use of memory information may have serious consequences. Therefore, better understanding of interaction of perception and memory in visual cognition is essential for the improvement of human interface.

REFERENCES

Brainard, D. H. (1997). The psychophysics toolbox. *Spatial Vision*, *10*, 443–446.

Busey, T. A., & Loftus, G. R. (1994). Sensory and cognitive components of visual information acquisition. *Psychological Review*, *101*, 446–469.

Chelazzi, L., Duncan, J., Miller, E. K., & Desimone, R. (1998). Responses of neurons in inferior temporal cortex during memory-guided visual search. *Journal of Neurophysiology*, *80*, 2918–2940.

Courtney, S. M., Petit, L., Maisog, J., Ungerleider, L. G., & Haxby, J. V. (1998). An area specialized for spatial working memory in human frontal cortex. *Science*, *279*, 1347–1351.

Courtney, S. M., Ungerleider, L. G., Keil, K., & Haxby, J. V. (1997). Transient and sustained activity in a distributed system for human working memory. *Nature*, *386*, 608–611.

Found, A., & Muller, H. J. (1996). Searching for unknown feature targets on more than one dimension: Investigating a "dimension weighting" account. *Perception and Psychophysics*, *58*, 88–101.

Kärnbach, C. (1990). A single-interval adjustment-matrix (SIAM) procedure for unbiased adaptive testing. *Journal of Acoustical Society of America*, *88*, 2645–2655.

Kahneman, D., Treisman, A., & Gibbs, B. J. (1992). The reviewing of object files: Object specific integration of information. *Cognitive Psychology*, *24*, 175–219.

Luck, S. J., & Vogel., E. K. (1997). The capacity of visual working memory for features and conjunctions. *Nature*, *390*, 279–281.

McMains, S. A., Fehd, H. M., Emmanouil, T.-A., & Kastner, S. (2007). Mechanisms of feature- and space-based attention: Response modulation and baseline increases. *Journal of Neurophysiology*, *98*, 2110–2121.

Moore, C. M., & Egeth, H. (1998). How does feature-based attention affect visual processing? *Journal of Experimental Psychology: Human Perception and Performance*, *24*, 1296–1310.

Pelli, D. G. (1997). The videotoolbox software for visual psychophysics: Transforming numbers into movies. *Spatial Vision*, *10*, 443–446.

Rensink, R. A. (2000). The dynamic representation of scenes. *Visual Cognition*, *7*, 17–42.

Saiki, J. (2003). Feature binding in object-file representations of multiple moving items. *Journal of Vision*, *3*, 6–21.

Saiki, J., & Miyatsuji, H. (2007). Feature binding in visual working memory evaluated by type identification paradigm. *Cognition*, *102*, 49–83.

Shih, S.-I., & Sperling, G. (1996). Is there feature-based attentional selection in visual search? *Journal of Experimental Psychology: Human Perception and Performance*, *22*, 758–779.

Todd, J. J., & Marois, R. (2004). Capacity limit of visual short-term memory in human posterior parietal cortex. *Nature*, *428*, 751–754.

Vickery, T. J., King, L.-W., & Jiang, Y.-H. (2005). Setting up the target template in visual search. *Journal of Vision*, *5*, 81–92.

Wheeler, M. E., & Treisman, A. (2002). Binding in short-term visual memory. *Journal of Experimental Psychology: General*, *131*, 48–64.

Wolfe, J. M., Horowitz, T. S., Kenner, N., Hyle, M., & Vasan, N. (2004). How fast can you change your mind? The speed of top-down guidance in visual search. *Vision Research*, *44*, 1411–1426.

Xu, Y., & Chun, M. M. (2006). Dissociable neural mechanisms supporting visual short-term memory for objects. *Nature*, *440*, 91–95.

VISUAL COGNITION, 2009, 17 (1/2), 232–253

Psychology Press
Taylor & Francis Group

Temporal binding favours the early phase of colour changes, but not of motion changes, yielding the colour–motion asynchrony illusion

Alex O. Holcombe
School of Psychology, University of Sydney, Sydney, Australia

How our binding mechanism judges features as simultaneous remains mysterious. When moving dots alternate in colour and motion direction, reports of the perceived colour and motion pairing reveal an asynchrony in temporal binding: The motion change best precedes the associated colour change by about 150 ms. Here the durations of the motion and colour were independently varied. Regardless of motion duration, pairing reports were most consistent when the midpoint of the motion interval occurred at a particular time relative to the colour, suggesting no differential weighting of early versus late portions of the motion interval. In contrast, as colour duration increased, the best time of its midpoint shifted later, indicating that it is best to align the early part of the colour with the motion. Thus, the colour–motion asynchrony phenomenon appears to result from the binding process favouring the early phase of the colour but not the early part of the motion.

Keywords: Binding; Asynchrony; Dynamics; Perception.

The billions of neurons in our brains operate largely in parallel. Functionally in vision this allows the concurrent labour of analysing the visual scene to be divided to some extent by features, with colour analysed separately from motion. How are these parallel analyses coordinated? With different features of multiple objects processed by different groups of neurons, there must be some scheme to determine which features belong to a particular object. Here in the present special issue of *Visual Cognition*, the papers are predominantly concerned with spatial binding. Spatial binding refers to the representation of which features are colocalized in space. Representation of location is embedded in the retinotopic organization of many visual cortical areas and therefore different features like colour and motion, although processed in

Please address all correspondence to Alex O. Holcombe, School of Psychology, University of Sydney, Sydney, NSW 2006, Australia. E-mail: alexh@psych.usyd.edu.au
I thank Daniel Linares for helpful discussion, Alex White, Colin Clifford, and Ed Vul for comments, and Australian Research Council grant DP0772037 for support.

© 2008 Psychology Press, an imprint of the Taylor & Francis Group, an Informa business
http://www.psypress.com/viscog DOI: 10.1080/13506280802340653

different areas, may share a common location tag. A particular location can be selected, thanks to the retinotopic organization of cortical areas, in multiple feature analysers such as a colour area and a motion area, allowing linkage of the colour and motion that belong to the same location (Clark, 2001; Treisman & Gelade, 1980). Spatial binding cannot be quite this simple due to the existence of spatially overlapping objects and the need for vision to fill in imperfect bottom-up information. However, that successful binding is neurophysiologically and psychophysically closely linked with intact spatial encoding provides some support for the location-tagging scheme (e.g., Neri & Levi, 2006; Ward, Danziger, Owen, & Rafal, 2002; Wu, Kanai, & Shimojo, 2004).

Temporal binding, or linking features that occur at a common time, may pose distinct problems for the visual system. For spatial binding, the common spatial organization (retinotopy or spatiotopy) provides a ready index but there is no evidence for strong maplike representations of temporal position (apart from in specialized detectors for motion). Without an obvious time tag in the visual system, some have suggested that we perceive as occurring together in time those features that are processed at the same time (Zeki, 2003, 2005, 2007; Zeki & Bartels, 1998). More specifically, the features encoded as together may reflect the time that the features become conscious in independent feature modules (Zeki, 2003, 2005, 2007; Zeki & Bartels, 1998), the time after identification they are accessed by attention (Botella & Eriksen, 1992; Keele & Neill, 1978), or the time they reach some binding stage or process (Arnold, Clifford, & Wenderoth, 2001; Clifford, in press). On each account, if the times until the critical process differ substantially for the two features that should be bound, then a temporal binding error occurs. Alternatively, features might be bound not based on when some aspect of their processing completes, but rather via a temporal tag, a counterpart to the location tag used in spatial binding. Nishida and Johnston (2002, in press) have suggested that features are assigned a temporal tag based on associated salient changes that are easy for the brain to detect, like sudden luminance changes. Such a change may create a temporal tag for the feature identification processes that follow the change. Whenever these separate feature identification processes complete, the system represents them as corresponding to the same stimulus time thanks to their shared temporal tag.

A particularly consistent temporal binding error, perhaps strong enough to be termed an illusion, was reported by Moutoussis and Zeki in 1997. In their display, a set of dots moved up and down, alternating every 308 ms. When the dots moved in one direction they were red, and when moving in the other direction they were green. In this condition of synchronous changes in colour and motion, although the motion and colour are perceived clearly, their pairing—whether when red, the dots are moving up or down—appears strange or inconsistent. This is most conspicuous when one compares the display to one in which the motion changes about 100 ms before the colour. Then, the pairing is much more clear. Moutoussis and Zeki measured this phenomenon by varying the temporal interval between motion change and colour change and asking observers to report the predominant pairing on each trial. To elicit a particular pairing, say red up, the timing interval was best set such that upward motion started about 80 ms before the dots turned red.

The authors explained this phenomenon by appealing to differences in processing time, concluding that motion takes about 80 ms longer to process than colour, explaining why giving the motion an 80 ms "head start" yields the best pairing percept (Moutoussis & Zeki, 1997). This theory, although still advocated (Zeki, 2003, 2005, 2007), has been difficult to reconcile with the findings that time to respond to a target motion is no different than response time for a particular colour and that synchrony judgements are veridical (Bedell, Chung, Ogmen, & Patel, 2003; Johnston & Nishida, 2001; Nishida & Johnston, 2002). However, Zeki is not alone in maintaining the basic asynchrony idea, with others suggesting that motion identity takes longer to reach the mechanisms involved in binding than does colour (Bedell et al., 2003; Clifford, in press).

In contrast, as mentioned earlier, Nishida and Johnston (2002, in press) proposed that the brain has a scheme to avoid asynchronies incurred by different processing times and that the Moutoussis and Zeki (1997) colour–motion asynchrony exploits a vulnerability in the scheme. They propose that the perceptual system aligns features based on temporal markers that usually reliably encode the onset and offset of a feature. Features perceived as bound are perceived as such because their temporal markers were detected at the same time by the system, rather than the features themselves being processed at the same time. The temporal markers are suggested to normally be the relative time of the response to the luminance or chromatic onsets and offsets that usually signal a feature change. Nishida and Johnston (in press) argue that identification of these usually has little temporal variability; hence, the transients can be used to estimate the time of a feature onset even when the identification of the feature itself is time-consuming or temporally variable. The Moutoussis and Zeki stimulus, however, cannot be bound accurately using this scheme. The reason is that although the colour changes are accompanied by colour transients that provide a reliable temporal marker, the times of the motion changes are not signalled by a colour or luminance transient. The absence of a temporal tag at onset then leads to the asynchrony.

The change in motion, or acceleration, is a second-order change that humans are poor at perceiving (Gottsdanker, 1956; Werkhoven, Snippe, & Toet, 1992) and thus according to Nishida and Johnston (2002) does not play much role in determining the features to bind. To test whether the salience of the change in features was indeed critical for binding, Nishida and Johnston modified the normally salient colour feature change. Instead of the colour changing suddenly from red to green, it changed gradually so that there was no discrete transient to signal the change. The asynchrony for best perceptual binding was then much smaller than before (Nishida & Johnston, 2002). This certainly implicates the transients but does not directly explain the consistent direction and magnitude of the original effect. In the original effect, why is the motion best begun 100 ms or so before the colour? Nishida and Johnston (in press) are not entirely explicit on this point but they suggest that the first-order change indicating the onset of a colour is matched to some subset of the many first-order changes in position that correspond to a particular motion. Most of these occur after the actual onset of the motion, so aligning them with a colour change would then result in asynchrony.

Clifford, Arnold, and Pearson (2003) also suggested the asynchrony might result from greater importance of the early part of the colour than for the early part of the motion. They suggested that the neural response to colour might adapt more quickly, which would result in the maximal correlation of the responses to colour and motion shifting such that colour is best begun after the motion. Although this is an adequate explanation of the original asynchrony phenomenon, this theory does not seem to explain the systematic changes in asynchrony when transients are either first order or second order.

Holcombe and Cavanagh (2008) provide additional evidence for the role of luminance or colour transients in determining the best relative timing for pairing the features. Their results show that unambiguous, attention-grabbing luminance transients can determine the best timing for pairing the features. Supporting the notion that it is not the processing of the features themselves but salient temporal markers that determine pairings, in their experiment the transients did not even belong to the colour or the motion but rather to a ring that encircled the stimulus at a variable time. Their experiment was thus able to dissociate the times of important transients from the times of the features themselves. Seven moving-dot patches were arrayed about fixation, each changing colour and motion every 471 ms. At some point during the trial, suddenly a ring appeared around one of the seven patches of dots. This cueing ring stayed on for the 471 ms duration of a single feature, and participants reported the feature pairing perceived while the ring was present. This was not subjectively difficult, and was perhaps aided by the strong exogenous cueing effect provided by the ring transients (Nakayama & Mackeben, 1989). Remarkably, pairing reports were best predicted by the timing of the ring relative to the colour, and the timing of the ring relative to the motion, quite apart from the timing of the colour relative to the motion. This indicates that the asynchrony phenomenon is not based on differential latency of the motion and colour themselves because the best stimulus asynchrony of colour and motion was shifted over a broad range by variation in the timing of the ring. Holcombe and Cavanagh suggested that the feature pairing is not determined until the ring summons attention, and attention then accesses whichever features are present at that time. In other words, there is no binding mechanism that correlates the exact temporal correspondence of the two features, but rather attention just accesses each feature independently, yielding the predominant colour and predominant motion during the cueing ring. Nishida and Johnston (in press) suggest that the transients of the features themselves are temporally correlated, whereas Holcombe and Cavanagh suggest that attention samples each feature independently at a time set by any transients available.

How attention would be expected to sample the features in the original Moutoussis and Zeki (1997) display is not clear. Holcombe and Cavanagh (2008) do suggest, however, that without a cueing ring, the transients in the colour–motion stimulus train may control access to the features, and that the inconspicuousness of the motion reversal causes the motion to be picked up later in the feature interval than is the colour.

In the present experiments, we tested whether early or late portions of the colour and motion intervals have differing importance when they are bound. To do this, the relative duration of the two features was varied, instead of presenting the two motions and two colours for equal durations as was done in previous literature. The theory of Nishida and Johnston (in press) appears to predict that the timing of the onset of the colour will be most important as they only mention the transients evoked by the onset of the colour and their illustration (their Figure 3) shows matching of the red onset transient with one of the position transients during the corresponding motion, without any depiction of a role for the offset. If the offsets are indeed less important than onsets, then the most consistent pairing should occur when onset of a particular colour has a particular timing relative to the onset of a motion. On the other hand, there is evidence that responses to feature offset are quicker, less stimulus-dependent, and sometimes less variable than responses to feature onset (Bair, Cavanaugh, Smith, & Movshon, 2002; Kreegipuu & Allik, 2007). Overall, then, it is far from clear to what extent humans when pairing features might rely on onsets, offsets, or the time in between.

In the original paper describing the colour–motion asynchrony, Moutoussis and Zeki (1997) conducted an experiment relevant to the issue of onsets and offsets. With their displays of dots alternating between red and green and upward and downward motion, in one experiment they deleted one half of each motion—for example, making the dots stationary during the first half of each motion. Apparently using one or two subjects, they then reported that the best time for the midpoint of the motion remained constant. However, no numbers were provided and the psychometric functions shown in their paper appear to contradict their claim. Judging by eye, the midpoint time did not remain constant, rather it shifted in the direction of preserving the motion onset time. This goes against their simple differential latency account as it suggests that the early part of the motion was favoured in determining the feature pairing. Deleting half of the motion in their case created a first-order transient at onset that may have then been favoured for binding. In a further experiment, they replaced half of each red interval with grey and also half of each green interval with grey. They reported that the best time of the colour midpoint was the same as with the original stimulus, although again no numbers are provided and their data appears inconsistent. For one subject, the psychometric function appears to show midpoint time was nearly preserved but fell slightly in the direction of preserving the colour onset. For the second subject, it appears that the colour midpoint time shifted substantially in favour of the colour onset. With these apparent inconsistencies and only two subjects, it would be premature to conclude anything about the relative importance of different parts of the motion and colour intervals. Here the goal was to vary durations of the features without introducing the new first-order transients that likely resulted after Moutoussis and Zeki deleted half the motion and half the colour.

We use a stimulus adapted from Moutoussis and Zeki (1997) by Holcombe and Cavanagh (2008). An array of seven dot patches (Figure 1, right) was presented, and in each patch the dots alternated asynchronously between inward and outward motion and between red, green, and sometimes blue. Blue was always irrelevant but was included for two purposes. First, to yield an irrelevant rhythm of transients across trials, which reduced the likelihood that observers might adopt any cognitive strategy related to the transients. This is a potential concern because previous work has shown participants are able to precisely judge the relative time of transients without asynchrony, even when in a feature pairing task they show a robust asynchrony (Bedell et al., 2003; Clifford et al., 2003). Second, the inclusion of irrelevant blue periods meant that participants could not expect a particular colour to occur immediately before or after the target red colour. This meant they were unlikely to violate the instructions and attend to a colour besides red.

We changed the time of the onsets and offsets by varying the duration of the three colours and of the two motions. If the onsets are more important than the offsets, then as the duration of the colour varies, the best timing of its onset should stay the same. Alternatively, the best relative timing for pairing reports might shift to preserve the time of the offset of colour relative

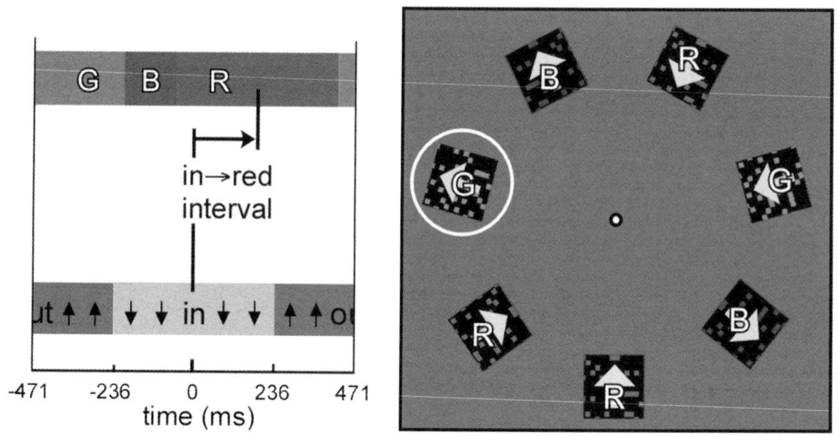

Figure 1. Left: Schematic depicting the relative timing of the midpoint of the inward period and the midpoint of the red period, the in→red interval. In Experiment 2, because motion was varied instead of colour the red→in interval was used, which is −1*(in→red interval). Right: A schematic snapshot of the stimulus, which contained 7 patches of dots alternating between inward and outward motion and between red, green, and blue. Each had a different phase and in→red interval. The target dot patch was designated by a ring that encircled it throughout the trial. To view this figure in colour, please see the online issue of the Journal.

to the motion. Finally, the best colour time might shift to preserve the relative time of its midpoint.

EXPERIMENT 1: VARYING THE DURATION OF RED

Methods

Participants. Four males and one female participated including the first author (AH), ages ranging from 21 to 34.

Stimulus. On a CRT controlled by a MacOS 9 computer with a custom program written using the C VisionShell library (Comtois, 2003), seven random-dot fields were arrayed around a circle, equally spaced (Figure 1). The centre of each 1.9° dot field was 5° from the white fixation point. Each dot field had a black background (<2 cd/m^2, but greater than scotopic levels), whereas the rest of the screen background was a dark grey (6 cd/m^2). Each dot field contained approximately 30 square dots each 0.15° wide dispersed randomly over the area, with sides of the dots oriented along the axis of motion. When the dots moved, new dots were revealed at the trailing edge, and dots at the leading edge disappeared, as if the dots were moving behind an aperture. The sides of the virtual aperture were aligned with the axis of motion. The dots alternated between moving inwards directly towards the fixation point and moving directly away, at 7.2°/s over a period of 942 ms (1.06 Hz), yielding approximately 471 ms per colour or motion. With the same period, they also alternated between red (14 cd/m^2, CIE $x = .63$, $y = .33$) and green (CIE $x = .29$, $y = .59$) and usually blue (CIE $x = .19$, $y = .13$), see Design and Procedure section for details of the alternation. The luminance for green and blue was set for each participant individually to match their approximate equiluminance point—determined by flickering the dot fields between red and green (or blue) at 8.5 Hz and adjusting the intensity of the green (or blue) to minimize the subjective intensity of the flicker (Wagner & Boynton, 1972).

To premask the stimulus train, the moving dot fields began at a random phase and were presented for one cycle at about 40% contrast flickering between red and green randomly with a probability of .5 on each frame. Then they began the appropriate colour alternation for that trial and gradually increased in contrast over the first 942 ms cycle. Subsequent to this premask period, the dots were presented at full contrast for two cycles. Finally, the dot fields disappeared in the same fashion that they had appeared—they gradually decreased in contrast over one cycle before flickering randomly between red and green for a cycle. The gradual ramping in and out avoided a sudden onset that might affect the asynchrony because of the apparent increase in temporal resolution that a sudden onset can engender (Beaudot, 2002; Dakin & Bex, 2002; Holcombe, Kanwisher, & Treisman, 1998). Figure 1 shows a schematic of the stimulus.[1]

Design and procedure. There were two important independent variables in this experiment. The first was the duration of the red, relative to that of the other colours. The period of the colour alternation was always 942 ms, and for a given trial the red occupied a variable portion of this, either 283 ms (30% of the cycle), 377 ms (40%), 471 ms (50%), 565 ms (60%), or 659 ms (70%). The rest of the cycle was occupied by green and blue, with the proportion of this remainder as blue taking a value of 0% (all green), 25%, 50%, or 75% on each trial. In half of the trials the blue period (if it existed) came before the green, and in half it occurred after. The second independent variable of primary interest was the time of the midpoint of the red interval relative to the midpoint of the inward motion, which we call "in → red interval" (Figure 1). The arrow in "in → red interval" signifies the direction time is measured, for example if red's midpoint occurred 50 ms after inward midpoint, the in → red interval is 50 ms. This varied over the whole range of possible temporal offsets. Before doing the experiment, it was thought that the relative timing of the red onset to the motion onset was of primary interest, so on each trial this was set to one of the following values (in ms): −353, −236, −118, 0, 118, 236, 353, or 471. The value of −471 was omitted because, due to the period being 942 ms, it is the same stimulus as 471 ms. For clarity, the data are analysed in terms of in → red interval. The particular values shift depending on the red duration, but still they fill the range of possible values with equal spacing, as can be seen by the data points in Figure 2. The variables were fully crossed and counterbalanced: (5 red durations) * (6 blue/green proportions and orders + 1 no-blue) * (8 relative timings) = 280 conditions in a block. Each subject participated in one block.

Observers were instructed to attend to the red intervals and determine the motion that was predominantly paired with it. When the in → red interval was 0 ms and red occupied 50% of the colour cycle, the features were exactly synchronized so that physically, red was paired only with inward motion. Observers pressed the "z" key if they perceived that red predominantly moved inward, and "x" if the red phase instead moved predominantly outward. For each red duration, two values for in → red should lead to the most unambiguous percepts, yielding the most consistent pairing reports. These are not expected to be the values where the stimulus was physically least ambiguous (0 and −471 ms), but instead to reflect the asynchrony.

[1] A demonstration of similar stimuli is available at http://www.psych.usyd.edu.au/staff/alexh/research/asynchronyVSS06/

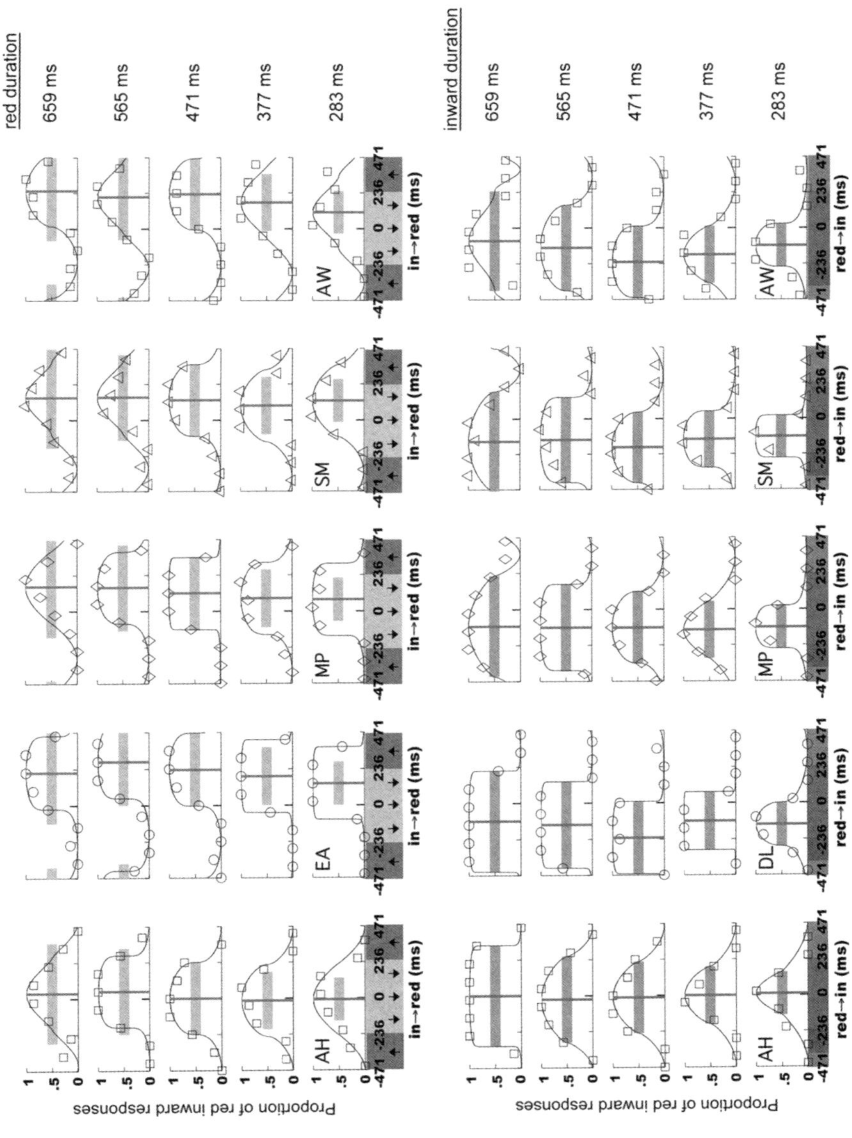

Figure 2 *(See next page for caption)*

One of the seven dot patches was chosen randomly on each trial as the target and indicated by a white ring (80 cd/m^2, diameter = 2.4°, thickness 0.22°), which encircled the target dot patch for the duration of the trial's stimulus train. The other six dot patches were set to random in → red intervals. This arrangement was identical to that used in Holcombe and Cavanagh (2008).

Participants sat approximately 1 m from the CRT. They participated in a variable number of practice trials until they were comfortable with the task. Participants fixated on the central point and were instructed to attend to the dot patch encircled by the ring. At any point during the stimulus train, participants could make their response. The participant's keypress terminated the trial immediately, even if the stimulus was still being presented.

Data analysis. Unlike in previous literature, the participant responses could not be modelled by a waveform such as a cosine wave, which has peak and trough of equal width, because in Experiment 2 (described later) the variation in the motion duration caused the relative width of the peak and trough to vary. For instance, if the best in → red time (α) were 0, rather than the in → red values spanning -236, 236 expected to yield in → red responses greater than 50% of the time, the motion duration (d) determined that instead the values spanning $-d/2$, $d/2$ did so instead. To create a psychometric function that would fit, the in → red values (x) corresponding to the peak were transformed into x' by linearly compressing them to fit in the domain under the top half of a cosine,

$$x' = \frac{\pi(x - a)}{d},$$

when $-d/2 < (x - a) < d/2$, with the remaining portion stretched to fill the domain of the trough

$$x' = \pi\left(\frac{(x - a) - .5d}{942 - d} + .5\right),$$

yielding pseudocosine waves with the appropriate duty cycle.

Figure 2 (previous page). Top: Probability of responding "red inward" as a function of in → red interval for each participant (columns) for each duration of red (rows). Vertical red lines show best in → red interval inferred from best-fitting psychometric function (black curves). Red rectangles depict the period red was presented at the best in → red interval. Bottom: Probability of responding "red inward" for each participant (columns) for each duration of inward motion (rows) as a function of red → in interval. Vertical red lines show best red → in interval inferred from best-fitting psychometric function (black curves). Grey rectangles depict the period inward was presented at the best red → in interval. As the duration of the inward motion increases, the range of times for which red is predominantly inward increases, and hence the peak of the psychometric function widens. To view this figure in colour, please see the online issue of the Journal.

For the data of Experiment 1, the duration d was always set to 471, yielding the degenerate case of an unmodified cosine curve. Another modification to the cosine, a variable exponent (β), was added to the peak and trough to capture the variation in the steepness of the psychometric functions. Finally, to better fit the data it was assumed that participants, due to keypress error and lapses in attention, made a random response on 0.8% of trials.

$$y = \frac{.99}{2}(\cos(x')^{1/b} + 1),$$

when $\cos(x') > 0$, to steepen the peak

$$y = \frac{.99}{2}(-(-\cos(x'))^{1/b} + 1),$$

otherwise, to steepen the trough, where y represents the proportion of red-inward responses. The parameters minimizing the sum of squared error difference between the stretched steepened cosine model and the actual responses were found using the Nelder-Mead simplex algorithm. The resulting fits are plotted as solid curves along with the data points (Figure 2).

Standard errors of the best-fitting in→red interval were determined by bootstrap (Efron & Tibshirani, 1993). In these experiments, the data in some conditions for some subjects were often at floor and ceiling, with inward-red responses forming 100% or 0% of the trials. In such cases, nonparametric bootstrapping yields inappropriately small confidence intervals. To avoid this, although the data were resampled 200 times as in nonparametric bootstrapping, rather than from the actual data, artificial data sets were generated from the best-fitting curve for that subject and condition. This yielded larger confidence intervals for the data near floor and ceiling while giving intervals similar to the nonparametric method in other cases. The confidence intervals are plotted in Figure 3 (Experiment 1) and Figure 4 (Experiment 2).

Results and discussion

The primary question was how the best timing of the red relative to inward motion would vary with the duration of the red. The effect of duration on best in→red interval is shown in the right panel of Figure 3. Each subplot shows the data for a single observer. The horizontal axis is time relative to the inward and outward motions, with the origin the midpoint of the inward motion. The five light red rectangles represent the best time of the red relative to the inward motion. First, consider the middle rectangles, corresponding to the condition when red had the same duration (471 ms) as the motions. This condition is like those of experiments in earlier literature. For four out of the five participants, a large asynchrony resulted, with the middle of the red best presented well after the midpoint of the inward motion. A striking exception to this was participant AH, the author, for whom the asynchrony was only 1 ms ($\pm$ 18, 95% CI). When conducting the experiments for his first paper on the asynchrony topic, AH had a robust asynchrony of about 100 ms (Holcombe & Cavanagh, 2008), which replicated in many pilot experiments. Recently, however, with the very same displays for which he once consistently had a $\sim$ 100 ms asynchrony, no asynchrony is obtained even though there is no conscious difference in the strategy being used. Furthermore, AH never participated in an experiment that provided feedback on individual trials. Possible implications of this plasticity for theories of the asynchrony are treated in the General Discussion.

Considering the other red durations besides the 471 ms condition, we distinguished between three different possible outcomes, depending on what aspect of the red feature was used for binding. One possibility was that regardless of the red duration, the best time for the red would be that which would preserve a constant interval between the red onset and the motion. Second was that binding involved matching of the colour offset, so that the offset of the red would always have a particular timing relative to the motion. Third was that either onsets and offsets were equally weighted for binding, or that the entire interval was equally important, in which case the midpoint of the red would have a constant time relative to the motion. This last possibility is the expectation from theories like differential latency (Moutoussis & Zeki, 1997; Zeki, 2007) that do not suggest any differential role of different parts of the interval. The data consistently show an intermediate result rather than any of these extreme scenarios. The midpoint shifts towards the direction of preserving the colour onset time, as can be seen in Figure 3. This was quantified by regressing the midpoints on red duration, scaled by the midpoint shift needed to keep onsets constant. For this regression, the constant colour onset time scenario (purple dashed line in Figure 3) predicts a regression coefficient of 1, constant colour offset times (green dotted line in Figure 3) would yield a coefficient of -1, and constant colour midpoint time corresponds to 0. The actual regression lines through the data points are plotted in red. The mean regression coefficient was significantly greater than zero, $t(4) = 5.3$, $p = .006$, at .44, which falls almost halfway between 0, the coefficient if the relative times of the midpoints were preserved and 1, that if the relative time of the onsets had been preserved. The .44 coefficient corresponds to a total average midpoint shift of 83 ms. This suggests that for feature pairing, the early portion of the colour is weighted more heavily than the portion near the end.

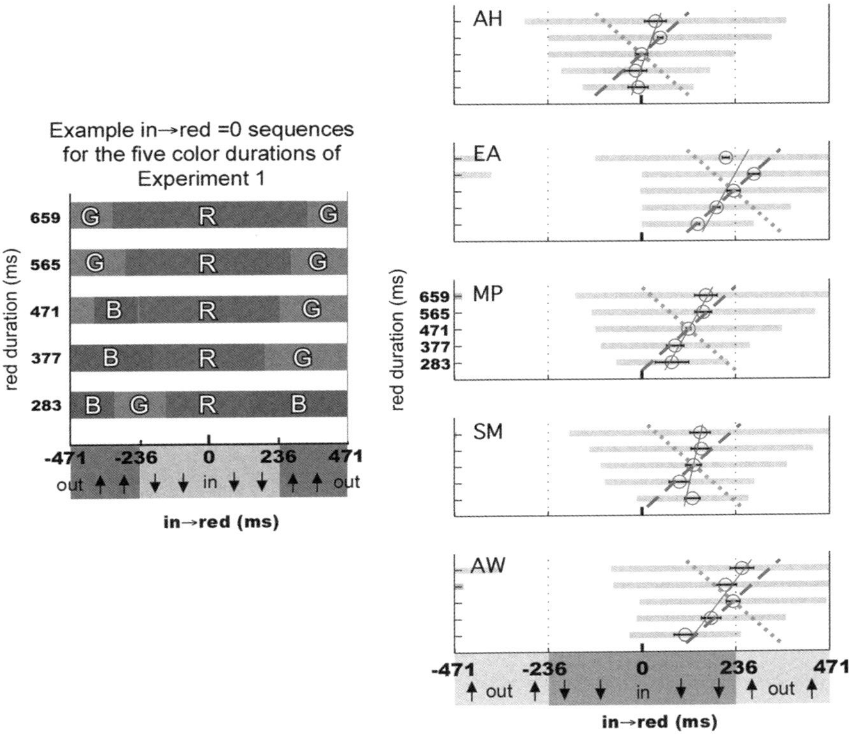

Figure 3. Left: The red durations of Experiment 1 are schematized (rows), each with an in→red interval of 0. Right: For each participant (initials), the red data circles show, for each red duration, the best time of the red midpoint relative to the inward midpoint. The red rectangles show the full range of times the stimulus was red for that in→red interval. Error bars show bootstrapped 95% confidence intervals. Green dotted lines show the result if best in→red interval had shifted to keep constant the relative timing of colour offset and motion (the red duration of 471 ms, the canonical stimulus, is used as the baseline). Purple dashed lines shows how in→red would have shifted if colour onset kept a constant timing relative to the motion. It can be seen from the data points and the line of best fit (red line) that neither is wholly true, but the data lean strongly towards preserving the onset time. To view this figure in colour, please see the online issue of the Journal.

EXPERIMENT 2: VARYING THE DURATION OF MOTION

Here the duration of the motion was varied to see whether the critical aspect of it was the beginning of the interval, the end, or something in between.

Methods

Participants. Four males and one female participated including the first author (AH) and three other participants from Experiment 1, age ranging from 21 to 34.

Stimulus. Same as Experiment 1 but with duration of red constant at 471 ms and proportion of inward motion taking one of five values: 283 ms (30% of the cycle), 377 ms (40%), 471 ms (50%), 565 ms (60%), or 659 ms (70%), and outward motion filling the remainder of the 942 ms feature period.

Design and procedure. Identical to Experiment 1 but with the critical variable the duration of the inward motion. Two of the participants ran in this experiment before running in Experiment 1.

Data analysis. Same as Experiment 1, with d (duration of motion) set appropriately to vary the duty cycle of the curvefit.

Results and discussion

The timing of the motion midpoint relative to the colour did not shift significantly, as can be seen in Figure 4. Regressing the best time of the motion midpoint relative to the colour (red lines) revealed that across subjects the mean motion midpoint shifted by only 2%, in the direction of preserving relative onset times, a tiny and nonsignificant, $t(4) = 0.33$, $p = .76$, fraction. Indeed, the shift was not large for any of the participants, as shown by the red regression lines in Figure 4. For two of the subjects the deviations from vertical were in one direction; in the rest they leaned the other way. Unlike for colour, then, reports of feature pairings do not favour the early part of the motion.

This conclusion rests on the presumption that the reason for the different results in Experiments 1 and 2 was the effect of each particular stimulus condition rather than the other conditions that it was intermixed with in a block. To test this, we can compare the results for the condition which was common to both experiments—when both features were presented for half a cycle. The average difference between the experiments in the best relative timing for the four who participated in both experiments was just 18 ms, not significant, $t(6) = 0.27$, $p = .8$, and very small in comparison to the 83 ms average effect of varying the colour duration.

EXPERIMENT 3: NO DIFFERENCE BETWEEN INWARD (FOVEOPETAL) AND OUTWARD (FOVEOFUGAL) MOTION

In the previous experiment, as the duration of inward motion increased, the duration of outward decreased. The intention was to reveal the relative importance of different parts of a motion interval. However, conceivably the two motions, inward and outward, might yield different asynchronies on

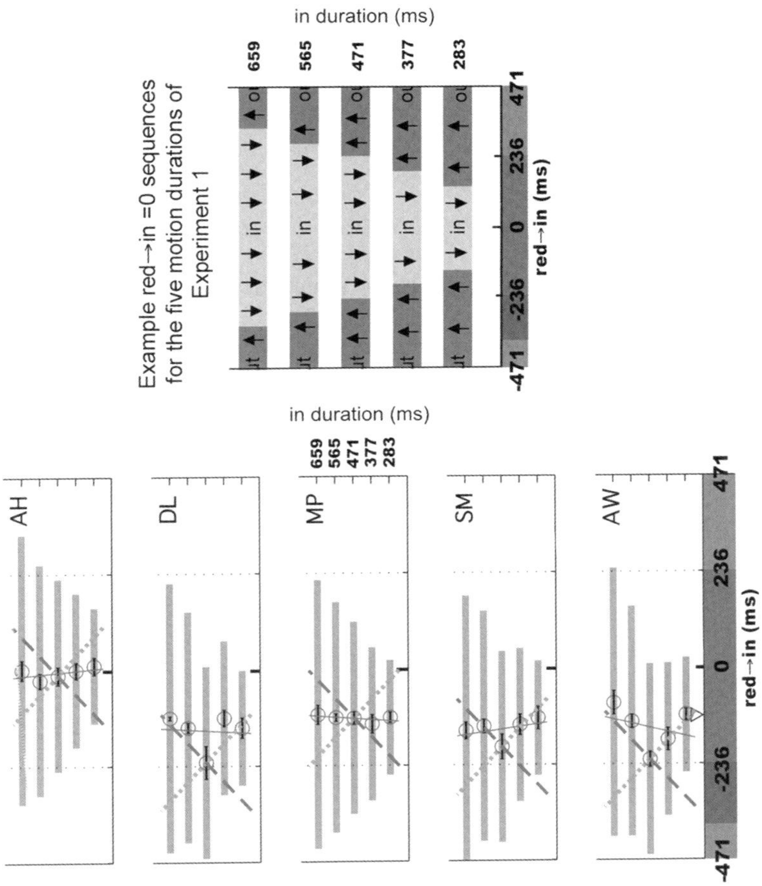

Figure 4 *(See next page for caption)*

their own. Changing their proportion as we did would then change the overall asynchrony quite apart from the point of the experiment. To check this, here the asynchronies for inward and outward motion were measured separately. In one condition, inward motion was alternated with dynamic noise and, in the other condition, outward motion was alternated with dynamic noise. In both cases the task was to report whether the dots, when red, were predominantly paired with inward motion, outward motion, or noise.

The concern that foveopetal (inward) and foveofugal (outward) motion would manifest different binding errors is motivated by previous differences found for the flash-lag effect (Mateef, Bohdanecky, Hohnsbein, Ehrenstein, & Yakimoff, 1991). If the flash-lag effect and asynchrony illusions are related, which is unknown at present, then a similar difference might occur in the current experiment.

Methods

Participants. Four of those who were in Experiment 2 participated.

Stimulus. Same as the previous experiments but with either inward or outward motion replaced by dynamic noise of similar temporal frequency content as the motion. The dots were randomly replotted every 33 ms.

Design and procedure. Identical to the previous experiments but with seven trials per motion type and timing combination, yielding a total of 112 trials.

Data analysis. Same as Experiment 1.

Results and discussion

The best timing of the colour midpoint relative to the motion midpoint (in→ red interval in the previous experiments) for each participant and type of

Figure 4 (previous page). Right: The various inward motion durations of Experiment 2 are schematized, each with the red→in interval of 0. The proportion of green and blue in the remainder was counterbalanced, and random values are shown in the timeline at bottom. Left: Each subplot shows the result for a different participant. The red data circles show, for each red duration, the best time of the inward motion midpoint relative to the red midpoint. The grey rectangles show the full interval of inward motion for that red→in interval. Error bars show bootstrapped 95% confidence intervals. Green dotted lines show the results if best in→red interval had shifted to keep constant the relative timing of colour offset and motion (the red duration of 471 ms, the canonical stimulus, is used as the baseline). Purple dashed lines show how in→red would have shifted if colour onset kept a constant timing relative to the motion. It can be seen from the data points and the line of best fit (red line) that neither is true, and different participants show opposite and small shifts in both directions. To view this figure in colour, please see the online issue of the Journal.

TABLE 1
Best timings of the colour relative to the motions in Experiment 3

Participant	*Inward*	*Outward*	*Difference*	*Baseline*
MP	87 ± 17 ms	52 ± 16 ms	−35 ms	119 ± 15 ms
AW	112 ± 18 ms	59 ± 16 ms	−53 ms	224 ± 19 ms
SM	59 ± 16 ms	73 ± 22 ms	14 ms	191 ± 30 ms
DL	49 ± 15 ms	59 ± 17 ms	10 ms	227 ± 40 ms

The "baseline" figures of the last column are the asynchrony measured for each subject in Experiment 2 when each motion was presented for 471 ms. The "outward" column shows the best time of red relative to motion for the outward motion condition, and the "inward" column the best time of red relative to the motion in the inward motion condition. Following the "±" is the 95% confidence interval from parametric bootstrapping. The numbers are smaller than the baseline, and inward and outward motion do not differ in any consistent way, as is evident from the "difference" column.

motion are tabulated in Table 1. For both kinds of motion, the asynchronies for each participant were much smaller than in the previous experiments with alternating motions. Various theories of the asynchrony could explain this, as it may be due either to lack of motion inhibition without opposing motions (Arnold & Clifford, 2002) or the presence of the motion streak cue (Amano, Johnston, & Nishida, 2007) here.

Most observers reported that, during each dynamic noise period, weak motion opposite to the previous motion's direction was perceived. The fact that this was not perceived when observers were asked to view a display with the dynamic noise in isolation indicates that it was a motion aftereffect, although probably of a nonclassical, rapid-induction variety (Kanai & Verstraten, 2005). Clearly, however, this motion was not strong enough to act similarly to the real motion—if it had, the asynchrony would not have been so dramatically reduced.

No consistent difference between the two types of motion was seen across participants, and a paired *t*-test was not significant, $t(3) = 0.96$, $p = .41$. This eliminates the potential confound in the previous experiment.

GENERAL DISCUSSION

The colour–motion asynchrony has been attributed to a difference in sensory latency between motion and colour (Moutoussis & Zeki, 1997; Zeki, 2003, 2007). But the data here support a different theory of the asynchrony—that it is caused by greater weighting of the early part of the colour. Here we found that the perception of feature pairings weights the early phase of an interval of colour more highly than other aspects, while not weighting differently the early and late parts of the motion.

This result is in good agreement with the theory of Nishida and Johnston (in press). In particular, Nishida and Johnston suggest that the middle portion of the motion interval is matched to a time closer to the onset or offset of the colour. There is another recent theory of the asynchrony (Clifford, in press), but it seems less relevant. This theory suggests that the asynchrony is caused by a difference in latencies, but rather than afferent latencies, a difference in latency of feedback of a new motion signal from late visual cortex to early visual cortex. Although that theory does not seem to explain the current results, in an earlier paper Clifford et al. (2003) suggested alternatively that the asynchrony might result from heavy weighting of the early portion of the colour, just as we have suggested here. Specifically, Clifford et al. proposed that early portions of colour would be differentially favoured due to a more rapid adaptation (reduction) of the neural response to colour. The present experiments do not speak to the reason for the greater weighting for early portion of the colour, be it difference in transients or difference in adaptation timescale. However, other literature already implicates involvement of transients (Nishida & Johnston, 2002), whereas we do not know of independent evidence for an adaptation or response difference between colour and motion.

A critical role for transients in binding is further supported by the results of Holcombe and Cavanagh (2008). Their experiments revealed that transients provided by an external cue can determine the best relative timing of the features. Hence, there is considerable support for the idea that different portions of the colour and motion features, perhaps their transients, drive the best timing for pairing rather than a difference in latency. However, the shift observed here in best colour timing was not as large as expected if the binding mechanism used only the onset of the colour, suggesting some involvement of other portions of the response to colour.

The plasticity in the asynchrony apparent in the data of AH is easier to explain for theories that include a role for attention. For such theories, there is at least the possibility of deploying attention in different ways, which could eliminate the asynchrony according to both the theories of Holcombe and Cavanagh (2008) and Nishida and Johnston (in press). The other theories of the asynchrony (Clifford, in press; Clifford et al., 2003; Zeki, 2007) have more difficulty explaining the elimination of the asynchrony. However, they could insist that the participant must be using synchrony judgements of the feature changes to do the task (although this would be in contradiction to his subjective experience), because synchrony judgements are already known to often be free of asynchrony (Bedell et al., 2003; Clifford et al., 2003; Nishida & Johnston, 2002).

Conceivably, it could be argued that the present experiments do not probe perceptual experience but instead reflect memory dynamics for the bindings presented. Plausibly for an extremely long 2-s duration of a feature like red (much longer than the present experiments), with inward motion duration of 1 s, then for every relative timing the participant is likely to experience red paired with both inward and outward motion. Ideally, the participant would take the bindings experienced and weight that experienced towards the beginning of the red equally to that experienced towards the end of the red. If that were the case, then the best relative timing would reflect the binding scheme used by the visual system. However, memory biases such as the primacy effect could cause the participant to not weight different portions of the red equally. But it is unlikely that memorial factors like this were the reasons for the results here. Memory biases should only emerge at long feature durations, whereas at short durations responses should be based entirely on the single percept experienced. If memory biases were beginning to contaminate responses, the regression coefficient should change as the feature duration got longer, which is not apparent in most of the data. Furthermore on the memory account it would be difficult to explain the difference in weighting the different aspects of colour and motion.

Another danger as feature duration increases is that more than one binding percept may occur during a single colour or motion interval. Theories such as ours that suggest a critical role for the early phase of the red should make clear that they refer to intervals on the order of the temporal resolution of the binding mechanism, which appears to be hundreds of milliseconds (Arnold, 2005; Bartels & Zeki, 2006; Cavanagh, Holcombe, & Chou, 2008; Holcombe & Cavanagh, 2001). If there is enough time for a second bound percept to be created, this likely would no longer be on the basis of the early phase of the colour and hence would dilute the greater weighting of early colour. Conceivably, this dilution may be occurring even with the present stimuli.

The actual mechanism that binds remains obscure, even if it is clear that it differentially weights different portions of colour and motions. Whether the system normally uses a binding scheme based on matching onset transients, or cross-correlating the neural response profile to the features, or one reflecting the dynamics of attentional access to the two features remains unsettled. Rather than cross-correlation of neural response profiles, we favour an account based on high-level, perhaps parietal and attentive processes accessing the features independently at a time mostly triggered by the onset transient in the case of the colour and for motion, a later portion when motion becomes more conspicuous. This is consistent with other evidence favouring a slow, high-level mechanism for the pairing of certain features like colour and motion (Cavanagh et al., 2008; Fujisaki & Nishida, 2007; Holcombe & Cavanagh, 2001, 2008).

REFERENCES

Amano, K., Johnston, A., & Nishida, S. (2007). Two mechanisms underlying the effect of angle of motion direction change on colour–motion asynchrony. *Vision Research*, *47*(5), 687–705.

Arnold, D. H. (2005). Perceptual pairing of colour and motion. *Vision Research*, *45*(24), 3015–3026.

Arnold, D. H., & Clifford, C. W. G. (2002). Determinants of asynchronous processing in vision. *Proceedings of the Royal Society of London, Series B*, *269*, 579–583.

Arnold, D. H., Clifford, C. W. G., & Wenderoth, P. (2001). Asynchronous processing in vision: Color leads motion. *Current Biology*, *11*, 596–600.

Bair, W., Cavanaugh, J. R., Smith, M. A., & Movshon, J. A. (2002). The timing of response onset and offset in macaque visual neurons. *Journal of Neuroscience*, *22*(8), 3189–3205.

Bartels, A., & Zeki, S. (2006). The temporal order of binding visual attributes. *Vision Research*, *46*, 2280–2286.

Beaudot, W. H. (2002). Role of onset asynchrony in contour integration. *Vision Research*, *42*(1), 1–9.

Bedell, H. C., Chung, S. T., Ogmen, H., & Patel, S. S. (2003). Color and motion: Which is the tortoise and which is the hare? *Vision Research*, *43*, 2403–2412.

Botella, J., & Eriksen, C. W. (1992). Filtering versus parallel processing in RSVP tasks. *Perception and Psychophysics*, *51*(4), 334–343.

Cavanagh, P., Holcombe, A. O., & Chou, W.-L. (2008). Mobile computation: Spatiotemporal integration of object properties. *Manuscript submitted for publication.*

Clark, A. (2001). Some logical features of feature integration. In W. Backhaus (Ed.), *Neuronal coding of perceptual systems* (pp. 3–20). Hackensack, NJ: World Scientific.

Clifford, C. W. G. (in press). Dynamics of visual feature binding. In R. Nijhawan & B. Khurana (Eds.), *Space and time in perception and action*. Cambridge, UK: Cambridge University Press.

Clifford, C. W. G., Arnold, D. H., & Pearson, J. (2003). A paradox of temporal perception revealed by a stimulus oscillating in colour and orientation. *Vision Research*, *43*, 2245–2253.

Comtois, R. (2003). *VisionShell PPC* [Software libraries]. Cambridge, MA: Author.

Dakin, S. C., & Bex, P. J. (2002). Role of synchrony in contour binding: Some transient doubts sustained. *Journal of the Optical Society of America, A: Optics, Image Science, and Vision*, *19*(4), 678–686.

Efron, B., & Tibshirani, R. J. (1993). *An introduction to the bootstrap*. Boca Raton, FL: Chapman & Hall.

Fujisaki, W., & Nishida, S. (2007). Feature-based processing of audio-visual synchrony perception revealed by random pulse trains. *Vision Research*, *47*(8), 1075–1093.

Gottsdanker, R. (1956). The ability of human operators to detect acceleration of target motion. *Psychological Bulletin*, *53*, 477–487.

Holcombe, A. O., & Cavanagh, P. (2001). Early binding of feature pairs for visual perception. *Nature Neuroscience*, *4*, 127–128.

Holcombe, A. O., & Cavanagh, P. (2008). Independent, synchronous access to color and motion features. *Cognition*, *107*(2), 552–580.

Holcombe, A. O., Kanwisher, N., & Treisman, A. (2001). The midstream order deficit. *Perception and Psychophysics*, *63*(2), 322–339.

Johnston, A., & Nishida, S. (2001). Time perception: Brain time or event time? *Current Biology*, *11*(11), R427–R430.

Kanai, R., & Verstraten, F. A. (2005). Perceptual manifestations of fast neural plasticity: Motion priming, rapid motion aftereffect and perceptual sensitization. *Vision Research*, *45*(25–26), 3109–3116.

Keele, S. W., & Neill, W. T. (1978). Mechanisms of attention. In E. C. Carterette & M. P. Friedman (Eds.), *Handbook of perception* (Vol. 9, pp. 3–47). San Diego, CA: Academic Press.

Kreegipuu, K., & Allik, J. (2007). Detection of motion onset and offset: Reaction time and visual evoked potential analysis. *Psychological Research, 71*(6), 703–708.

Mateeff, S., Bohdanecky, Z., Hohnsbein, J., Ehrenstein, W. H., & Yakimoff, N. (1991). A constant latency difference determines directional anisotropy in visual motion perception. *Vision Research, 31*(12), 2235–2237.

Moutoussis, K., & Zeki, S. (1997). A direct demonstration of perceptual asynchrony in vision. *Proceedings of the Royal Society of London, Series B, 264*, 393–399.

Nakayama, K., & Mackeben, M. (1989). Sustained and transient components of focal visual attention. *Vision Research, 29*(11), 1631–1647.

Neri, P., & Levi, D. (2006). Spatial resolution for feature binding is impaired in peripheral and amblyopic vision. *Journal of Neurophysiology, 96*(1), 142–153.

Nishida, S., & Johnston, A. (2002). Marker correspondence, not processing latency, determines temporal binding of visual attributes. *Current Biology, 12*(5), 359–368.

Nishida, S., & Johnston, A. (in press). The time marker account of cross-channel temporal judgements. In R. Nijhawan & B. Khurana (Eds.), *Space and time in perception and action*. Cambridge, UK: Cambridge University Press.

Treisman, A., & Gelade, G. (1980). A feature integration theory of attention. *Cognitive Psychology, 12*, 97–136.

Wagner, G., & Boynton, R. M. (1972). Comparison of four methods of heterochromatic photometry. *Journal of the Optical Society of America, 62*(12), 1508–1515.

Ward, R., Danziger, S., Owen, V., & Rafal, R. D. (2002). Deficits in spatial coding and feature binding following damage to spatiotopic maps in the human pulvinar. *Nature Neuroscience, 5*, 99–100.

Werkhoven, P., Snippe, H. P., & Toet, A. (1992). Visual processing of optic acceleration. *Vision Research, 32*(12), 2313–2329.

Wu, D. A., Kanai, R., & Shimojo, S. (2004). Vision: Steady-state misbinding of colour and motion. *Nature, 429*(6989), 262.

Zeki, S. (2003). The disunity of consciousness. *Trends in Cognitive Science, 7*(5), 214–218.

Zeki, S. (2005). The Ferrier Lecture 1995 behind the seen: The functional specialization of the brain in space and time. *Philosophical Transactions of the Royal Society of London, Series B: Biological Sciences, 360*(1458), 1145–1183.

Zeki, S. (2007). The disunity of consciousness. *Progress in Brain Research, 168*, 11–268.

Zeki, S., & Bartels, A. (1998). The asynchrony of consciousness. *Proceedings of the Royal Society B: Biological Sciences, 265*(1405), 1583–1585.

VISUAL COGNITION, 2009, 17 (1/2), 254–272

Psychology Press
Taylor & Francis Group

Building visual representations: The binding of relative spatial relations across time

Jennifer D. Ryan
Rotman Research Institute, and Departments of Psychology and Psychiatry, University of Toronto, Toronto, ON, Canada

Christina Villate
Rotman Research Institute, Toronto, ON, Canada

In this study, the construction of, and subsequent access to, representations regarding the relative spatial and temporal relations among sequentially presented objects was examined using eye movement monitoring. Participants were presented with a series of single objects. Subsequently, a test display revealed all three objects simultaneously and participants judged whether the relative relations were maintained. Eye movements revealed the binding of relations across study images; eye movements transitioned between the location of the presented object and the locations that were previously occupied by objects in prior study images. For the test displays, changes in the relative relations were accurately detected. Eye movements distinguished intact displays from those in which the relations had been altered. Order of fixations to objects in test images mimicked the temporal order in which objects had been studied, but disruption of temporal order was observed for manipulated images. The present findings suggest that memory representations regarding the visual world include information about the relative spatial and temporal relations among objects. Eye movements may be the conduit by which information is integrated into a lasting representation, and by which current information is compared to stored representations.

Keywords: Binding; Visual memory; Eye movements; Spatial relations; Temporal relations.

We can typically remember the series of turns required in taking the shortest route to work, and we can return to our car in the car park at the end of the

---

Please address all correspondence to Jennifer D. Ryan, Rotman Research Institute, 3560 Bathurst St., Toronto, ON, Canada M6A 2E1. E-mail: jryan@rotman-baycrest.on.ca

We wish to thank Noah Ivers and Grace Leung for their assistance. Funding was provided by the Natural Sciences and Engineering Research Council of Canada (NSERC) and the Canada Research Chairs Program.

© 2008 Psychology Press, an imprint of the Taylor & Francis Group, an Informa business
http://www.psypress.com/viscog DOI: 10.1080/13506280802336362

day. As a result, we tend to believe that a considerable amount of information is extracted when viewing the external world and is subsequently kept in veridical form in a lasting memory representation (Levin, Momen, Drivdahl, & Simons, 2000; Wells & Olson, 2003). However, when such beliefs were put to empirical testing, a range of theories regarding the nature of memory representations emerged—from the notion that information can be readily extracted from a single glance and held in memory for a prolonged period of time (Biederman, Rabinowitz, Glass, & Stacy, 1974) to the idea that little to no information is actually maintained across time and eye fixations (O'Regan, 1992). Thus, over the past few decades, research has strived to answer the following question: What is maintained over time in memory? The current work aims to contribute to this vast literature by exploring the extent to which the spatial and temporal relations among objects can be maintained in memory, and how such representations are constructed.

Research suggests that memory representations regarding visual displays include information regarding the spatial locations of objects. For instance, visual search performance was faster for displays that were repeated across trials compared to novel displays (Chun & Jiang, 1998; Peterson & Kramer, 2001), suggesting the remembered spatial locations of display elements were used to guide visual search. Additional evidence comes from studies in which viewers' eye movements were attracted to regions within scenes that had undergone a change in the location or presence of an object from a prior viewing (Hollingworth, Williams, & Henderson, 2001; Parker, 1978; Ryan, Althoff, Whitlow, & Cohen, 2000; Ryan & Cohen, 2004). The fact that the eyes were attracted to previously occupied regions reveals that memory for object locations had been maintained in memory. Additionally, Meegan and Honsberger (2005) observed that spatial information could be recalled from a prior learning episode even when it was not required for successful task performance to occur; when participants were enquired about the identity of a previously studied object, their eye movements were attracted to the (now empty) region of a display that had previously contained the object in question (see also Spivey & Geng, 2001). These findings demonstrate that spatial information regarding objects was maintained in memory, but questions remained regarding the nature of such spatial information. That is, the spatial information that is maintained in memory could include the metric locations in x,y,z-coordinate space of each object (i.e., absolute locations) and/or it could include the position of each object that is coded with respect to the other objects, but is not tied to a static frame of reference (i.e., relative location).

Findings from Olson and Marshuetz (2005) suggest that relative, rather than absolute, spatial relations are maintained in visual memory representations (see also Irwin, 1991). Participants were presented with displays of a face amongst objects during a study phase and were subsequently asked to make recognition decisions regarding the identity of the face when the multi-object displays were re-presented following a delay. Recognition decision times were slowed when changes were introduced to the absolute and relative spatial positions of the objects, but not when the absolute positions were altered and the relative positions among the objects remained unchanged. This demonstrated that changes to the relative, but not absolute, locations of objects interfered with decisions regarding object identity. Had no spatial information been retained, no interference would have been expected. In addition to demonstrating that relative locations were maintained in memory, the Olson and Marshuetz study further demonstrated that relative spatial locations were accessed even when the task does not require such information. In considering findings such as these, Hollingworth (2007) has suggested that the relative spatial relations that are maintained in memory may provide the foundation of visual representations upon which further information is embedded, such as object identity information.

Although these studies speak to issues surrounding the nature of memory representations, they do not address questions concerning the manner by which such representations are constructed. That is, how are spatial relations maintained in memory? One possibility is that the relations among the objects are extracted from a single composite representation of a static visual display (cf. Irwin, 1991). That is, displays may be encoded and subsequently retrieved as a whole, and, from this whole, particular details regarding spatial location may be queried. Alternatively, each object within a visual display may be encoded and maintained separately in memory. In this case, the spatial relations among the objects may be bound across time, thereby forming links among distinct objects (Cohen & Eichenbaum, 1993). Studies that present the to-be-bound information within a single display cannot address whether relations among single objects are subsequently extracted from a single composite or are bound across time in memory. One aim of the current work was to address whether relations among sequentially presented objects can be bound across time.

If spatial relations can be bound across time in memory, information regarding the temporal order by which objects were viewed (e.g., X was viewed prior to viewing Y) may be maintained as well. Findings from research on the *scanpath hypothesis* speak to issues surrounding the maintenance of temporal relations in visual representations. Work on the scanpath hypothesis sought to determine whether the order by which objects are initially sampled is reenacted during subsequent viewings (Noton & Stark, 1971; Stark & Ellis, 1981). Although exact repetitions of scanning have not been found, there were indications that some sequential order of scanning was retained across repetitions of a visual display (Brandt & Stark, 1997; Laeng & Teodorescu, 2002; Walker-Smith, Gale, & Findlay, 1977).

These results point to the possibility that temporal order information may be maintained across viewings. A second aim of the current work was to assess whether the temporal relations among sequentially presented objects was maintained in memory.

Thus, the goal of the current work was to investigate the construction and maintenance of visual memory representations regarding the (spatial and temporal) relations among sequentially presented objects. In the present study, participants viewed three novel objects, overlaid onto a unique background while eye movements were monitored. The novel objects were presented singly across three study images, on the same background. Subsequently, a test display presented all three objects simultaneously. In the test displays, all three objects moved to a different absolute spatial location. However, their relative locations either remained intact or the position of one object was altered with respect to the other two objects. Participants were asked to indicate whether the relative relations were maintained from the study to the test displays. Given that each to-be-bound object was presented alone, the present paradigm required the binding of relations to be achieved solely within the confines of memory rather than extracted during perceptual processing (Yamamoto & Shelton, 2007).

As noted earlier, eye movements can provide an index of access to stored memory representations (e.g., Ryan et al., 2000). Here, the use of eye movement monitoring can reveal the online updating of memories during the study phase of the present paradigm. Therefore, we can use this tool to inform us about the manner by which representations are *constructed*. Specifically, if relational representations are constructed in memory during viewing of the study images, eye movements should transition between the presented object and any (now empty) locations that had been previously occupied. If observed, this would suggest that the construction of a relational representation would inherently entail combining stored information with current perceptual input. Moreover, such findings would lend credence to research suggesting that eye movements may have a critical role in the construction of a memory representation (Brockmole & Irwin, 2005). That is, eye movements may be the conduit by which retrieved information from memory is bound with current perceptual input. Conversely, if eye movements do not transition to previously occupied locations during viewing of the study images, this finding would provide evidence that eye movements are not the underlying mechanism by which relational representations are constructed.

To provide evidence that the relative relations among sequentially presented objects were *maintained*, we used verbal reports and measures derived from eye movement monitoring to distinguish between intact and manipulated test displays. Verbal reports revealed whether participants knew, in general, that a change had occurred. Eye movement monitoring revealed whether participants had knowledge regarding the specific location of change within the test displays. Specifically, if relative relations were maintained, the eyes should be attracted to either the now-empty region in which the object should have been located had all the relations remained intact, or the now-filled region to which the object had been relocated (e.g., Ryan & Cohen, 2004). This would result in an increase in viewing of those regions for manipulated images compared to intact images. Note that in all test trials, all objects underwent a change in absolute spatial location. As a result, local changes in luminance or spatial frequency could not alone support either verbal or eye movement performance; rather only information regarding the relative relations could be used to distinguish intact from manipulated displays.

By virtue of exploring whether relative spatial relations among sequentially presented objects are maintained in visual memory representations, the present paradigm allows us to explore whether temporal relations are maintained within a lasting representation, as well. If temporal order is maintained, we would expect participants to sample the objects during the test display in an order that is consistent with the order in which the objects were revealed during the study images. Further, we can observe the extent to which changes in the relative spatial relations among the objects disrupts the temporal order of fixations. Thus, although we never directly asked the participants to comment on whether temporal information was maintained in memory, findings from their eye movement scanning patterns will nevertheless reveal whether such temporal relations have been maintained.

All together, the current work will outline the manner by which memory representations regarding the visual world are constructed and whether they include information about the relative spatial and temporal relations among sequentially presented objects. Using eye movements as a marker of access to previously stored representations in memory, this work may additionally lend support to an age-old view that perception of a multi-object display or event is achieved through binding in memory (James, 1890/1983).

Figure 1 (opposite). Examples of stimuli and procedures for (a) intact and (b) manipulated trials. For each trial, three study images depicting one object were presented for 3000 ms each, followed by a visual mask for 2000 ms. The test image (5000 ms) for all trials presented the three previously viewed objects in new absolute spatial locations. For intact images, the relative relations among the objects were maintained as revealed across the study images. For manipulated images, one object changed in its relative relations to the other objects. To view this figure in colour, please see the online issue of the Journal.

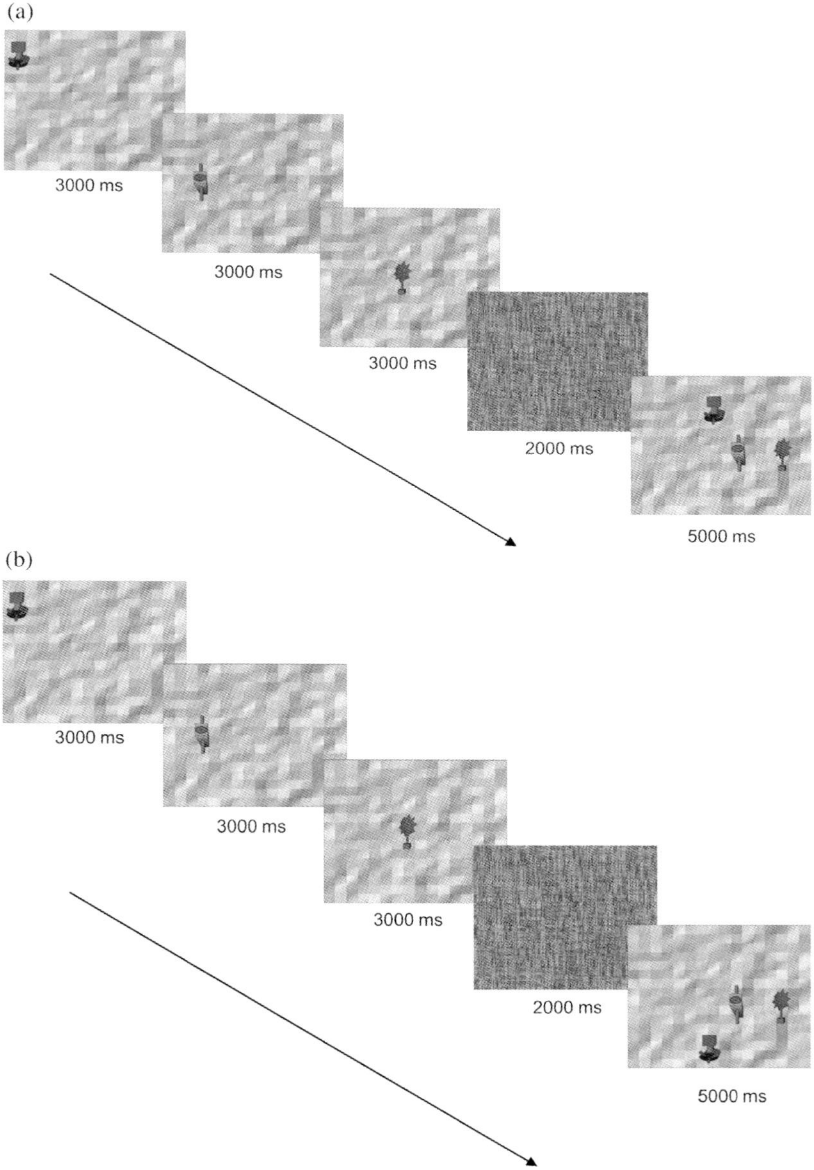

Figure 1. (*See opposite page for caption*)

METHOD

Participants

Sixteen healthy adults (12 female) with normal or corrected-to-normal vision participated in exchange for monetary compensation. The participants had an average age of 24.94 years (range 20–31) and an average education of 17.25 years (range 13–22).

Stimuli and design

Stimuli consisted of coloured images (1024 × 768 pixels) and novel objects created using Corel Draw v.12. Images were grouped into sets that were distinguished by a unique patterned background and three objects. The novel objects were designed to minimize resemblance to real-world objects, discourage use of associated verbal labels to aid in remembering the relative locations (e.g., "the cat is to the left of the boy") and were among the set used in prior work (Ryan, Leung, Turk-Browne, & Hasher, 2007). The study images each presented a single object in a unique spatial location; three study images were presented for each set. The test displays consisted of all three novel objects presented simultaneously in new absolute spatial locations, but the relative relations among the objects either remained intact (*intact* trials; see Figure 1a), or the relative relations among the objects were altered for one of the objects with respect to the other two (*manipulated* trials; see Figure 1b). Sets were counterbalanced across participants, and alternate study images were created, so that intact test trials for one participant became the manipulated trials for another. Each test image then was seen equally often as an *intact* or *manipulated* image. This allowed eye movement comparisons to be made across physically identical stimuli; the only difference was in the participants' prior viewing history.

Procedure

Participants were presented with 24 sets of images (12 intact, 12 manipulated) in random order. For each set, participants viewed the three study images for 3 s each. After the presentation of the three objects, a visual mask was presented for 2 s, followed by either the intact or manipulated image, which was displayed for 5 s (see Figure 1). Participants were instructed to remember the relative relations among the objects and to indicate whether the relative relations among the objects were maintained across study and test images. Button presses (left, right) were counterbalanced across participants. Written informed consent was obtained before testing, and verbal debriefing was provided upon completion.

Apparatus

Stimuli were presented on a 19-inch Dell M991 monitor that subtended approximately 33.4 degrees of visual angle from a distance of 25 inches. Eye movements were measured with a SR Research Ltd. Eyelink II eyetracker and sampled at a rate of 500 Hz with a spatial resolution of 0.1 degrees. A 9-point calibration was performed; calibration was repeated if the error at any point was more than 1°, or if the error for any the points was greater than 0.5°.

Data analysis

For the study images, regions of interest were created which outlined the region surrounding the presented object and the regions surrounding the previously presented or the to-be-presented objects (see Figure 2). For the test images, regions of interest were outlined surrounding each of the three objects, and the empty region, which, for *manipulated* images, corresponded to the location that would have been occupied if all the relative relations were intact. Various measures were derived from the eye movement data that described viewing to regions of interest, including: Viewing time, number of fixations, and number of transitions.

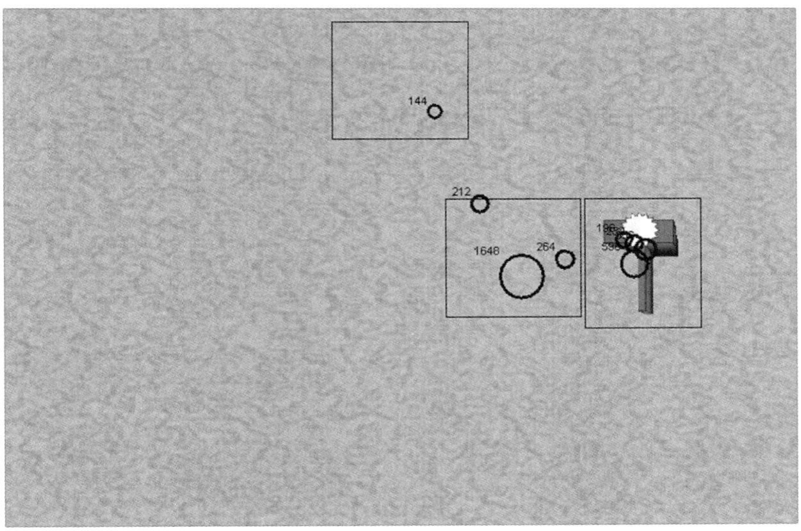

Figure 2. Viewing behaviour on a third study image for a representative participant. Fixations (noted by circles that vary in size according to duration) and fixation durations are noted. Eye movements are primarily directed towards the region surrounding the object, but fixations are also directed to the other regions of interest that represent the locations of the objects from the prior two study images. To view this figure in colour, please see the online issue of the Journal.

RESULTS

Behavioural responses

Due to programming error, one study image was not displayed on one "intact" trial for each of five participants. Therefore, a total of five "intact" trials were removed from all subsequent analyses. No response was recorded for three intact trials and twelve manipulated trials, but redundant verbal reports were taken. Participants responded that the relations were "intact" on 90% of the intact trials (range: 67–100%) and responded that the relations were ""manipulated" on 87% (range: 67–100%) of the manipulated trials. Average corrected recognition accuracy for manipulated trials ("manipulated" responses for manipulated minus intact responses) was 77% (range: 34–100%).

Study displays

Repeated-measures ANOVAs examined viewing to the three regions of interest (one filled, two empty) representing the locations of the to-be-bound objects, separately for the first, second, and third study images. There were significant differences in viewing of the three regions of interest in each of the study images (see Table 1A for means and relevant statistics).

TABLE 1A
Means (*SD*) and statistical results for measures of viewing directed to regions of interest of the study images

Display type	*Region of interest*	*Duration of viewing time*	*Number of fixations*	*Number of transitions*
Study 1	1 (filled)	2375.77 (166.88)	5.89 (1.19)	1.23 (0.17)
	2 (empty)	21.48 (20.88)	0.09 (0.09)	0.09 (0.08)
	3 (empty)	22.16 (12.38)	0.09 (0.05)	0.09 (0.04)
$F(2, 30)$		3094.10*	378.21*	803.23*
Study 2	1 (empty)	754.22 (201.23)	1.58 (0.50)	1.12 (0.29)
	2 (filled)	2253.67 (349.43)	4.81 (1.05)	1.36 (0.33)
	3 (empty)	9.89 (16.83)	0.02 (0.04)	0.02 (0.03)
$F(2, 30)$		395.74*	225.21*	234.70*
Study 3	1 (empty)	113.67 (102.84)	0.30 (0.30)	0.25 (0.26)
	2 (empty)	828.21 (231.79)	1.44 (0.43)	1.10 (0.28)
	3 (filled)	2037.19 (401.90)	4.24 (0.76)	1.47 (0.36)
$F(2, 30)$		192.87*	259.54*	288.61*

*$p \leq .01$.

Unsurprisingly, viewing was directed primarily to the object-filled region of interest for each of the images.

During the viewing of the first study image, little to no viewing was directed to the empty regions of interest for which no object had yet been presented, and viewing did not differ between the two empty regions of interest, all $ts(15) < 0.2$, $p > .85$. However, during viewing of the second study image, significantly more viewing was directed to the previously occupied empty region of interest compared to the as-yet-unoccupied empty region of interest (see Table 1A), as revealed by planned *t*-tests between the two empty regions of interest: Viewing time, $t(15) = 15.29$, $p < .001$; number of fixations, $t(15) = 12.39$, $p < .001$; number of transitions, $t(15) = 15.32$, $p < .001$. Critically, both regions were empty and one would not expect viewing to be directed to empty regions. However, one region had previously contained an object; therefore, we take the increased viewing to the region of the previously presented first object to reflect the influence of memory.

Viewing was directed to all three regions in the third study image (see Figure 2), but significantly more viewing was directed to the empty area of the second object compared to the empty region that marked the location of the first object (see Table 1A), as revealed by planned *t*-tests between the two empty regions of interest: Viewing time, $t(15) = 9.91$, $p < .001$; number of fixations, $t(15) = 10.99$, $p < .001$; number of transitions, $t(15) = 13.99$, $p < .001$. Both regions were empty and both had contained an object previously, yet, more viewing was directed to the recently occupied region, perhaps reflecting differences in memory strength between the two objects.

We compared viewing between the first and third study images to additionally test for memory for previously observed object locations. The region denoting the location of the second studied object was empty in the first and third study images; however during viewing of the first study image, viewers did not know the location of the upcoming second object, whereas during viewing of the third study image, viewers could maintain memory for the previously observed second object. The region is identical; the only difference is in the participant's prior viewing history. Results showed that significantly more eye movements were directed to the empty area of the second object during the third versus the first study image: Duration of viewing, $t(15) = 13.86$, $p < .001$; number of fixations, $t(15) = 13.00$, $p < .001$; number of transitions, $t(15) = 16.38$, $p < .001$, suggesting that memory for previously observed objects resulted in increased eye movement behaviour directed towards the empty region.

It should be noted that in all of the above analyses, increased viewing to the now-empty, but previously occupied, region could represent a holdover effect from the prior study image. That is, upon presentation of a new object, viewers may maintain fixation on the now-empty location before moving their eyes to the new object. This may lessen the memory demands of maintaining an active representation of the previously observed object–location relation, and yet permit the relative binding of relations among objects to occur. To address this, we removed the first fixation from analyses if the first fixation was in the region of the first object during viewing of the second study image and, likewise, if the first fixation was in the region of the second object during viewing of the third study image. This had no effect on the pattern of results observed as described earlier (see Table 1B).

Likewise, when the first fixation was not considered in the third study image if it had remained in the region of the second study object, there was still an increase in viewing directed to the region of the second study object for the third versus the first study image: Duration of viewing, $t(15) = 7.44$; number of fixations, $t(15) = 5.70$; number of transitions, $t(15) = 6.09$; all $ps < .001$. This again reveals that memory for the previously observed objects underlies increased eye movements directed to empty regions.

Test displays

Viewing of critical regions. To reveal detection of relational changes, we examined viewing of two different critical regions of the intact and manipulated test displays—the object-filled and the empty region. The filled critical region contained the object, which had undergone a manipulation in

TABLE 1B
Means (*SD*) and statistical results for measures of viewing directed to regions of interest of the study images; the data from the first fixation of the second and the third study image were removed if the fixation had remained in a previously occupied region of interest

Display type	*Region of interest*	*Duration of viewing time*	*Number of fixations*	*Number of transitions*
Study 2	1 (empty)	187.24 (147.35)	0.73 (0.49)	0.86 (0.71)
	2 (filled)	2253.67 (349.43)	4.81 (1.05)	1.36 (0.33)
	3 (empty)	9.89 (16.83)	0.02 (0.04)	0.02 (0.03)
$F(2, 30)$		412.23*	250.88*	53.27*
$t(15)$	1 vs. 2	17.66*	15.09*	4.19*
$t(15)$	2 vs. 3	4.74*	17.93*	16.78*
$t(15)$	1 vs. 3	25.82*	5.72*	4.77*
Study 3	1 (empty)	113.67 (102.84)	0.30 (0.30)	0.25 (0.26)
	2 (empty)	224.63 (115.53)	0.67 (0.43)	0.56 (0.33)
	3 (filled)	2037.19 (401.90)	4.24 (0.76)	1.47 (0.36)
$F(2, 30)$		246.77*	293.62*	308.22*
$t(15)$	1 vs. 2	3.34*	4.40*	5.27*
$t(15)$	2 vs. 3	15.96*	17.34*	17.82*
$t(15)$	1 vs. 3	16.06*	18.14*	27.94*

*$p \leq .01$.

its relations relative to the other two objects; the empty critical region would have contained the object had the relative relations remained intact.

There were marginal to significant effects of display type on the measures of viewing to the empty critical region due to greater sampling of the empty critical region of manipulated displays compared to the identical empty critical region of intact displays (see Table 2 for relevant means and standard deviations): Duration of viewing time, $F(1,\ 15) = 4.03$, $p = .06$; number of fixations, $F(1,\ 15) = 14.00$, $p < .01$; number of transitions, $F(1,\ 15) = 11.40$, $p < .01$. There were no significant effects of display type on any of the measures that examined viewing to the object-filled critical region (see Table 2), all $Fs(1,\ 15) < 1.48$, all $ps > .2$. Altogether, a manipulation to the relative relations among the objects generally resulted in increased viewing to the empty region which should have contained an object had the relative relations remained intact.

Order of fixation. If memory for the temporal relations among the objects is maintained, eye movement scanning of the test displays should mimic the temporal order of object presentation during the study images. Therefore, the location of the subsequent fixation directed to any one of the objects was examined based on which object was currently fixated. Totals were accumulated across participants. Instances in which the current or subsequent fixation landed outside of the object-filled regions were not included. Given that single fixations to any of the presented objects were quantified (rather than gazes made to an object), refixations onto the same object were considered as well as subsequent fixations that landed on a different object. A chi-square test contrasted the observed frequency with which the subsequent fixation landed on Object 1, Object 2, or Object 3 depending on whether the current fixation was on Object 1, Object 2, or

TABLE 2
Means (*SD*) regarding viewing directed to critical regions

Critical region	*Display type*	*Duration of viewing time*	*Number of fixations*	*Number of transitions*
Empty	Intact	75.07 (66.29)	0.17 (0.14)	0.13 (0.12)
	Manipulated	136.96 (99.98)	0.43 (0.27)	0.30 (0.20)
	$F(1, 15)$	4.03*	14.00**	11.40**
Filled	Intact	1164.59 (246.38)	3.39 (0.57)	2.26 (0.47)
	Manipulated	1239.07 (289.16)	3.59 (0.86)	2.12 (0.41)
	$F(1, 15)$	0.75	0.88	1.22

*$p < .1$, **$p \leq .01$.

TABLE 3
Frequency of fixations for intact and manipulated trials

Current object	*Next object*	*Observed fixations*	*Expected fixations*	*Residual*
Intact trials				
1	1	151	109.74	41.26
	2	194	173.66	20.34
	3	77	138.59	−61.59
2	1	157	162.79	−5.79
	2	248	257.62	−9.62
	3	221	205.59	15.41
3	1	80	115.46	−35.46
	2	172	182.72	−10.72
	3	192	145.82	46.18
Manipulated trials				
1	1	154	138.27	15.73
	2	182	168.09	13.91
	3	108	137.64	−29.64
2	1	174	168.17	5.83
	2	205	204.43	0.57
	3	161	167.40	−6.40
3	1	108	129.55	−21.55
	2	143	157.49	−14.49
	3	165	128.96	36.04

Object 3 compared to the expected frequencies as determined through crosstabulations.

Chi-square tests revealed significant differences between observed and expected frequencies for intact, $\chi^2(4, N = 1492) = 73.13$, $p < .001$, and manipulated trials, $\chi^2(4, N = 1400) = 24.76$, $p < .001$, when examined separately. Examination of the residuals for the intact and manipulated trials (Table 3) revealed commonalities: Refixations onto the same object were more frequent than expected for Objects 1 and 3, and subsequent fixations tended to be more frequently directed to the object that was closer in temporal order (e.g., more fixations subsequently directed to Object 2 than Object 3 when the current fixation is Object 1; fewer transitions between Objects 1 and 3 than would otherwise be expected). When Object 2 was fixated on an intact trial, the subsequent fixation was more likely to go to Object 3, and less likely to go to Object 1, than what would otherwise have been expected; the reverse pattern was observed for manipulated trials. Thus, the fact that viewers tended to direct their subsequent fixation to the object that was closer in temporal order suggests that memory for the temporal relations had been accessed. Moreover, it appears that manipulations to the relative relations resulted in changes in the temporal scanning order.

DISCUSSION

The current work examined the binding and maintenance of relative relations among objects across time and the role of eye movements in the construction of such relations. Our findings have implications for understanding the nature of scene representations; namely that representations for scenes may be similar to memory representations for an "event" or "episode" in that they all may be comprised of a series of relative spatial and temporal relations among objects. Moreover, eye movements may be the conduit by which information is bound into a lasting representation, and by which current information is compared to stored representations.

Our findings from the study phase demonstrated that locations of objects were integrated with respect to one another in memory. Our findings from the test phase revealed that the representations of relative spatial and temporal relations were maintained over time. Participants were highly accurate in distinguishing intact from manipulated images via verbal reports, and eye movements were directed towards the location of manipulated images that would have contained an object had the relative spatial relations been maintained, compared to the same (unmanipulated) region of intact trials. Additionally, eye movements revealed some preservation of temporal order in scanning behaviour and the presence of a manipulation may have disrupted the eye movement reenactment of temporal order. Temporal disruption in scanning may occur prior to, and give rise to, conscious awareness of change; this possibility remains to be explored in further work.

The previously noted findings of accurate verbal reports and changes in eye movement scanning reveal access to representations that included information regarding the relative relations among objects that were subsequently compared to the external displays (Mitroff, Simons, & Levin, 2004; Parker, 1978; Ryan & Cohen, 2004). These findings are consistent with recent work from Yamamoto and Shelton (2007) in which participants learned the spatial layout of sequentially presented objects either through visual or tactile/proprioceptive exposure. Participants' memory for the relations among objects was subsequently assessed by having participants imagine a directional heading and point to the location of a target object. Regardless of modality of exposure, participants were able to learn the relative locations among objects and judge the appropriate target location with reasonable accuracy.

The current findings may provide insight into the nature of visual representations and the role of eye movements in constructing such representations. Here, participants were required to bind relations across, rather than within, displays and thus the stimuli used in the present study could be considered as a series of "events" rather than images per se. However, it is possible that for static images, as well as events, information is integrated across space and time. That is, when viewing static images, under particular conditions, the relations among objects may be bound across time rather than extracted from a single composite. For instance, if the image contains numerous objects or contain objects that are a considerable distance from one another, it may be necessary to invoke multiple fixations across the display, and inspect objects with foveal vision to obtain more detailed information than what can be perceived from peripheral vision. Once fixations move from one location to another, information must be integrated within the confines of memory (Brockmole, Wang, & Irwin, 2002). The same occurs for events or episodes that encompass multiple objects that are revealed, or change, over an extended period of time, such as when navigating through the external environment. In this manner, visual representations may be similar to, if not the same as, memory representations for an event/episode (Burgess, 2002; Cohen & Eichenbaum, 1993; Tulving, 2002)—in all instances, the spatial and temporal relations among the objects must be integrated in memory. One prediction that emerges from this view is that the hippocampus, a medial temporal lobe structure that is critically involved in the binding of distinct objects to form memories of events and episodes (Cohen & Eichenbaum, 1993), would contribute to the development of scene representations, even when a static image is presented. In support of this, findings reveal that amnesic patients with hippocampal damage are impaired on verbal report and eye movement indices regarding memory for the relations among objects within a static scene, even when memory for the scene relations is examined over a brief delay (Hannula, Tranel, & Cohen, 2006; Olsen, Page, Moore, Chatterjee, & Verfaellie, 2006; Ryan et al., 2000; Ryan & Cohen, 2004). These findings suggest that visual representations consist of spatial relations among the objects within a scene, and that the hippocampus contributes to the development of visual representations in a manner similar, if not identical to, memory representations for events or episodes.

Considering a visual representation to be similar to memory for an event can offer an alternate interpretation for the resampling of a location that has already been foveated. Previously, it has been proposed that little to no detail is maintained within a lasting representation, therefore, refixations reflect the reencoding of information that was otherwise poorly maintained (O'Regan, 1992). Transitions to an already sampled region may serve to recall that information from memory, or at least maintain it in an active state, so that it may be bound together with the target of the subsequent fixation. Numerous refixations between distinct regions may allow multiple combinations of relations to be integrated within a single representation and permit the entire set of relations to be stored as a single "event" or "episode". Therefore, eye movements may serve to bind the relations among objects and refixations may be the outward manifestation of the binding process.

Eye movements serve to direct attention to particular regions within a display such that specific details regarding a single object may be extracted from foveal vision and maintained within the focus of attention (Hollingworth, 2004; Hollingworth & Henderson, 2002; Irwin, 1991, 1992; Irwin & Zelinsky, 2002; Loftus, Nelson, & Kallman, 1983; Zelinsky & Loschky, 2005). But, as comprehension of a multi-object display requires distributed eye movements, information that is received from each successive fixation must be bound in memory[1] to construct a larger representation (Brockmole, Irwin, & Wang, 2003; Brockmole et al., 2002). Eye movements may reveal the activation of stored information, and serve to link memorial information with current perceptual input (Brockmole & Irwin, 2005). Thus, eye movements may have a critical role in the construction and/or modification of memory representations. Evidence in support of this idea comes from findings in which recognition memory was aided by free scanning behaviour (Henderson, Williams, & Falk, 2005), and was positively related to the number of fixations made (Loftus, 1972).

Support for the notion that eye movements serve to bind information across time comes from behavioural, electrophysiological, and neuroimaging studies on visual attention, imagery and memory. Brandt and Stark (1997) noted that eye movement patterns elicited during imagery of a previously studied (but now absent) array largely resembled the eye movement pattern observed during viewing when the array was present, suggesting that eye movements serve to activate portions of the remembered scene and arrange those activated portions into their proper location within the (imagined) scene. The electrophysiological and neural responses observed when participants were performing spatial attention tasks were similar to responses observed when participants were performing spatial working memory tasks, suggesting that the covert (or here, overt) allocation of attention may mediate the rehearsal of previously studied spatial relations (Awh, Anllo-Vento, & Hillyard, 2000; Awh, Smith, & Jonides, 1995). Altogether, this work reveals that the allocation of attention and eye movement behaviour may serve to initially bind, and subsequently (re)construct, the relative relations among objects within a visual representation.

One final remark concerns the notion of temporal relations. Although the discussions of spatial and temporal relations have been considered separately, spatial and temporal relations may be treated similarly within visual representations in memory. The spatial relations among objects may not be

[1] Here, we take *memory* to refer either to the contents of a shorter or longer term store as both may contribute to changes in eye movement scanning behaviour (Brockmole & Irwin, 2005; Ryan & Cohen, 2004).

maintained in coordinate (x,y,z) or metric space, but rather, may be simply expressed as a set of relative categorical relations that are perhaps, but not necessarily, based in language (e.g., "*X* is to the left of *Y*."; Pani, 2000). Maintaining spatial information as a set of categorical relations may allow information to be bound across displays that differ in spatial dimensions without altering the nature of the existing representation itself. This may explain why integrating information across displays of differing spatial scales or orientations affords no temporal cost relative to integrating information across displays in which the spatial dimensions remain unchanged (Brockmole & Wang, 2003). Jiang, Olson, and Chun (2000) similarly noted that object change detection was not affected by expanding the spatial scale of the array from the study to the probe image, suggesting that change detection is aided by the comparison of stored relative spatial relations against current perceptual information and further, that change detection performance may be disrupted when the use of stored relative spatial relations is prevented (Jiang et al., 2000). In the same vein as spatial relations, stored temporal relations may be relative categorical relations (e.g., "*X* is before *Y*.") that are used to compare against perceptual input for the purpose of detecting changes in the environment. There may be no useful distinction between temporal and spatial relations; a notion that has been expressed by philosophers, physicists, and psychologists, alike (see Hawking, 1988, and James, 1890/1983, for reviews). In that regard, visual representations may simply be a series of relations among objects that are integrated in memory.

REFERENCES

Awh, E., Anllo-Vento, L., & Hillyard, S. A. (2000). The role of spatial selective attention in working memory for locations: Evidence from event-related potentials. *Journal of Cognitive Neuroscience*, *12*(5), 840–847.

Awh, E., Smith, E. E., & Jonides, J. (1995). Human rehearsal processes and the frontal lobes: PET evidence. *Annals of the New York Academy of Sciences*, *769*, 97–117.

Biederman, I., Rabinowitz, J. C., Glass, A. L., & Stacy, E. W. (1974). On the information extracted from a glance at a scene. *Journal of Experimental Psychology*, *103*(3), 597–600.

Brandt, S. A., & Stark, L. W. (1997). Spontaneous eye movements during visual imagery reflect the content of the visual scene. *Journal of Cognitive Neuroscience*, *9*, 27–38.

Brockmole, J. R., & Irwin, D. E. (2005). Eye movements and the integration of visual memory and visual perception. *Perception and Psychophysics*, *67*, 495–512.

Brockmole, J. R., Irwin, D. E., & Wang, R. F. (2003). The locus of spatial attention during the temporal integration of visual memories and visual percepts. *Psychonomic Bulletin and Review*, *10*(2), 510–515.

Brockmole, J. R., & Wang, R. F. (2003). Integrating visual images and visual percepts across time and space. *Visual Cognition*, *10*, 853–873.

Brockmole, J. R., Wang, R. F., & Irwin, D. E. (2002). Temporal integration between visual images and visual percepts. *Journal of Experimental Psychology: Human Perception and Performance*, *28*(2), 315–334.

Burgess, N. (2002). The hippocampus, space and viewpoints in episodic memory. *Quarterly Journal of Experimental Psychology, 55A*, 1057–1080.

Chun, M. M., & Jiang, Y. (1998). Contextual cueing: Implicit learning and memory for visual context guides spatial attention. *Cognitive Psychology, 36*, 28–71.

Cohen, N. J., & Eichenbaum, H. (1993). *Memory, amnesia, and the hippocampal system.* Cambridge, MA: MIT.

Hannula, D. E., Tranel, D., & Cohen, N. J. (2006). The long and the short of it: Relational memory impairments in amnesia, even at short lags. *Journal of Neuroscience, 26*(32), 8352–8359.

Hawking, S. (1988). *A brief history of time.* New York: Bantam Books.

Henderson, J. M., Williams, C. C., & Falk, R. J. (2005). Eye movements are functional during face learning. *Memory and Cognition, 33*(1), 98–106.

Hollingworth, A. (2004). Constructing visual representations of natural scenes: The roles of short- and long-term visual memory. *Journal of Experimental Psychology: Human Perception and Performance, 30*, 519–537.

Hollingworth, A. (2007). Object-position binding in visual memory for natural scenes and object arrays. *Journal of Experimental Psychology: Human Perception and Performance, 33*, 31–47.

Hollingworth, A., & Henderson, J. M. (2002). Accurate visual memory for previously attended objects in natural scenes. *Journal of Experimental Psychology: Human Perception and Performance, 28*, 113–136.

Hollingworth, A., Williams, C. C., & Henderson, J. M. (2001). To see and remember: Visually specific information is retained in memory from previously attended objects in natural scenes. *Psychonomic Bulletin and Review, 8*(4), 761–768.

Irwin, D. E. (1991). Information integration across saccadic eye movements. *Cognitive Psychology, 23*(3), 420–456.

Irwin, D. E. (1992). Memory for position and identity across eye movements. *Journal of Experimental Psychology: Learning, Memory, and Cognition, 18*, 307–317.

Irwin, D. E., & Zelinsky, G. J. (2002). Eye movements and scene perception: Memory for things observed. *Perception and Psychophysics, 64*, 882–895.

James, W. (1983). The principles of psychology. Cambridge, MA: Harvard University Press. (Original work published 1890)

Jiang, Y., Olson, I. R., & Chun, M. M. (2000). Organization of visual short-term memory. *Journal of Experimental Psychology: Learning, Memory, and Cognition, 26*(3), 683–702.

Laeng, B., & Teodorescu, D. (2002). Eye scanpaths during visual imagery reenact those of perception of the same visual scene. *Cognitive Science, 26*, 207–231.

Levin, D. T., Momen, N., Drivdahl, S. B., & Simons, D. J. (2000). Change blindness blindness: The metacognitive error of overestimating change detection ability. *Visual Cognition, 7*(1–3), 397–412.

Loftus, G. R. (1972). Eye fixations and recognition memory for pictures. *Cognitive Psychology, 3*, 525–551.

Loftus, G. R., Nelson, W. W., & Kallman, H. J. (1983). Differential acquisition rates for different types of information from pictures. *Quarterly Journal of Experimental Psychology, 35*, 187–198.

Meegan, D. V., & Honsberger, M. J. M. (2005). Spatial information is processed even when it is task-irrelevant: implications for neuroimaging task design. *Neuroimage, 25*, 1043–1055.

Mitroff, S. R., Simons, D. J., & Levin, D. T. (2004). Nothing compares 2 views: Change blindness can occur despite preserved access to the changed information. *Perception and Psychophysics, 66*(8), 1268–1281.

Noton, D., & Stark, L. W. (1971). Scanpaths in saccadic eye movements while viewing and recognizing patterns. *Vision Research, 11*, 929–942.

Olson, I. R., & Marshuetz, C. (2005). Remembering "what" brings along "where" in visual working memory. *Perception and Psychophysics*, *67*, 185–194.

Olson, I. R., Page, K., Moore, K. S., Chatterjee, A., & Verfaellie, M. (2006). Working memory for conjunctions relies on the medial temporal lobe. *Journal of Neuroscience*, *26*, 4596–4601.

O'Regan, J. K. (1992). Solving the "real" mysteries of visual perception: The world as an outside memory. *Canadian Journal of Psychology*, *46*, 461–488.

Pani, J. R. (2000). Cognitive description and change blindness. *Visual Cognition*, *7*, 107–126.

Parker, R. E. (1978). Picture processing during recognition. *Journal of Experimental Psychology: Human Perception and Performance*, *4*, 284–293.

Peterson, M. S., & Kramer, A. F. (2001). Attentional guidance of the eyes by contextual information and abrupt onsets. *Perception and Psychophysics*, *63*(7), 1239–1249.

Ryan, J. D., Althoff, R. R, Whitlow, S., & Cohen, N. J. (2000). Amnesia is a deficit in relational memory. *Psychological Science*, *11*, 454–461.

Ryan, J. D., & Cohen, N. J. (2004). The nature of change detection and on-line representations of scenes. *Journal of Experimental Psychology: Human Perception and Performance*, *30*(5), 988–1015.

Ryan, J. D., Leung, G., Turk-Browne, N. B., & Hasher, L. (2007). Assessment of age-related changes in inhibition and binding using eye movement monitoring. *Psychology and Aging*, *22*, 239–250.

Spivey, M. J., & Geng, J. J. (2001). Oculomotor mechanisms activated by imagery and memory: Eye movements to absent objects. *Psychological Research*, *65*, 235–241.

Stark, L. W., & Ellis, S. R. (1981). Scanpaths revisited: Cognitive models direct active looking. In D. F. Fisher, R. A. Monty, & J. W. Senders (Eds.), *Eye movements: Cognition and visual perception* (pp. 193–226). Hillsdale, NJ: Lawrence Erlbaum Associates, Inc.

Tulving, E. (2002). Episodic memory: From mind to brain. *Annual Review of Psychology*, *53*, 1–25.

Walker-Smith, G. J., Gale, A. G., & Findlay, J. M. (1977). Eye movement strategies involved in face perception. *Perception*, *6*, 313–326.

Wells, G. L., & Olson, E. A. (2003). Eyewitness testimony. *Annual Review of Psychology*, *54*, 277–295.

Yamamoto, N., & Shelton, A. L. (2007). Path information effects in visual and proprioceptive spatial learning. *Acta Psychologica*, *125*, 346–360.

Zelinsky, G. J., & Loschky, L. C. (2005). Eye movements serialize memory for objects in scenes. *Perception and Psychophysics*, *67*, 676–690.

VISUAL COGNITION, 2009, 17 (1/2), 273–291

Psychology Press
Taylor & Francis Group

Two forms of scene memory guide visual search: Memory for scene context and memory for the binding of target object to scene location

Andrew Hollingworth
Department of Psychology, University of Iowa, Iowa City, IA, USA

The role of scene memory in visual search was investigated in a preview-search task. Participants saw a preview of a real-world scene prior to searching through that scene for a target object. Compared with a no preview baseline, search was facilitated following a preview scene that did not contain the ultimate target object, indicating that memory for the general context and layout of a scene exemplar facilitates later search. In addition, search was more efficient when the preview scene contained the ultimate target object than when it did not, demonstrating that memory for the specific binding of objects to locations facilitates later search. Both forms of memory were explicitly available for participant report.

Keywords: Visual search; Visual memory; Scene memory; Eye movements; Attention.

Recent research has demonstrated that people can generate robust visual memory representations of natural environments, retaining information about the visual features of objects in a scene (Castelhano & Henderson, 2005; Hollingworth, 2004, 2005b; Hollingworth & Henderson, 2002; Melcher, 2006; Tatler, Gilchrist, & Land, 2005; Tatler, Gilchrist, & Rusted, 2003) and the locations of those objects (Brockmole, Castelhano, & Henderson, 2006; Brockmole & Henderson, 2006a, 2006b; Hannula, Tranel, & Cohen, 2006; Hollingworth, 2005a, 2007). Such capability raises the question of the function of this visual memory: For what real-world, behavioural purposes is visual memory for natural scenes utilized?

Please address all correspondence to Andrew Hollingworth, Department of Psychology, University of Iowa, 11 Seashore Hall E, Iowa City, IA 52242-1407, USA.
E-mail: andrew-hollingworth@uiowa.edu

The present research was supported by NIH grants R03MH65456 and R01EY017356. Parts of this study were reported at the Munich Visual Search Symposium, Munich, Germany, 2003, and the fourth annual meeting of the Vision Sciences Society, Sarasota, Florida, 2004.

© 2008 Psychology Press, an imprint of the Taylor & Francis Group, an Informa business
http://www.psypress.com/viscog DOI: 10.1080/13506280802193367

One plausible function for scene memory is the guidance of visual search through a scene (Brockmole & Henderson, 2006b; Chun & Jiang, 1998; Henderson, Weeks, & Hollingworth, 1999). Almost all real-world tasks require visual search of some sort. For example, when cooking a meal, one must search for many of the items (ingredients, utensils) that are necessary to complete the task (Land & Hayhoe, 2001). More generally, almost every behavioural operation requires attending to (and typically fixating) the target of the behaviour. If the relevant target object is not attended beforehand or does not recruit attention to itself directly, a visual search operation is necessary to orient attention and the eyes to that object. Thus, visual search is a fundamental process underlying object selection, and understanding visual search in real-world environments is therefore critical to understanding how humans are able to behave intelligently in the service of top-down goals (such as making a meal).

Memory for the visual form of objects could facilitate search by specifying the perceptual features that discriminate the target from distractors (Desimone & Duncan, 1995; Hollingworth, Richard, & Luck, 2008). Search for a pen is likely to be more efficient if one remembers that the pen is blue, as search can be limited to blue items. Perhaps more importantly, memory for the spatial properties of scenes could guide attention efficiently to a location that is known to, or is likely to, contain the relevant object.

Research over the last decade has probed various circumstances under which memory for the spatial properties of scenes guides visual search. First, memory for scenes and objects in general (e.g., that pedestrians tend to appear on pavements and pictures on walls) can guide attention and the eyes to locations within a scene where the target object is likely to appear (Henderson et al., 1999; Neider & Zelinsky, 2006; Torralba, Oliva, Castelhano, & Henderson, 2006), even for scenes that participants have never viewed before. Second, repeated search through a particular scene exemplar generates more efficient search when the position of the target object remains constant, both for naturalistic scene stimuli (Brockmole et al., 2006; Brockmole & Henderson, 2006a, 2006b; Summerfield, Lepsien, Gitelman, Mesulam, & Nobre, 2006) and for scenes composed of randomly arrayed collections of simple objects (Chun & Jiang, 1998). Finally, a brief preview of a scene facilitates subsequent search through that scene when the search stimulus is degraded so that only the currently fixated portion of the scene is visible (Castelhano & Henderson, 2007).

My goal in the present study was to examine the means by which visual memory for a particular scene exemplar facilitates subsequent search through that scene. The present experiments served to isolate two forms of scene memory that might plausibly guide search: (1) Memory for the general context and layout of the scene and (2) memory for the particular binding of target object to scene location. Memory for the context of the scene (e.g., that the kitchen counter extends across the left side of the image) combined with knowledge of the target object (that toasters tend to appear on kitchen counters) could serve to direct attention to the region of the scene where the target is likely to appear (the left side). In addition, one's memory for the actual, observed location of the target could serve to guide attention directly to that location in the scene.

To tease apart these two mechanisms, I used a preview-search paradigm, manipulating scene information contained in the preview before search through that scene. The basic method is illustrated in Figure 1. Participants saw a preview image of a scene (or no preview image in the control condition). This was followed by a target-probe object, which was displayed in isolation in the centre of the screen, indicating the object that was to be found during search. Next, participants saw a search scene. The target object was always present in the search scene, and it was either identical to the target probe or mirror reversed. Participants' task was to find the target in the search scene as quickly as possible and respond to indicate whether it was the same as the target probe or mirror reversed. This forced participants to search through the scene and fixate the target, because they needed to acquire fairly precise information from the target to assess its left/right (l-r) orientation. Search efficiency was measured using standard search RT data and eyetracking data.

There were three preview conditions. In the *no preview* condition, participants did not see a preview of the scene prior to search. In this case, participants could have used knowledge about scenes and objects in general to guide search (for example, directing attention and the eyes to the lower regions of the exercise room scene where a pair of sneakers were likely to appear; Torralba et al., 2006), but they did not have an existing visual memory representation of the particular scene exemplar through which they were searching. In the *target-absent preview* condition, participants saw a preview of the scene, but it did not contain the ultimate target object. In this case, participants could remember the general context and layout of the preview scene. If search were more efficient in the target-absent preview condition than in the no preview condition, this would indicate that participants can use memory for scene context to guide attention and the eyes to plausible target locations. Finally in the *target-present preview* condition, participants saw a preview of the scene, and the preview contained the target object in the same location as it would appear in the search scene. When the target appeared in the preview scene, its l-r orientation was the same as the target probe but was uncorrelated with the orientation of the target in the search scene. Thus, participants could not respond on the basis of memory for the orientation of the target in the preview scene; they were forced to find the target in the search scene. If search were more efficient in the target-present preview condition than in the target-absent preview

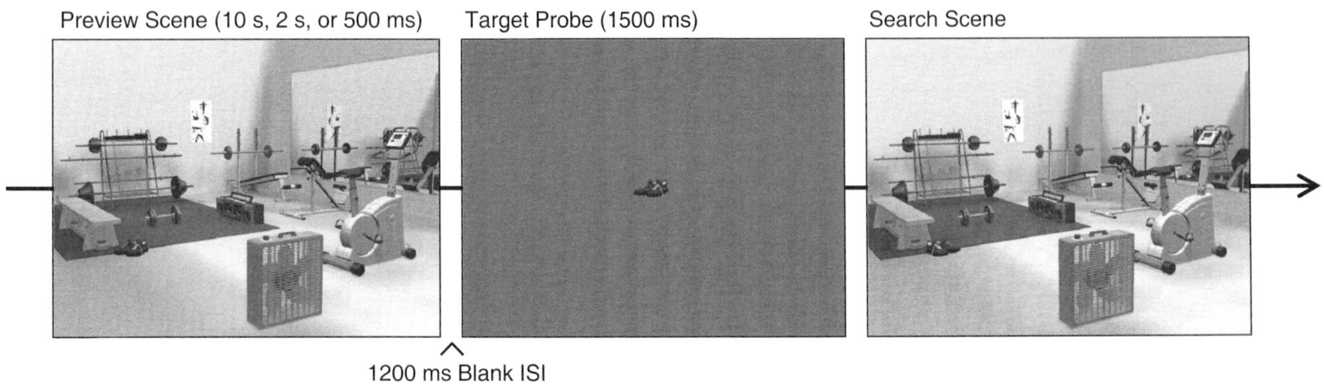

Figure 1. Sequence of events in a trial. Participants saw a preview of a scene (pictured) or no preview (not pictured), followed by a target probe and a search scene. Participants searched through the scene to find the target object and responded to indicate whether its orientation in the search scene was the same as the orientation of the target probe (in this example, the correct response was "no"). To view this figure in colour, please see the online issue of the Journal.

condition, this would indicate that memory for the specific binding of target object to scene location facilitates search, as the two conditions differed only in the presence of the target in the preview scene.

The present study complements and extends existing research on the role of scene memory in visual search. Studies examining the phenomenon of contextual cueing have already demonstrated that memory for a particular target location can facilitate search (Brockmole & Henderson, 2006b; Chun & Jiang, 1998). However, contextual cueing depends on repeated search, and in the standard version of the contextual cueing task, significant facilitation is observed only after multiple repetitions of a particular search context. In the present study, the effect of scene memory was examined on the very first search through the scene. Because participants had no previous search trials for a particular scene item, they could not know the location of the target object during learning, and therefore the best strategy was to encode the locations of multiple objects from the preview scene. If robust facilitation were observed in the target-present preview condition, this would indicate that participants encoded a scene representation that maintained the binding of multiple object exemplars to scene locations (Hollingworth, 2007) and that could be used flexibly to facilitate search depending on the particular object that was the ultimate target of search. Such a result would also demonstrate single-trial learning of scene information functional in search, in contrast with the incremental learning over multiple trials of repetition in traditional contextual cueing studies.

In addition, an advantage in the present study for the target-present preview condition over the target-absent preview condition requires memory for the *binding* of particular objects to scene locations. In contrast, contextual cueing requires only memory for location. In contextual cueing tasks, the identity of the target varies across repeated search trials (as do the identities of the distractors, typically), and thus the information functional in facilitating search is limited to spatial properties of the search arrays and the target location. In the present study, however, learning only the spatial properties of the scene would be insufficient to generate an advantage for the target-present preview condition over the target-absent preview condition, because the two conditions were identical in their spatial properties (except for the presence of one additional occupied location in the former condition). In addition, learning the visual forms or identities of the objects in the preview scene without remembering their locations would also be insufficient to generate an advantage for the target-present preview condition. The 1500 ms presentation of the target probe ensured that, in all conditions, participants had an accurate search target template. And memory for the l-r orientation of the target in the preview scene could not influence performance directly, because the orientation of the target in the preview and search scenes was uncorrelated. Thus, an advantage for the target-present preview condition over the target-absent preview condition could plausibly arise only if participants remembered the specific binding between the visual properties and/or identity of object that was to be the target and its location within the scene (Hollingworth, 2005a, 2007).

Finally, the present preview manipulations are similar to those used in a study by Castelhano and Henderson (2007). In that paper, participants saw a brief, 250 ms preview of a scene, followed by a label describing the target object and a search scene. Participants' task was to orient the eyes to the target object and fixate it. Castelhano and Henderson were interested in the effects of a scene preview independently of the visual information that could be extracted from the scene during search. Thus, during search, only a very small portion of the search scene was visible, corresponding roughly to the foveal region at the centre of gaze. Although this "moving window" approach was necessary to answer Castelhano and Henderson's central research question, this method has limited applicability to understanding search under natural conditions, in which one has access to information across the visual field. In particular, degraded perceptual information during search may have caused participants to depend more heavily on memory than they would have if the search scene had been fully visible (Oliva, Wolfe, & Arsenio, 2004). In the present experiments, the search task could be performed solely on the basis of perceptual information acquired from the search scene, allowing for a more stringent test of the utility of memory in guiding visual search.

In a manner similar to the present study, Castelhano and Henderson (2007) included two preview conditions, one in which the preview scene contained the ultimate search target object and another in which the preview did not. A scene preview facilitated search in both of these conditions compared with a no preview control. There was a numerical trend towards more efficient search when the preview scene contained the search target than when it did not, but this effect did not approach statistical significance. Thus, one cannot determine from the Castelhano and Henderson data whether memory for the specific binding of target object to scene location generates search facilitation beyond that attributable to familiarity with the general context of the scene.

The present study consisted of two main experiments. Experiment 1a and 1b included only the target-present preview condition and the no preview condition to establish and quantify the basic preview effect. In addition, the length of the preview was varied to determine whether participants accumulate visual information from the preview scene over extended viewing. Experiment 2 added the target-absent preview condition so as to isolate the effects of memory for general scene layout and memory for the binding of target object to scene location.

EXPERIMENTS 1A AND 1B

Two preview conditions were contrasted: Target-present preview and no preview. In Experiment 1a, the preview duration was 10 s. In Experiment 1b, the preview duration was 2 s or 500 ms. Given evidence that scene structure and identity can be extracted from a very brief view of a scene (e.g., Castelhano & Henderson, 2007; Potter, 1976), facilitation of search was expected at all preview durations. In addition, given evidence that visual memory for individual objects accumulates over the course of multiple seconds of scene viewing (Hollingworth, 2004; Hollingworth & Henderson, 2002; Tatler et al., 2003), it was expected that the amount of facilitation would be larger with longer preview duration.

Method

Participants. In all experiments, participants were recruited from the University of Iowa community. Each participant completed only one experiment. All participants reported normal, uncorrected vision. They either received course credit or were paid. Sixteen participants completed Experiment 1a, and twenty-four completed Experiment 1b.

Stimuli. Scene stimuli were rendered from 48 3-D models of real-world environments. An additional eight scenes were used for practice trials. In each scene model, a single target object was chosen. Two versions of the scene were rendered that differed only in the l-r orientation of the target object. For the target probe images, the target object was rendered at screen centre against a neutral green background (its appearance at screen centre was identical to its appearance embedded within the preview scene). Scene stimuli subtended $19.5^\circ \times 26.1^\circ$. Target objects had a mean width of 3.0° and mean height of 2.3°.

Apparatus. Stimuli were presented on a 17-inch computer monitor with a refresh rate of 120 Hz. Stimulus presentation was synchronized with the monitor's refresh cycle. Responses were collected by a serial button box. Stimulus presentation and response collection were controlled by a PC-compatible computer running E-Prime software. Eye position was monitored by a video-based, ISCAN ETL-400 eyetracker sampling at 240 Hz. A chin and forehead rest was used to maintain a constant viewing distance of 70 cm and to minimize head movement.

Procedure. The sequence of events in a trial is illustrated in Figure 1. In Experiment 1a, each trial was initiated by the experimenter after eyetracker calibration was checked. This was followed by a 1000 ms central fixation cross.

In the 10 s preview condition, the preview scene was then displayed for 10 s. In the no preview condition, instead of the preview scene, an otherwise blank screen with the words "No preview" was displayed for 2 s. Next, there was a blank, 1200 ms delay. The target-probe image (target object at screen centre) was then presented for 1500 ms. Finally, the search scene was displayed until response. Participants pressed one of two buttons to indicate whether the target object in the search scene was the same as the target probe or mirror reversed.

The sequence of events in Experiment 1b was the same, except a message appeared before the preview scene for 2 s informing the participant about the length of the preview ("2 second preview", "½ second preview", or "No preview"). The message was followed either by a preview scene for 2 s, a preview scene for 500 ms, or no preview.

Participants were instructed that they would or would not be given a preview of each scene before searching through it to find a particular object. They were told that after the preview, they would see the search target at the centre of a blank image. When the search scene appeared, they were to find this object in the scene and respond to indicate whether its orientation was the same as or different from the orientation of the target presented in isolation before the search. They were further instructed that the orientation of the target in the preview scene did not predict the orientation of the target in the search scene, and thus they must find the target in the search scene and respond on the basis of its orientation. Finally, they were instructed to respond as quickly and as accurately as possible.

When the participants arrived, they first gave informed consent, followed by instructions and eyetracker calibration. In Experiment 1a, participants completed a practice block of eight trials, evenly divided among the main conditions. Participants then completed 48 experiment trials, six in each of the eight conditions created by the 2 (10 s preview, no preview) × 2 (target same/different orientation) × 2 (initial target orientation) design.

In Experiment 1b, participants completed a practice block of six trials, evenly divided among the main conditions. Participants then completed 48 experiment trials, four in each of the 12 conditions created by the 3 (2 s preview, 500 ms preview, no preview) × 2 (target same/different orientation) × 2 (initial target orientation) design.

Each participant viewed each of the 48 scene items on one trial; there was no scene repetition. Across participants, condition-item assignments were counterbalanced by Latin square so that each scene item appeared in each condition an equal number of times. Trial order was determined randomly. The entire session required approximately 45 min.

Data analysis. Eyetracking data analysis was conducted offline using dedicated software. A velocity criterion (eye rotation > 31°/s) was used to define saccades. These data were then analysed with respect to the target object region. Target regions were rectangular, 0.65° degrees larger on each side than the smallest rectangle encompassing the target object.

Results

Data for Experiments 1a and 1b are reported in Tables 1 and 2, respectively. The initial orientation of the target object did not produce any reliable effects, and the analyses collapsed this factor. In addition, the match between target probe and search target (same orientation, different orientation) also did not produce any reliable effects, and the analyses collapsed this factor as well.

Eye movement analysis. The data of interest reflected the efficiency with which the eyes were directed to the target object region. Thus, trials on which the participant did not fixate the target prior to response were eliminated. In Experiment 1a, the target region was fixated prior to response on 96.2% of trials. In Experiment 1b, the target region was fixated prior to response on 95.7% of trials. Trials were also excluded from eyetracking analysis if the participant provided an incorrect manual response (see later). Altogether, 6.3% of the trials was eliminated from Experiment 1a and 6.9% from Experiment 1b.

Eye movement scan paths for one of the scene items in Experiment 1a are shown in Figure 2. The top panel depicts the scan paths during search for the eight participants who had a 10 s preview of the scene prior to search. The bottom panel depicts the scan paths of the eight participants who did not have a preview of the scene prior to search.

Elapsed time to target fixation. The primary eyetracking measure of search efficiency was the elapsed time from the onset of the search scene

TABLE 1
Experiment 1a search data

	Preview condition	
	10 s preview	*No preview*
Elapsed time to target fixation (ms)	390	591
Path ratio	1.22	1.65
Manual reaction time (ms)	1232	1487
Manual response accuracy (%)	93.3	95.0

TABLE 2
Experiment 1b search data

	Preview condition		
	2 s preview	*500 ms preview*	*No preview*
Elapsed time to target fixation (ms)	441	489	608
Path ratio	1.31	1.47	1.62
Manual reaction time (ms)	1241	1299	1539
Manual response accuracy (%)	91.1	95.3	94.9

to the beginning of the first fixation on the target region.[1] In Experiment 1a, there was a reliable effect of scene preview, $F(1, 15) = 53.8$, $p < .001$, with shorter elapsed time to target fixation in the 10 s preview condition than in the no preview condition. In Experiment 1b, there was also a reliable effect of scene preview, $F(2, 46) = 10.7$, $p < .001$. Elapsed time to first fixation in both the 2 s preview condition and 500 ms preview condition was reliably shorter than that in the no preview condition, $F(1, 23) = 28.0$, $p < .001$, and $F(1, 23) = 8.87$, $p = .007$, respectively. Elapsed time did not reliably differ in the 2 s and 500 ms preview conditions, $F(1, 23) = 1.50$, $p = .23$, but the numerical trend was towards shorter elapsed time with longer preview duration.

Elapsed time to target fixation was related to eye movement behaviour during the scene preview. The target object was fixated during the 10 s preview on 92% of trials, during the 2 s preview on 54% of trials, and during the 500 ms preview on 5% of trials. In the 5 s preview condition (which included a significant proportion of both preview-fixated and preview-unfixated trials), mean elapsed time to target fixation during search was 351 ms when the target had been fixated during study, and 570 ms when the target was not fixated during study.

Path ratio. Path ratio (Henderson et al., 1999) provides a converging measure of search efficiency. Path ratio is the length of the actual eye movement scan path from scene centre to target object fixation (summing the straight-line distances of each of the saccades) divided by the absolute, Euclidean distance from scene centre to target. A path ratio of 1 would indicate that the eyes were oriented on a direct path to the target. Path ratios greater than 1 indicate an indirect path. These data are reported in Tables 1 and 2. In Experiment 1a, there was a reliable effect of scene preview, $F(1, 15) = 41.9$, $p < .001$, with a shorter mean path in the 10 s preview condition

[1] An equivalent pattern of results was observed for the number of fixations on the scene prior to target fixation.

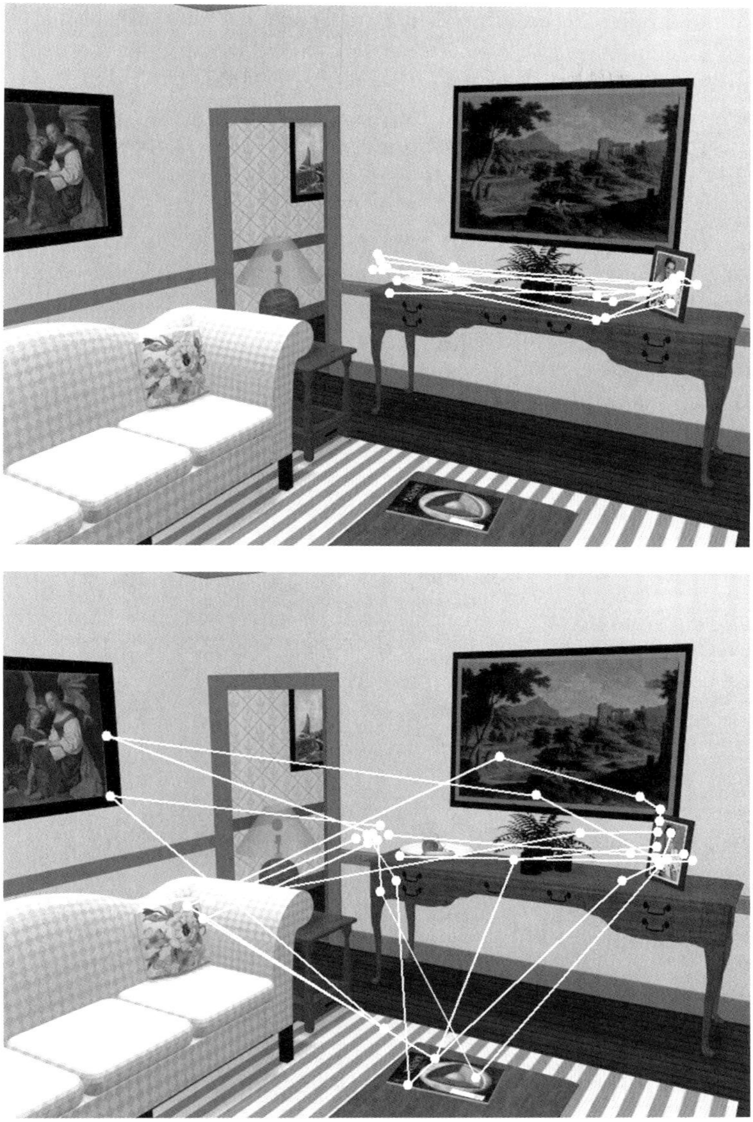

Figure 2. Experiment 1a. Eye movement scan paths for all 16 participants over one of the scene items. Dots represent fixations and lines saccades. The first fixation on the scene tended to lie at the centre of the image. The target object was the framed photograph, and all participants fixated the target prior to manual response. The top panel shows the scan paths of the eight participants who saw this item in the 10 s preview condition. The bottom panel shows the scan paths of the eight participants who saw this item in the no preview condition. To view this figure in colour, please see the online issue of the Journal.

than in the no preview condition. In Experiment 1b, there was also a reliable effect of scene preview, $F(2, 46) = 6.65$, $p = .003$. Path ratio was shorter in the 2 s preview condition than in the no preview condition (1.62), $F(1, 23) = 13.5$, $p = .001$, and there was a trend towards shorter path in the 500 ms preview condition than in the no preview condition, $F(1, 23) = 3.46$, $p = .08$. Finally, there was also a trend towards a shorter path in the 2 s preview condition than in the 500 ms preview condition, $F(1, 23) = 3.15$, $p = .09$.

It is useful to compare these path ratio data with those from Brockmole and Henderson (2006a). Brockmole and Henderson examined eye movements in a contextual cueing paradigm using small letter targets embedded within photographs of real-world scenes. Path ratio significantly declined with scene repetition. However, even after nine previous searches through a scene, path ratio was no lower than 1.8, on average. The significantly shorter path ratios in the present study (even in the no preview condition) are likely to have been caused by multiple factors, including: The use of relatively large, natural objects that could be detected in the periphery; the 1500 ms presentation of the target probe before search, which provided a precise visual search template; and the placement of objects in contextually appropriate locations.

Manual RT analysis. In Experiment 1a, there was a reliable effect of preview, $F(1, 15) = 31.3$, $p < .001$, with shorter mean correct RT in the 10 s preview condition than in the no preview condition. In Experiment 1b, there was also a reliable effect of scene preview, $F(2, 46) = 11.5$, $p < .001$. RT in both the 2 s preview condition and 500 ms preview condition was reliably shorter than that in the no preview condition, $F(1, 23) = 19.8$, $p < .001$, and $F(1, 23) = 8.69$, $p = .007$, respectively. RT did not reliably differ in the 2 s and 500 ms preview conditions, $F(1, 23) = 1.72$, $p = .20$, but the numerical trend was again towards shorter RT with longer preview duration.

Accuracy analysis. In Experiment 1a, there was no effect of preview on the accuracy of the manual response, $F < 1$. In Experiment 1b, there was a trend towards an effect of preview, with lower accuracy in the 2 s preview condition (91.1%) than in the 500 ms preview condition (95.3%) and no preview conditions (94.9%), $F(2, 46) = 2.73$, $p = .08$. Lower accuracy in the 2 s preview condition, which had the fastest RTs in Experiment 1b, raises the possibility of a speed–accuracy tradeoff, potentially complicating interpretation of the RT data in that condition. However, the significant effects of preview in the 500 ms and 10 s preview conditions cannot be attributed to speed–accuracy tradeoff, and these two durations framed the 2 s duration. In addition, the eyetracking data are not compromised by manual response accuracy, because they measure a discrete event, target fixation, that can be analysed independently of the participant's criterion for generating a manual response.

Discussion

Experiments 1a and 1b showed that a scene preview facilitates search even when the scene is fully visible during the search and participants could perform the task without consulting memory. These results are broadly inconsistent with claims that participants fail to consult memory when search can be accomplished on the basis of visual inspection of the scene (Oliva et al., 2004; Wolfe, Klempen, & Dahlen, 2000). In addition, the effect of the preview tended to be larger as preview duration increased, suggesting that during the preview, participants accumulated visual information relevant to the subsequent search. With a 10 s preview of the scene, participants came to fixate the target object only 390 ms after the onset of the search scene, which was quite remarkably efficient considering that when viewing the preview scene, they did not know which of the objects would be the target. Even a very brief preview of 500 ms was sufficient to facilitate subsequent search through the scene, consistent with the finding of Castelhano and Henderson (2007).

EXPERIMENT 2

In Experiment 2, the preview duration was set at 10 s, and a target-absent preview condition was added to isolate the effects of (1) memory for general scene context and (2) memory for the binding of target object to scene location, both of which could have facilitated search in Experiments 1a and 1b.

Method

Participants. Twenty-four participants completed the experiment.

Stimuli and apparatus. The stimuli and apparatus were the same as in Experiments 1a and 1b, except for the target-absent preview scenes. These scenes were identical to the target-present preview scenes, except the target object was removed before rendering the image. The software automatically filled in the scene information that had been occluded by the target object.

Procedure. The events in a trial were the same as in Experiment 1a. When viewing a scene preview, participants did not know whether the target object was present in the scene or not present in the scene. Participants were informed that some preview scenes would contain the target object and some would not. Participants completed a practice block of six trials, evenly divided among the main conditions. Participants then completed 48 experiment trials, four in each of the 12 conditions created by the 3 (preview type) $\times$ 2 (target same/different orientation) $\times$ 2 (initial target orientation) design. The entire session required approximately 45 min.

Results

Data from Experiment 2 are reported in Table 3. Neither the initial orientation of the target object nor the match between target probe and search target produced a reliable effect, and the analyses collapsed these factors.

Eye movement analysis. On 2.9% of the trials, participant responded without fixating the target, and these were eliminated from the eyetracking analysis. Trials were also excluded from eyetracking analysis if the participant provided an incorrect manual response. Altogether, 6.2% of the trials was eliminated.

Elapsed time to target fixation. There was a reliable effect of scene preview on elapsed time to target fixation, $F(2, 46) = 12.6$, $p < .001$, with shorter elapsed time in the target-present preview condition than in the target-absent preview condition, $F(1, 23) = 5.62$, $p = .03$, and shorter elapsed time in the target-absent preview condition than in the no preview condition, $F(1, 23) = 6.20$, $p = .02$.

Path ratio. There was a reliable effect of scene preview on path ratio, $F(2, 46) = 8.28$, $p < .001$. There was not a significant difference between path ratios in the target-present preview and target-absent preview conditions, $F(1, 23) = 1.96$, $p = .18$, though the numerical trend was towards a shorter path in the target-present preview condition. Path was shorter in the target-absent preview condition than in the no preview condition, $F(1, 23) = 5.4$, $p = .02$.

Manual RT analysis. Consistent with the eyetracking analysis, there was a reliable effect of preview on correct RT, $F(2, 46) = 12.6$, $p < .001$, with shorter RT in the target-present preview condition than in the target-absent preview condition, $F(1, 23) = 7.20$, $p = .01$, and shorter RT in the target-absent preview condition than in the no preview condition, $F(1, 23) = 5.75$, $p = .03$.

TABLE 3
Experiment 2 search data

	Preview condition		
	Target-present preview	*Target-absent preview*	*No preview*
Elapsed time to target fixation (ms)	404	492	576
Path ratio	1.29	1.41	1.62
Manual reaction time (ms)	1207	1425	1546
Manual response accuracy (%)	94.4	95.7	92.4

Accuracy analysis. Accuracy on the search task did not vary as a function of preview condition, $F(2, 46) = 1.59$, $p = .22$.

Discussion

Search was more efficient in the target-present preview condition than in the target-absent preview condition, which in turn was more efficient than search in the no preview condition, both for correct RT and for elapsed time to target fixation. Memory for general scene context and memory for the specific binding of target object to scene location guided search.

One of the issues that arises when examining the role of scene memory in search is the extent to which the learning is implicit or explicit. In experiments examining contextual cueing, the contextual learning that facilitates search is typically implicit, at least for arrays of simple stimuli (Chun & Jiang, 1998). For real-world scenes, repeated search generates memory for target location that is explicitly available (Brockmole & Henderson, 2006b). To test whether the learning in the present experiments was explicit, I conducted an additional experiment ($N = 12$). The method was identical to that in Experiment 2, except instead of searching for the target object, participants had to estimate the position of the target in the scene. Specifically, participants saw a preview scene (or no preview scene in the no preview condition). Next, the target probe was presented at screen centre. The target probe was removed, and a blank screen was displayed with a mouse cursor. Participants moved the cursor and clicked to mark their estimate of the position of the target object in the scene. This experiment was a replication of Hollingworth (2005a) but using the present set of scene stimuli and a 10 s preview duration (instead of 20 s) so as to allow direct comparison with the present Experiment 2.

In the target-present preview condition, participants were instructed to click on the location in the blank image where the target object had appeared in the preview scene. In the target-absent preview condition, participants were instructed to place the mouse cursor at the position where the target object would have appeared in the preview scene had it been present. Finally, in the no preview condition, participants were instructed to imagine a scene that could contain the target object and choose a position where that object might likely appear. Even with no preview, participants could use knowledge about objects and scenes in general (e.g., that paintings tend to appear higher in scenes than do shoes) to guide placement.

On each trial, position error was calculated as the Euclidean distance (in degrees of visual angle) between the participant's position estimate and the centre of the target object as it appeared in the actual scene. Mean error was reliably lower in the target-present preview condition (3.79°) than in the target-absent preview condition (4.82°), $F(1, 11) = 11.7$, $p = .006$, and error was reliably lower in the target-absent preview condition than in the no preview condition (7.81°), $F(1, 11) = 72.1$, $p < .001$. These data replicate the results of Hollingworth (2005a). Participants had explicit access to both forms of memory that were functional in guiding search in Experiments 1 and 2. Memory for general scene context allowed them to select a plausible target location that was quite close to the actual location of the target when it appeared in the scene, and memory for the specific binding of target object to location enabled even more accurate estimates. Although the present results do not rule out effects of implicit learning on search in Experiments 1 and 2, the most parsimonious account is that explicit learning of scene context and target position was functional in guiding attention and the eyes to the target location.

GENERAL DISCUSSION

In the present experiments, the role of visual memory in search through natural scenes was examined using a preview-search task. Before searching for a particular object in a scene, participants were or were not provided a preview of the scene. The visual memory representation derived from the scene preview significantly facilitated later search through that scene, even though the task could have been performed by a purely visual search process that did not consult memory. Effects of a preview were observed on the very first search through the scene. Therefore, repeated search and target detection (as in contextual cueing experiments) is not necessary to facilitate search in natural scenes. Further, the effect of a preview increased with longer preview durations, consistent with evidence that participants accumulate visual scene information over the course of viewing a scene (Hollingworth, 2004; Hollingworth & Henderson, 2002; Melcher, 2006; Tatler et al., 2003, 2005). Finally, effects of scene memory were observed both on manual search RT and eye movement measures of search efficiency. The latter data add to a large body of literature demonstrating that eye movements when viewing natural scenes are strongly driven by—and often dominated by—cognitive factors, such as memory and top-down goals (Brockmole & Henderson, 2006a, 2006b; Castelhano & Henderson, 2007; Henderson, Brockmole, Castelhano, & Mack, 2007; Henderson et al., 1999; Neider & Zelinsky, 2006; Summerfield et al., 2006; Torralba et al., 2006; Yarbus, 1967).

The main goal of the study was to tease apart two means by which scene memory could facilitate visual search. First, memory for the general context and layout of a scene could guide attention and the eyes to scene regions where the target object was likely to be found. Second, memory for the specific binding of target object to scene location could guide attention and the eyes to the remembered location of that object. To assess the former type of memory, the target-absent preview condition used a scene preview that did not contain the ultimate target object. This preview allowed participants to encode information about the scene context but not information about the specific location of the target. In the target-present preview condition, the target object was present in the preview scene, allowing the encoding of both scene context and target location. Search was more efficient in the target-present preview condition than in the target-absent preview condition, which was in turn more efficient than search in the no preview control condition. Thus, both forms of memory facilitated search.

In the present task, participants could not have known which of the objects in the preview scene would be the target. Thus, the task demanded that they remember the binding of multiple individual objects to scene locations from the preview. Evidence of more efficient search in the target-present preview condition than in the target-absent preview condition therefore demonstrates that the scene memory representation functional in guiding search is not limited to spatial layout, but also preserves information about the form and/or identity of the objects occupying those locations. In addition, such object-to-location binding is likely to be specific to the particular scene in which the object appeared (Hollingworth, 2007).

Finally, both types of scene memory were explicitly available for participant report. Accuracy in a position-estimation task mirrored the results observed in visual search. This finding is consistent with contextual cueing studies using real-world scene stimuli, in which memory for target location is also explicitly available (Brockmole et al., 2006; Brockmole & Henderson, 2006b). Explicit learning of the structure of natural scenes contrasts with implicit learning of spatial structure in contextual cueing studies using random arrays of simple stimuli (Chun & Jiang, 1998). The present results do not rule out a contribution from implicit learning, but they do raise the possibility that traditional search arrays fail to instantiate important features of the behavioural task under investigation (real-world search for natural objects). More generally, as the visual search literature evolves from using search as a methodological tool (e.g., for understanding binding in early vision; Treisman & Gelade, 1980) to investigating search in its own right as an important real-world behaviour, research stimuli and tasks must replicate core properties of that real-world behaviour, including the use of scene stimuli that instantiate the spatial structure and semantic coherence of natural environments.

REFERENCES

Brockmole, J. R., Castelhano, M. S., & Henderson, J. M. (2006). Contextual cueing in naturalistic scenes: Global and local contexts. *Journal of Experimental Psychology: Learning, Memory and Cognition*, *32*(4), 699–706.

Brockmole, J. R., & Henderson, J. M. (2006a). Recognition and attention guidance during contextual cueing in real-world scenes: Evidence from eye movements. *Quarterly Journal of Experimental Psychology*, *59*(7), 1177–1187.

Brockmole, J. R., & Henderson, J. M. (2006b). Using real-world scenes as contextual cues for search. *Visual Cognition*, *13*(1), 99–108.

Castelhano, M. S., & Henderson, J. M. (2005). Incidental visual memory for objects in scenes. *Visual Cognition*, *12*(6), 1017–1040.

Castelhano, M. S., & Henderson, J. M. (2007). Initial scene representations facilitate eye movement guidance in visual search. *Journal of Experimental Psychology: Human Perception and Performance*, *33*(4), 753–763.

Chun, M. M., & Jiang, Y. (1998). Contextual cueing: Implicit learning and memory of visual context guides spatial attention. *Cognitive Psychology*, *36*, 28–71.

Desimone, R., & Duncan, J. (1995). Neural mechanisms of selective visual attention. *Annual Review of Neuroscience*, *18*, 193–222.

Hannula, D. E., Tranel, D., & Cohen, N. J. (2006). The long and the short of it: Relational memory impairments in amnesia, even at short lags. *Journal of Neuroscience*, *26*(32), 8352–8359.

Henderson, J. M., Brockmole, J. R., Castelhano, M. S., & Mack, M. (2007). Visual saliency does not account for eye movements during search in real-world scenes. In R. van Gompel, M. Fischer, W. Murray, & R. Hill (Eds.), *Eye movements: A window on mind and brain* (pp. 537–562). UK: Elsevier: Oxford.

Henderson, J. M., Weeks, P. A., & Hollingworth, A. (1999). The effects of semantic consistency on eye movements during complex scene viewing. *Journal of Experimental Psychology: Human Perception and Performance*, *25*(1), 210–228.

Hollingworth, A. (2004). Constructing visual representations of natural scenes: The roles of short- and long-term visual memory. *Journal of Experimental Psychology: Human Perception and Performance*, *30*(3), 519–537.

Hollingworth, A. (2005a). Memory for object position in natural scenes. *Visual Cognition*, *12*, 1003–1016.

Hollingworth, A. (2005b). The relationship between online visual representation of a scene and long-term scene memory. *Journal of Experimental Psychology: Learning, Memory and Cognition*, *31*(3), 396–411.

Hollingworth, A. (2007). Object-position binding in visual memory for natural scenes and object arrays. *Journal of Experimental Psychology: Human Perception and Performance*, *33*(1), 31–47.

Hollingworth, A., & Henderson, J. M. (2002). Accurate visual memory for previously attended objects in natural scenes. *Journal of Experimental Psychology: Human Perception and Performance*, *28*(1), 113–136.

Hollingworth, A., Richard, A. M., & Luck, S. J. (2008). Understanding the function of visual short-term memory: Transsaccadic memory, object correspondence, and gaze correction. *Journal of Experimental Psychology: General*, *137*, 163–181.

Land, M. F., & Hayhoe, M. (2001). In what ways do eye movements contribute to everyday activities? *Vision Research*, *41*, 3559–3565.

Melcher, D. (2006). Accumulation and persistence of memory for natural scenes. *Journal of Vision*, *6*(1), 8–17.

Neider, M. B., & Zelinsky, G. J. (2006). Scene context guides eye movements during visual search. *Vision Research*, *46*(5), 614–621.

Oliva, A., Wolfe, J. M., & Arsenio, H. C. (2004). Panoramic search: The interaction of memory and vision in search through a familiar scene. *Journal of Experimental Psychology: Human Perception and Performance*, *30*(6), 1132–1146.

Potter, M. C. (1976). Short-term conceptual memory for pictures. *Journal of Experimental Psychology: Human Learning and Memory*, *2*, 509–522.

Summerfield, J. J., Lepsien, J., Gitelman, D. R., Mesulam, M. M., & Nobre, A. C. (2006). Orienting attention based on long-term memory experience. *Neuron*, *49*(6), 905–916.

Tatler, B. W., Gilchrist, I. D., & Land, M. F. (2005). Visual memory for objects in natural scenes: From fixations to object files. *Quarterly Journal of Experimental Psychology: Human Experimental Psychology*, *58A*(5), 931–960.

Tatler, B. W., Gilchrist, I. D., & Rusted, J. (2003). The time course of abstract visual representation. *Perception*, *32*(5), 579–592.

Torralba, A., Oliva, A., Castelhano, M. S., & Henderson, J. M. (2006). Contextual guidance of eye movements and attention in real-world scenes: The role of global features in object search. *Psychological Review*, *113*, 766–786.

Treisman, A., & Gelade, G. (1980). A feature-integration theory of attention. *Cognitive Psychology*, *12*, 97–136.

Wolfe, J. M., Klempen, N., & Dahlen, K. (2000). Postattentive vision. *Journal of Experimental Psychology: Human Perception and Performance*, *26*, 693–716.

Yarbus, A. L. (1967). *Eye movements and vision*. New York: Plenum Press.

VISUAL COGNITION, 2009, 17 (1/2), 292

Psychology Press
Taylor & Francis Group

Corrigendum

Please note that in this issue, 17(1&2), of *Visual Cognition*, in the paper by George Alvarez and Todd Thompson entitled "Overwriting and rebinding: Why feature-switch detection tasks underestimate the binding capacity of visual working memory", there is an error on p. 149.

An alert reader brought the authors' attention to the error in the Methods section on p. 149, under *Data Analysis*, *Capacity K*. The error occurs in equations (7) and (8), in which the portions reading "$(2*N+1)$" should read "$(2*N-1)$".

While the equation was written incorrectly in the text, the correct equation was used in the analyses reported in the paper, and so none of the results reported in the paper are incorrect. Note also that equation 8 is the equation for computing the K value in a switch detection task (K_{switch}), rather than a 4 alternative forced choice task (K_{4AFC}). Correct versions of equations 7 and 8 are included below.

Correction

$$\mathrm{O} = -(K^2) + (2*N-1)*K - 2*T*(\mathrm{HIT}-\mathrm{FA}) \tag{7}$$

In this form ($\text{zero} = \mathrm{a}K^2 + \mathrm{b}K + \mathrm{c}$), we can solve for K using the quadratic equation, as follows:

$$\begin{aligned} &\mathrm{a} = -1 \\ &\mathrm{b} = 2*N - 1 \\ &\mathrm{c} = -2*T*(\mathrm{HIT}-\mathrm{FA}) \\ &K_{\text{switch}} = [-\mathrm{b} + /-\mathrm{sqrt}(\mathrm{b}^2 - 4*\mathrm{a}*\mathrm{c})]/(2*\mathrm{a}) \end{aligned} \tag{8}$$

© 2009 Psychology Press, an imprint of the Taylor & Francis Group, an Informa business
http://www.psypress.com/viscog DOI: 10.1080/13506280802646562

Subject Index